CRITICAL TO CARE: THE INVISIBLE WOMEN IN
HEALTH SERVICES

Who counts as a health care worker? The question of where we draw the line between health care workers and non-health care workers is not merely a matter of academic nicety or a debate without consequences for care. It is a central issue for policy development because the definition often results in a division among workers that serves to undermine care.

Critical to Care uses a wide range of evidence to reveal the contributions that those who provide personal care, who cook, clean, keep records, and do laundry make to health services. As a result of current reforms, these workers are increasingly treated as peripheral even though the research on what determines health demonstrates that their work is essential. The authors stress the invisibility and undervaluing of 'women's work' as well as the importance of context in understanding how this work is defined and treated.

Through a gendered analysis, *Critical to Care* establishes a basis for discussing research, policy, and other actions in relation to the daily work of thousands of marginalized women and men.

PAT ARMSTRONG is a professor in the Department of Sociology at York University and holds a CHSRF/CIHR Chair in Applied Health Services and Nursing Research.

HUGH ARMSTRONG is a professor in the School of Social Work and the Institute of Political Economy at Carleton University.

KRISTA SCOTT-DIXON is an independent scholar and consultant living in Toronto.

Critical to Care

The Invisible Women in Health Services

PAT ARMSTRONG
HUGH ARMSTRONG
KRISTA SCOTT-DIXON

UNIVERSITY OF TORONTO PRESS
Toronto Buffalo London

© University of Toronto Press Incorporated 2008
Toronto Buffalo London
www.utppublishing.com
Printed in Canada

ISBN 978-0-8020-9333-2 (cloth)
ISBN 978-0-8020-9608-1 (paper)

Printed on acid-free paper

Library and Archives Canada Cataloguing in Publication

Armstrong, Pat, 1945–
    Critical to care : the invisible women in health services / Pat
Armstrong, Hugh Armstrong, Krista Scott-Dixon.

Includes bibliographical references and index.
ISBN 978-0-8020-9333-2 (bound). – ISBN 978-0-8020-9608-1 (pbk.)

    1. Allied health personnel – Canada.   2. Allied health
personnel – Canada – Social conditions.   3. Women employees –
Canada – Social conditions.   4. Medical care – Canada.
I. Armstrong, Hugh, 1943–   II. Scott-Dixon, Krista, 1973–   III. Title.

R692.A75 2008   305.43'6107370971   C2008-901279-8

This book has been published with the help of a grant from the Canadian
Federation for the Humanities and Social Sciences, through the Aid to
Scholarly Publications Programme, using funds provided by the Social
Sciences and Humanities Research Council of Canada.

University of Toronto Press acknowledges the financial assistance to its
publishing program of the Canada Council for the Arts and the Ontario
Arts Council.

University of Toronto Press acknowledges the financial support of its
publishing activities of the Government of Canada through the Book
Publishing Industry Development Program (BPIDP).

Contents

List of Figures and Tables   ix

Acknowledgments   xi

1 Introduction   3
  Critical to Care: Invisible and Undervalued   4
  Counting the Work and the Workers   6
  Determining Who Counts   7
  Identifying Contributions to Care   8
  Making Gender Matters Visible   9
  Exposing Health Hazards at Work   9
  Establishing the Context: Further Explanations   10
  Developing Options   11
  Building on the Past, Moving to the Future   12

2 Counting the Work and the Workers   14
  Clerical Work   19
  Assisting Occupations in Health Care   36
  Visiting Homemakers, Housekeepers, and Related Occupations   42
  Cleaning/Housekeeping, Laundry, and Food Services   44
  Security Work   52
  Managers   52
  Unpaid Ancillary Work   56
  The Composite Picture   59

3 Determining Who Counts   62
  Feminist Political Economy   63
  The Determinants of Health   66

4 Identifying Contributions to Care   75
The Specificity of Health Care   75
The Origins of Ancillary Work   82
Conclusions   87

5 Making Gender Matters Visible   88
Women's Care Work   88
Skills and Care   91
  Defining Skills   92
  Gender Skills   93
  Health Care Skills   96
  Regulation and Training   103
Resistance   105
  Moving into the Labour Force   105
  Unions and Professions   109
  Women's Individual Responses   116
Conclusions   119

6 Exposing Health Hazards at Work   121
Infection and Respiratory Diseases   123
Lifting, Bending, Twisting, and Musculoskeletal Injuries   124
Chemicals, Needles, and Cuts   126
Lack of Employment Security and Control   127
Workplace Organization   130
Workplace Violence, Bullying, Sexual Harassment, and Racism   135
Lack of Respect   138
Conclusions   138

7 Challenging the Construction of Ancillary Work   140
International Contexts and Trends   140
  Rising Health Care Expenditures   140
  New Public Management   143
  Health Care as an Opportunity for Profit   146
  Global Markets and Workers   150
The Health Policy Context in Canada   152
  Public Health Care in Canada   153
  Privatization   156
  Integration and Teamwork   160
  Evidence-Based Decision Making   162
  Accountability   164

Public Health   167
Regionalization and Decentralization   168
Conclusions   169

8 Developing Options   170
Implications for Policy, Research, and Action   171
First, We Need an Active State   172
Second, We Need Better Management   175
Third, We Need to Promote Unions and Other Forms of Collective Organization   177
Fourth, We Need More and Better Research   180
Conclusions   181

Appendix: A Guide to Canadian Data on Ancillary Workers in the Health Care Sector   183
Introduction: Interpret Data with Care!   183
Methodology and General Overview   184
Notes on the Labour Force Survey   185
Notes on Census Data   185
Defining Ancillary Occupations in Health Care   186
The Importance of Industry   189
Form of Employment   191
Immigrant and Visible Minority Status   193

References   195

Index   219

List of Figures and Tables

Figures

Figure 2.1   Canada's health care industries, by Statistics Canada occupational groups   17

Figure 2.2   Clerical occupations in health care and social assistance industries, by sex   33

Figure 2.3   Education levels for men and women in secretarial and other clerical occupations   34

Figure 2.4   Ages of men and women in secretarial and clerical occupations   35

Figure 2.5   Clerical occupations by full-time/part-time status: health care and social assistance industries and all other industries   35

Figure 2.6   Median hourly wage for women workers in clerical occupations: health care and social assistance industries and other industries   37

Figure 2.7   Visiting homemakers, housekeepers, and related occupations in health care and social assistance industries, by sex   44

Figure 2.8   Rates of part-time employment in childcare/home support occupations (aggregate category): health care and social assistance industries and all other industries   44

Figure 2.9   Highest educational attainment in the chefs-and-cooks occupational group, health care and social assistance industries, by sex   49

Figure 2.10   Rates of part-time employment in the food services and cleaning services occupations   51

Figure 2.11   Age in management occupations, by sex   54
Figure 2.12   Highest educational attainment in management occupa-
              tions, health care and social services industries, by
              sex   55
Figure 2.13   Participation in unpaid ancillary-type tasks, by sex   58
Figure 5.1   Women's rate of labour force participation   106
Figure 5.2   Union coverage in ancillary occupations in health
              care   112

Tables

Table 2.1   Median hourly wage for men and women in management
              occupations   56
Table 2.2   Time spent on unpaid ancillary-type tasks by participat-
              ing adults, by sex   59
Table A.1   List of ancillary occupations   188
Table A.2   List of health care and social assistance industry
              categories   190

Acknowledgments

This book, like other academic books, builds on the work of those far too numerous to mention. The pages and pages of references list many of them, and we are grateful to all of them for their work. But we would like to identify some individuals and groups not mentioned or not very visible there.

First, we would like to thank Lynn Spink, whose extraordinary skills and compassion are revealed in the excellent interviews for this book. We would also like to thank the women who took the time during what for them is often an endlessly tiring day to share with us descriptions of their work, descriptions that make bloodless categories come alive for readers.

Second, we are grateful to the National Networks on Environments in Women's Health (NNEWH), the organization that commissioned a paper from us on ancillary work, and particularly to the National Coordinating Group on Health Care Reform and Women (now Women and Health Care Reform) for the provocative feedback on a very early version of that paper. We benefited greatly from input provided at the workshop on ancillary work organized by the Group, where people from the policy, research, and practitioner communities shared their ideas and struggled through the issues. Karen Grant, a long-time and invaluable member of Women and Health Care Reform, came up with the title for that report and we have used it here for a book that has come a long way from the report.

Third, in addressing the issues raised by the three anonymous reviewers, we improved the text significantly, although not always in the directions they suggested. We are grateful as well to Stephen Koto-wych from the University of Toronto Press for his efficient, effective, and supportive guidance through the production of this book, and to Maureen Epp for her thorough copy-editing.

Fourth, Pat and Hugh Armstrong would like to thank those they have worked with in research groups over the years. We have learned a great deal working with Ivy Lynn Bourgeault, Jacqueline Choiniere, Eric Mykhalovskiy, Jerry P. White, and Joel Lexchin in particular, in a team that explored many aspects of women's work in health care together. Leah Vosko, Kate Laxer, and others in the Community/University Research Alliance project on precarious employment stimulated collective thinking about work that contributed in important ways to the argument we make in this book. So did Leah's Gender and Work Data Base, which introduced us to Krista Scott-Dixon. Ellen Balka's Innovation in the New Economy project brought us together again with Karen Messing, whose work is central to our conceptualization of health hazards women face in health care work. Our various projects with Tamara Daly have been an essential source of material for this book, as the many quotes from them suggest. Although our daughters no longer provide research assistance, they do constantly assist us in other ways, such as buying computers and showing us how to work them. And they, along with our extended family and friends, put up with our work overload.

Finally, Krista Scott-Dixon would like to thank Walter Giesbrecht, data librarian at York University, for his invaluable guidance on survey peculiarities, data access, and insider factoids about Statistics Canada. Walter is almost single-handedly responsible for Krista coming out of the qualitative closet as a number lover.

CRITICAL TO CARE

1 Introduction

Who counts as a heath care worker? The question seems straightforward, but the answer is far from simple. And it is far from irrelevant either to those working in care or to those needing care.

Virtually everyone would agree that doctors and nurses are health care workers. However, even here there may be disagreement. Do we include as doctors those who practise chiropractic and homeopathy? Do we include nursing aides, assistants, and orderlies when we talk about nurses? When it comes to other jobs created by developments in technology and in the division of labour, there is even less consensus. Are cleaners and dietary workers, personal care providers and ward clerks health care workers? Increasingly, many of these jobs in the health care sector whose status is controversial are described as ancillary.

The (Romanow) Commission on the Future of Health Care in Canada (2002, 6), for example, makes a distinction between those who provide direct care and those who are engaged in ancillary services. While not offering a clear definition of ancillary services, the Commission's report (hereafter referred to as the Romanow Report) describes them as services 'such as food preparation, cleaning and maintenance.' Clerical workers and laundry workers would also seem to fit in with this understanding of ancillary work, given that they too do not provide 'direct' care. Neither do most managers and technicians. But the lines between 'direct' and 'non-direct' work in health care remain blurred. For instance, some of those who provide homemaking services do food preparation and cleaning but may also provide some direct care. At the same time, personal care providers who work in homes and hospitals often clean and prepare food, thus fitting into both categories as well. And nurses who are mainly managers may sometimes give medication and even prepare food or clean.

The question of where we draw the line between health care workers and non–health care workers is not just a matter of academic nicety, a debate without consequences for care. It is a theoretical question that requires us to think systematically about the meaning of health care and of health care work, as well as about the intersection of gender, racialization, and class in specific places at particular times. It is also an empirical question, although this too requires us to raise important theoretical issues about what counts and how it is counted. As Deborah Stone (1988, 30), the noted American feminist puts it, no number is innocent. Drawing the line between health care workers and non–health care workers, postmodernists in particular would emphasize, involves the subjective and experiential as well as the empirical and the theoretical. How those doing the work define their work matters.

But the question of who is defined as a health care worker does not stop at the level of thinking, measuring, and feeling. It reaches right into the spaces where people seek, find, and provide health care. It is a central issue for policy development in health care, because a narrow definition reflects and reinforces practices that allow workers in health care to be divided into two camps, with each camp treated differently and unequally. Defining some health sector workers as external to health care work, or 'out of care,' often means that too little attention is paid to their role in the success of interventions, in recovery, in sustaining health, and in preventing illness or disability, with negative consequences for health and care. Even less attention may be paid to their relations with other workers and to their own health, with negative consequences for services as well as for workers.

Critical to Care: Invisible and Undervalued

This book is about those defined in many policy circles as ancillary workers. Combining feminist political economy with a social determinants of health approach, our first argument is that all those jobs described as ancillary are critical to care, and that those with jobs defined as ancillary are health care workers. Our starting point for defining ancillary jobs is the Romanow Report's distinction between direct and non-direct, or ancillary, health care work. We include as ancillary workers not only the dietary, housekeeping, and maintenance staff listed in the Romanow Report, but also the clerical, laundry, security, and managerial staff working in health services who are seldom defined as providing direct care. We also extend the list to personal care providers and homemakers, who are sometimes understood to be involved in direct care and sometimes considered ancillary. Our intention is to be inclusive in ways that ensure that all those involved in providing health services are considered when we look at care. The logic of this argument would lead us to use another term for these workers. We explored other labels, such as 'support workers,' but our consultations with workers and academics on this issue have led us to retain the term 'ancillary' here in order to relate our work to current debates.

With the exceptions of management, maintenance, and security work, these jobs are done mainly by women. And it is the female-dominated jobs that are most frequently defined as ancillary. Such work is traditionally women's work, although it is sometimes also done by some marginalized and a few powerful men. Moreover, many of the women who do this work are recent immigrants and/or are racialized. Associated as it is with women's work in the home, the skills, effort, responsibilities, and working conditions involved in ancillary work remain invisible and undervalued. This invisibility and undervaluing contributes to the phenomenon of defining ancillary work as 'out of care' and equating it with the hotel services that are dismissed as requiring few skills and little effort or responsibility. Women's lack of power contributes to this process, and this is especially the case for the most marginalized women. Our second argument, then, is that gender is a particularly critical factor in understanding the definition and related conditions of this work.

Finally, we argue that ancillary work and the changes it is undergoing can be understood only within the context of global and national developments in economies, states, and health services. The issues are not only institutional or even just Canadian ones. Nor can they be addressed exclusively at the local level or simply in terms of health care.

These three arguments – namely, the contribution ancillary work makes to health care, the invisibility and undervaluing of this as women's work, and the importance of context in understanding influences on this work – are woven throughout the book. These arguments influence how we count ancillary workers as well as how we represent their work. Our analysis is a gendered analysis, taking into account not only the similarities among women but also their differences.

We argue as well that the definition of the work as ancillary and not part of health care has significant consequences for both those employed in care and those needing care. It is reflected in, and reflects, policy and practices. As Eric Olin Wright (2006, 95) so clearly explains, 'The starting point for an emancipatory social science is not simply to show that there is suffering and inequality in the world, but to demonstrate that the explanation for these ills lies in the specific properties of existing institutions and social structures, and to identify the ways in which they systematically cause harm to people.' Thousands of women undertake ancillary work each day. Indeed, depending on where we draw the line, ancillary workers may account for the majority of those who work in the health and social service sector. The way the work is defined and organized has an impact far beyond the harm to workers. It shapes the nature of health care itself. Our objective, like Wright's, goes beyond exposing the harm. We seek to provide a basis for discussion of the implications for research, policies, and practices.

Counting the Work and the Workers

In chapter 2, we draw a portrait of the work and the workers. This portrait is informed by a theoretical framework that directs us to include as health care workers the wide range of people employed in the health care sector, as we explain in the subsequent chapter. The portrait is a Canadian one, although the patterns are very similar throughout North America. Equally important, this theoretical framework guides us to explore the data on gender and on other social phenomena such as racialization and immigration. Our theoretical basis also means that we are interested in where people work as well as in what they do in their jobs, because many aspects of work are specific to times and workplaces.

The portrait is primarily based on Statistics Canada data mined by Krista Scott-Dixon. But statistics produce a limited picture, in part because there are real limits to the data produced by national statistical agencies and in part because numbers are so remote from the people who actually do the work. To provide some flavour of what is involved in doing the jobs and to make workers' experience matter in our analysis, we have turned to a number of additional sources. First, we draw on interviews done for other Armstrong projects, ones conducted with a range of other researchers. Second, we include material from the handful of other Canadian researchers who have talked with workers in these jobs. And third, we report on interviews conducted for this book. Together, these various sources give some life to the numerical data, but much more needs to be done if we are to get a full picture of the work and the workers' experiences, as we explain in the final chapter.

It is always difficult to determine how to order the development of an argument, and we have struggled over where to locate this portrait. On the one hand, our theoretical framework suggests that theory guides how we count and what we count. And most scholarly books begin with theory, mainly for this reason. It would make sense, then, to make theory our next chapter. However, we want to make the workers and their work the centre of our discussion. Moreover, we want to have readers know whom we are talking about when we set out our theoretical guide and make our argument. After considerable debate, we have decided to offer the portrait first and explain the how and why of this portrait next. Readers may want to do the reverse.

Determining Who Counts

Although theory guides what we see along with how we see and understand, like the British historian E.P. Thompson (1978), we understand all research as a dialogue between theory and evidence that allows evidence to constantly inform theory. Feminist political economy provides our theoretical frame, but it is a frame that evolves with the evidence.

Political economy theory itself takes multiple forms and remains a work in progress. Nevertheless, each strand-in-motion shares some common assumptions. Global processes, states, markets, institutions, ideas, discourses, civil society, and households are understood as integrally related rather than as separate variables. They are shaped by how people provide for their needs, by the means of producing and reproducing, as well as by collective and individual efforts to resist. Analysis begins, then, with how people come together to provide food, shelter, jobs, and babies, and how they make change. These forces, institutions, relations, and practices are historically specific, varying with time and place. What sociologist Dorothy Smith (1990) calls the relations of ruling are classed, gendered, and racialized, to name only the more prominent aspects of inequality. These relations pervade households and formal economies, public and private spaces.

It is not only power but also contradictions that are critical to understanding both historical developments and daily life. Contradictions are about opposing forces and internal tensions, some possible to eliminate and others integral to social relations. And it is not only economics, but also ideas, discourses, and practices developed over time that matter.

The differences among political economists emerge in the ways these basic assumptions are understood and applied. Here our emphasis is on the visible and invisible forces at work in defining and structuring health care, and on how these forces work in gendered and racialized ways within and outside the formal economy.

Political economy has played a central role in the development of what has come to be known as a 'social determinants of health' approach, although it could more accurately be called a 'social and economic determinants' approach. From this perspective, health is critically influenced by social and physical environments and by social and economic relations, structures, and technologies, as well as by genetic makeup and health care services (Farmer 2005). Class, racialization, and gender matter in health and care. The approach we take here differs from many current versions of the increasingly popular social determinants of health approach in two significant ways.

First, our emphasis is on the importance of these determinants *within* health care rather than on their influence on health. Our emphasis rests on their significance both for those needing care and for those involved in the provision of health care services. Although the health of all people is shaped by their environments, relations, and the structures in which they work and play, those who are ill, under treatment, or disabled are particularly vulnerable to unhealthy conditions. Equally important, the health of workers is shaped by their work environments. And what affects their health affects the health of those in their care. For these and other reasons, we reject arguments that, in attempting to pit the determinants of health against health care, call for reduced spending on care. Moreover, we also understand health care as a relationship between health care workers and those with health care needs that cannot easily be reduced to a series of specified tasks and allotted to narrow time frames (Armstrong and Armstrong 2004b).

Second, these determinants are understood by us as being themselves shaped by global, national, regional, local, individual, and institutional forces in interconnected and often contradictory ways. This understanding contrasts with those who treat the determinants more as independent variables and more as the result of individual or national choice. Chapter 3 explores in more detail the way feminist political economy informs this book, and then discusses the determinants of health at greater length.

Identifying Contributions to Care

In chapter 4, we set out the implications of applying this feminist political economy approach within health care services, seeking to reveal the ways in which ancillary work is critical to care. In thinking about how feminist political economy and the social determinants of health apply within care, it is important to begin by recognizing the features that make services in care different from other services, such as those offered in hotels.

The brief history of nursing work that follows is intended to demonstrate that ancillary work was once part of nursing. It is still done by nurses if and when it is not done by others, precisely because it is so critical to care. In short, this chapter is designed to establish the characteristics of care that make it a unique service and that make ancillary services integral to care.

Making Gender Matters Visible

Chapter 5 explores the gendered nature of ancillary work. Our examination of the historical division of labour is designed to show that health care and ancillary work have traditionally been done by women within and outside the household. One legacy of this division is the blurred boundary between direct care and ancillary work, a blurring that indicates the integral relationship between the two kinds of labour. Another legacy is the invisibility and undervaluing of the skills, effort, responsibilities, and conditions involved in doing the work.

As women have entered the labour force in large numbers, they have made some significant gains through unions and professional organizations as well as through their efforts to influence legislation and regulation. Rising female labour force participation rates, along with professionalization and unionization, have helped improve conditions in care work. Registered nurses in particular have been able to make many of their skills visible and valued, in part by shedding at least some of the tasks traditionally associated with women and the home. But the definition and valuing of skills remains a profoundly gendered process rather than a simple measurement of technical competence and a rewarding of objectively assessed effort and expertise. Here we set out some of the skills, efforts, and responsibilities involved in ancillary work, in an attempt to highlight both how gender has obscured them and how more research is needed on the nature and conditions of this work.

Exposing Health Hazards at Work

This leads us to address the health hazards built into ancillary work. Just as the skills are all too frequently rendered invisible by gender, so too are many of the hazards women frequently face in the relations and conditions of this work. Health care work has the highest rates of illness and injury of any occupational group. Part of the explanation for this pattern can be found in what Karen Messing (1998b) calls 'one-eyed science': approaches to health that are gender biased and that fail to recognize the health hazards of women's work.

These hazards are important to us all. For one thing, poor conditions for workers mean poor conditions for care. For another, high illness and injury rates mean high costs in training, recruitment, recovery, and replacement.

In sum, chapters 5 and 6 set out ancillary work as women's work, exploring the ways in which female dominance contributes to the value attached to the jobs and the hazards faced in the work, and examining the ways in which women have challenged these patterns.

Establishing the Context: Further Explanations

Chapter 7 looks at the contexts in which ancillary work is developing and changing, in order to understand other forces that are shaping ancillary work in health care. Health care has become a global issue. One reason for this global interest is what is often presented as an alarming rise in health care expenditures. The solution offered is mainly better government management, usually understood as the adoption of practices taken from the for-profit sector, and the shedding of government services, usually through contracting out to for-profit firms. Another reason for global interest is the opportunity for profit in an area traditionally without many investor-owned services. The movement known as 'New Public Management' and the concomitant shift to for-profit health services are both being promoted through international trade agreements and other sources of pressure on national governments. And there is pressure to open borders, not only to international services but to international workers as well.

Ancillary services are particularly vulnerable to these pressures, given their assumed similarity to existing food and accommodation services in the international for-profit sector and the notion that few skills are required. However, we argue that government health care expenditures are not out of control, and that the most rapidly rising costs are those in the for-profit sectors, especially in pharmaceuticals and technologies. This suggests that the model should not be the for-profit sector, especially when we take the evidence on the determinants of health into account. Moreover, little can be saved by reducing expenditures on the lowest-paid workers, the ones who do ancillary work.

Yet international pressure, along with considerable local support, is moving Canadian health care in this direction.

In a number of ways, health care reforms are a local version of international developments, albeit played out in a particular way. The Canadian public health care system was introduced in the wake of similar programs in other countries, although it certainly has its own unique features. We set out a brief history of public health care in order to show how the structure of the system makes it vulnerable to the kinds of privatization underway, and how privatization influences ancillary work.

This privatization takes at least six forms that are increasingly common throughout the world. Some services have been contracted out to the private sector, while some services have been duplicated by the for-profit sector. Responsibility for health care payment has been shifted to the individual, as has the responsibility for care work and for staying healthy. Within the remaining public sector, for-profit managerial techniques have been adopted and public–private partnerships established, making the public sector harder to distinguish from for-profit firms. Together these processes make health care decision making more a private than a public concern.

Ancillary workers have been particularly vulnerable to several forms of privatization, with negative consequences for their pay, job security, and conditions of work. Other health care reforms, such as regionalization, may also promote or at least allow the privatization of ancillary services. Under regionalization, each local decision-making body seeks to reduce costs in the most immediate form possible, and the cost savings that come from contracting ancillary work out to firms that pay less seems attractive. Privatization can also make teamwork more difficult, even as teams are being promoted in health care. And privatization is being undertaken without much research on the consequences for public health and care, in spite of the current emphasis on evidence-based decision making. In summary, international pressures and local health care reforms are creating pressure to change the management and delivery of ancillary services in ways that are undermining both the stated purposes of many reforms and the conditions for the ancillary workers.

Developing Options

Finally, the last chapter looks at implications for policy, research, and other actions, stressing the issues for women as a group and for different groups of women. In order to recognize and value the contribution ancillary work makes to health care, we first need an active state that supports a public health care system based on non-profit delivery and is dedicated to ensuring decent employment for the entire health care team. This means developing better mechanisms for accountability and better means for promoting equity, including a gender analysis of all practices.

Second, we need better management. Such management should not only understand how the determinants of health apply within health care but should also be well versed in the roles gender and racialization play. This means ensuring employment security, along with decent conditions of work and for participation in work.

Third, we need to promote unionization and ensure that these unions are responsive to their various members, especially in ways that recognize their skills. Unions are the most effective device to ensure better conditions and participation, but new measures are necessary to encourage their growth and development under changing work organization. Along with unions, we need better and better-enforced labour standards in order to protect those who remain outside unions. We need other forms of collective organizing and some individual ones as well.

Fourth, we need more and better research that gets translated into practice. This means making gender a central component in all research, research that begins by recognizing the critical part ancillary work plays in health care.

According to the World Health Organization (WHO 2006, 4), such workers 'provide an invisible backbone for health systems; if they are not present in sufficient numbers and with appropriate skills, the system cannot function.' And, we would add, without adequate conditions of work, ancillary workers cannot function and care is compromised in ways that are harmful to the economy as well as to individuals seeking care.

Building on the Past, Moving to the Future

This book began some decades ago when Pat Armstrong and Hugh Armstrong started to look at women's work in health care. The first study was based on a single hospital and included the entire range of women's work there. Several years later, the Armstrongs established a research team that produced a series of books that drew primarily on interviews with people who did the kind of work classified here as ancillary. More recently, Pat became involved in Leah Vosko's research team on precarious employment. As part of that project, Pat and Kate Laxer produced an article using statistical data to compare the workers described by the Romanow Report as direct and ancillary (Armstrong and Laxer 2006). Leah also set about constructing the Gender and Work Data Base. Managed by Krista Scott-Dixon, the data base includes a module on the health industry created by Pat, Hugh, and Kate that emphasizes how important it is to define all those employed in the health sector as health care workers. When the National Coordinating Group on Health Care Reform and Women, along with the National Network on Environments and Women's Health, organized a workshop on ancillary work, they commissioned Hugh and Pat to prepare a background paper and Krista to prepare a statistical profile. Finally, Pat and Hugh have been working with unions and with Nordic academic partners to survey workers employed in long-term care facilities. This book builds on all this work and owes a significant debt to those involved along the way as researchers, research participants, and commentators on our work.[1] The book moves beyond our previous work to present new data, an integrated analysis of ancillary work, and an argument for reforming health care in all our interests.

---

1 The research projects involved ethics review and informed consent by participants. A full description can be found in the sources for previously published work. The quotes cited as LTCa (2006) are from comments written in on a survey conducted with workers in long-term care facilities for a CIHR-funded project carried out by Pat Armstrong, Hugh Armstrong, and Tamara Daly, with survey ethics approval received by the York Institute for Social Research on behalf of the research team. The interviews conducted specifically for this book (LTCb 2006) received ethics approval at York University, with Pat Armstrong as the faculty supervisor of the research.

2 Counting the Work and the Workers

She has a care aide certificate from a college, and she worked for years providing palliative home care. In recent times, this meant working through a series of private agencies. She came to know many of her patients well, often working extra, unpaid hours because they were so alone. She left the job for several reasons. Every time someone died she went through two losses: the loss of someone she had come to know well, and the loss of a job. She found both highly stressful. The private agencies that employed her would often phone, leaving a message about the death and the funeral, but offering no condolences or other recognition of the relationship. Her employers were managers without health care training who were primarily interested in the business. Frequently, there were no other assignments immediately available so she would have to search out work with other agencies. One agency would send her to prospective wealthy clients, taking advantage of her certification as well as her race. She was white, and often these clients wanted a white care aide. Once the client was signed up, a different care aide was sent. The new one frequently had no formal training and was often from a racialized group. In the end, the job was too hard on her family, as well as on her. She quit to take another job.

Now she works as a unit aide in a hospital. The job involves a wide range of activities, from replacing refuse bags on patient tables and chatting with families to cleaning shelves and responding to nurses' requests. She is casually employed, working weekends and replacing sick or vacationing workers during the week. She seldom knows her schedule in advance and often works seven or eight days in a row. She works at an amalgamated hospital, which means she is at the bottom of the list in terms of both assignments and opportunities to switch to full-time work. At least the union makes sure she is on the list and receives above-minimum wages.

The union has also protected her from an abusive supervisor, handling her grievance and ensuring action. With children at home, she finds it difficult to juggle the demands of family work with her irregular paid work.

In the same hospital, another unit aide started working part-time in housekeeping at age 16, when she arrived in Canada from the Caribbean. She has now worked her way up to full-time hours on regular shifts. Such promotions through the ranks are no longer possible, because housekeeping is now contracted out. So are food services. As a result, women who have worked all their lives in the kitchen lost their jobs. The same thing happened in the laundry, where the hospital lost the services of a woman who not only ensured the linen was clean but also that it was repaired. In each of these transitions, the workers first learned of the changes by rumour and then by notice of layoff. But the layoffs happened after one kitchen worker slipped on a spill in the hall and a laundry worker was stuck by a needle left in the linen.

A clerical worker managed to keep her job, but staffing in her area has been cut back significantly at the same time as people are being moved more quickly in and out of the hospital. The pace of work has become faster, and there are fewer other workers available. As a result, she rarely takes breaks or time off for lunch. She regularly has to learn new computer programs, deal with anxious families, and assist many people seeking admission who are both frail and unable to read or write either official language. A medical error resulted in a big investigation into her record keeping. Although she was absolved of blame, the investigation has made her nervous about her work. Now her wrists are bothering her, and she fears another outbreak like SARS. Few people seem to wash their hands when they come to the hospital now, and it could start all over again.

The food services manager at the hospital works for a private firm that has contracts in a range of facilities. She does not get paid what she could expect elsewhere as a manager and has to answer to both the business that employs her and to the hospital. She often has to take work home and work on the weekend without being paid overtime, making it hard on her young family and on her housework. While she would prefer to work directly for the hospital and make friends with the staff, everything else she has tried has been part-time. And with her family back in India and her husband unemployed, she has little choice about what kind of paid work she takes.

This is a composite picture, based on encounters we have had with workers in health care rather than on any individual's actual life. The picture is intended to offer some idea of the complex skills, conditions, and relations involved in some ancillary jobs. Developing a fuller portrait of ancillary workers is no simple task. The people we seek to capture in this chapter are often missing from the multitude of reports and statistics on health human resources. These health care workers cook and serve food; they clean and keep records; they bathe, feed, and comfort; they do laundry, maintenance, and security work. Some also hold managerial jobs. They work in hospitals and long-term care facilities, in homes and in offices, in courts and in governments. Most of those who do maintenance and security work are men, while the overwhelming majority of those who cook and clean, provide home support, serve food, and keep records are women. It is the female majority who are the focus of this book, but it is also important to understand what jobs men do in health care. Our theoretical framework, as we explain in the next chapter, leads us to define the people who do this work as health care workers, distinguishing us from most other data analysts.

According to Statistics Canada, almost one in ten Canadians in the labour force is employed in health and social services. Almost one in five employed women works in this sector. Yet Statistics Canada's 2005 Labour Force Survey reports that only 46 per cent of those employed in the health and social assistance sector are in health occupations (see figure 2.1).

Although they are employed by organizations defined as providing care, almost half of the employees are not counted as health care workers. The difference between those counted as working in health care and those counted as health care workers is explained in part by the difference in the two main ways Statistics Canada categorizes people in the labour force, and in part by the assumptions buried within these categories.

One way Statistics Canada categorizes people in the labour force is based on where they work, on what are called industrial categories. Health and social services is defined as an industry. This industry includes people employed in hospitals and long-term care facilities, as well as those who work in homes, clinics, courts, and government offices defined as providing health and social services. Until recently, all those employed in workplaces defined as providing health or social services were counted as being in the industry. Now, with the adoption of the North American Industrial Classification System (NAICS), the industry is defined more in terms of the employer and less in terms of location. This has the effect of moving some people previously counted

Figure 2.1 Canada's health care industries, by Statistics Canada occupational groups, 2005

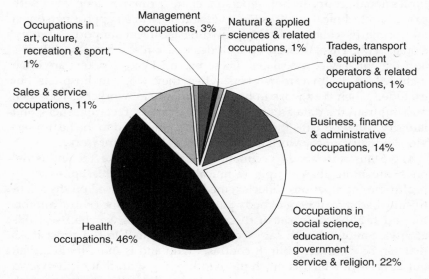

Occupations in art, culture, recreation & sport, 1%

Management occupations, 3%

Natural & applied sciences & related occupations, 1%

Trades, transport & equipment operators & related occupations, 1%

Sales & service occupations, 11%

Business, finance & administrative occupations, 14%

Health occupations, 46%

Occupations in social science, education, government service & religion, 22%

Source: Statistics Canada 2005c.

as working in health care into another industry if their work is contracted out to a for-profit provider. For example, housekeeping services in a hospital that are under contract to a for-profit company may be counted as part of the food and accommodation industry rather than as part of health and social services. In the process, housekeepers are relabelled as service associates. This new way of sorting the health care industry suggests that industrial categories are about more than simply seeing the data in another way. The categories reflect and reinforce new ways of organizing work, moving some people out of health care and defining them as non–health care workers in doing so.

The second way Statistics Canada sorts people in the labour force is based on what people do, on occupational categories. Diane Galarneau explains that for Statistics Canada, 'health care workers can be divided into three major categories: professional, technical personnel, and support personnel' (2003, 16). Health professionals are those 'primarily concerned with diagnosing and treating health problems in humans and animals and with providing related services such as pharmacy, nutrition, speech therapy, physiotherapy and occupational therapy' (17). Both registered nurses and licensed practical nurses are included in this professional group. Technical personnel are 'primarily concerned with providing technical services to professionals' while support personnel are 'primarily concerned with providing technical support to profes- sionals' (17). This latter group includes assistants and aides, orderlies and patient service associates. These personal care workers are often included as health care workers when they work in hospitals but excluded when they work in homes as home care workers. Also often missing from the data are the cooks and cleaners, record keepers, and laundry workers. Thus there can be people employed in the health ser- vices industry whose work is not defined as health care work.

The Statistics Canada occupational categories, like the industrial ones, are more than simple technical groupings. This approach to health care occupations reflects a medical model focused on the scien- tifically based treatment of body parts, with doctors the central author- ity and health care a set of discrete activities. As we shall see, this approach allows health care work to be separated into distinct tasks that can be contracted out. It contrasts with and is more limited than our approach, which is much more in keeping with that of the World Health Organization's recent report entitled *Health Workers*, which defines them as 'all people engaged in actions whose primary intent is to enhance health' (WHO 2006, 1). For the World Health Organization, and for us, this means including all paid workers in places primarily focused on improving health.

The other major source of data on health care workers, the Canadian Institute for Health Information, also relies on occupational data nar- rowly defined. *Canada's Health Care Providers* (CIHI 2005a and 2002) reports data on nurses, doctors, and some others such as denturists, health record administrators, and technicians. Its publication entitled *Health Personnel Trends in Canada* acknowledges that its focus 'on only regulated health professions excludes unregulated health professions, and informal caregivers' (CIHI 2004). But the data on health occupa- tions puts only 5 per cent of the labour force in health occupations, leav- ing out approximately another 5 per cent counted by Statistics Canada as working in the health and social service sector as well as ignoring all the unpaid providers, most of whom are women. In its most recent publication on human health resources (HHR), CIHI acknowledges that without 'the broad range of health care providers' included in the WHO approach, 'the health care system would not exist.' CIHI then goes on to declare that 'in order to put some boundaries around the broad topic of HHR,' it is largely restricting its report to a narrower definition of health care providers, with the effect of excluding most ancillary workers (CIHI 2007, 25).

The categories used by the major statistical agencies along with the assumptions buried within these categories limit the data available on ancillary work. So too does the lack of detail resulting from the small sample sizes that necessarily leave out some workers or lump them with others. For example, the data from Statistics Canada tell us nothing about the approximately 1000 people, most of whom are Aboriginal, who work as community health representatives (McCulla 2004, 14). Nevertheless, it is possible to highlight some of the most significant patterns in terms of the work and the workers. The following portraits are based primarily on an analysis of Statistics Canada occupational and industry data, supplemented by interview data intended to provide some idea of what is involved in the work. The statistics are as detailed as possible, in part because greater detail often reveals greater differences and larger inequalities. But they should be treated with some caution, because small numbers sometimes distort patterns. This is particularly the case when it comes to data on those identifying as visible minority. This chapter uses data in an attempt to fill the gap in attention paid to these workers. However, only some of the data can be found in this chapter. Those seeking more details and further data behind many of the numbers presented in the following pages can find them in the appendix.

Clerical Work

Statistics Canada provides a definition of clerical work in health care, but its brief, terse definition fails to capture the range and complexity of the work and the content that is specific to health care. So we talked with a woman who works in a children's ward of a multi-sited hospital. She has been a ward clerk for 30 years, making her an expert on the job. We reproduce virtually the full transcript of the interview below, with only some brief commentary, in order to allow the ward clerk to develop a fuller picture of this ancillary job.

The interview began with a question about what she does when she goes into the hospital in the morning. Her answer reveals not only that this work is very much about health care, but also that she is at the centre of a complicated and hectic system that requires both knowledge of health care needs and skills for dealing with patients, families, administrators, and providers.

ANSWER: Well it's very busy first thing in the morning, and you've got a lot of patients coming in. I work on a pediatrics floor. Very busy. So you have all the tonsil patients coming in for their tonsil surgery. It could be tonsil patients, it could be hernia repairs, but all the day surgery patients are coming in and you have to register them. So you have a list of day surgery patients. You have to make sure the information is correct. You have to register them into the system so that they can have their lab ... if any lab work needs to be done, any tests need to be run before their surgery, and have all their charts ready to go to the OR. So you might have up to 20 charts that you have to have ready to go first thing in the morning, and you have to register all those people.

INTERVIEWER: You're working at a desk, a reception area?

ANSWER: Yeah, right in the main part of the nursing station.

INTERVIEWER: Are there other clerks working with you?

ANSWER: There's just one clerk. And so you're very busy. And you're actually the hub of the floor. You have to know everything that's going on on the floor, because everybody is coming and asking you where is so and so, when are they going for their surgery ...

INTERVIEWER: Who is everybody?

ANSWER: All the nursing staff. Not just nursing staff. You're going to have doctors come in and ask you where the patient is, when the test is going to be done; you can have housekeeping staff ... [asking] has the patient left yet? Have they been discharged yet? Do we need to make the bed yet? You have porters coming up and asking, where is the patient? We need to take them, we're here to pick them up for their test. So really, you are the information centre of the floor. You need to know all the information about all the patients and everything that's going on ... because everybody is coming at you, asking you for the information.

INTERVIEWER: You said this is a pediatric floor, so there are youngsters there with their parents?

ANSWER: Yes.

INTERVIEWER: And do they ask you questions also?

ANSWER: Oh, parents are at the desk all the time. And you're dealing with a lot of family ... a lot of family situations on a pediatric floor. Of course parents are extremely stressed out. It's probably one of the most emotional areas because, you know, parents of a child, they're always afraid and you have to give a lot of comfort. And if it's even just saying, you know, I'll get back to you; I'll find out what you need and get back to you ... Sometimes parents can be a little unreasonable, but they're just very upset and so you're dealing with that all the time.

INTERVIEWER: So you have to be a social worker as well?

ANSWER: You do. I think there's a little bit of everything mixed in there.

INTERVIEWER: Give me an example – let's say a parent is bringing a child in for a tonsillectomy in the day. What are the things that you would have to record on the piece of paper that you are given? So you arrive at work, and do you have a pile of folders knowing who is coming in?

ANSWER: I do. So we get the list the day before, but that's actually the day they arrive for their surgery [which] is their second visit. The first visit is a pre-operative visit where you take down, you do what's called a pre-admission. So you take all their medical information: Do they have allergies? Is their address correct? Is this the right doctor?

INTERVIEWER: So they see you for that first visit as well?

ANSWER: They see me initially, first before they even seen the nurse. I make sure that they get registered, pre-registered, and make sure that their allergies are documented, that their right hospital number, their hospital card is valid; that everything – their insurance, everything – is correct on their forms. Then we send that pre-operative chart with the patient down to the nurse, and then the nurse goes over all the medical information. And that's their first visit. The second visit, when they're coming in in the morning, you verify again, make sure this is the right patient, this is your patient, your child, make sure [about] the allergies again, ask about the allergies and the address and the health card, and then you send them down to the day surgery area where they get ready for their surgery.

INTERVIEWER: And do you ever see them again, or is that the end of your ...

ANSWER: Oh no. You see them. Parents come out all day long. They may say, you know, can Johnny have some more Coke or a popsicle, if the nurse has stepped out of the room for the moment. So you're always the go-between. Now they may even ask you even just to call a family member to come. Can you call my husband to come and pick us up? There is a phone for parents, but sometimes it's in use so

we do a lot of things for the families. If a child is very ill, we'll call
other family members to come in to be with the parents.

In one sense, this is a specialized ward that requires specific knowledge of children's needs, their families, and their care providers. In
another sense, this ward involves constantly changing demands and a
wide range of issues. *

INTERVIEWER: What would be the age range of children who you
    would see?
ANSWER: From zero to 16.
INTERVIEWER: And how many patients in a day ... how many beds are
    there?
ANSWER: Well, pediatric floor is a little different. It goes up and down
    with the seasons. Winter is a very heavy season when you've got a
    lot of asthmatic kids coming in with flu, so that's a very heavy sea-
    son. Now we used to go up to 65 patients but it's been cut drastically
    in the last few years. There is better care with asthmatics so you
    don't see as many. I would say maybe in the winter, an average of 20
    kids. That's in-patients. But then you have all your day surgery and
    your pre-op patients as well that you see in a day. So you might have
    anywhere, I would say, from 10 to 20 day surgeries a day, and pre-op
    clinic would be the same. You would have anywhere from 10 to 20
    pre-op patients coming in.
INTERVIEWER: And at the same time, there are some patients who have
    been there for some time and will be there for some time?
ANSWER: Yes.
INTERVIEWER: How many beds would that be?
ANSWER: As I said, it could go up to 20, 25. Now we also have desig-
    nated five psychiatric beds. This is for children in crisis. Psychiatric
    patients. And that could be any age. Usually, you know ... we've had
    as young as five and right into the teen years. So we have a lot of eat-
    ing disorders and, you know, children in crisis, suicidal ... So those
    patients are constant care patients, one-on-one nursing.
INTERVIEWER: How many other staff are on the floor? RNs [registered
    nurses], personal support workers, those people?
ANSWER: We have no personal support workers. It's all RNs. There
    used to be RPNs [registered practical nurses] on the floor but with
    the cut in beds that the government has done, there has to be a cer-
    tain number of RNs on the floor in case a child arrests [i.e., goes into

cardiac arrest], so they keep the numbers down to a minimum of three RNs on the floor.

INTERVIEWER: So three RNs and you?

ANSWER: Right. And as the patients increase, the in-patients, they would increase the number of RNs.

INTERVIEWER: Who supervises your work? Who do you report to? Give me an idea of the structure.

ANSWER: Usually I would report to a team leader on the floor ...

INTERVIEWER: And that would be an RN team leader?

ANSWER: Yes. And there's also a program director that you report to.

INTERVIEWER: You've described your responsibilities for out-patients. Tell me, do you have on hand, do you have any reason to refer to files of overnight patients?

ANSWER: Yes. Now we do all the patient charts whether they're day surgery, pre-op, or in-patients. We prepare all the charts. We register all the patients. So that means we admit all the patients. We take the same information as we do for an out-patient as an in-patient.

INTERVIEWER: And when you say 'we,' on this floor you're doing it?

ANSWER: I'm doing it. But there would be an evening ward clerk as well.

INTERVIEWER: But you're working alone during the day?

ANSWER: We're always working alone. We prepare all the charts. Not only do we prepare all the charts, we do all the doctors' orders.

While her work involves many of the skills commonly associated with clerical work, it also involves specialized skills related to health care. Moreover, mistakes can have major consequences, there is often time pressure, and all the documents must remain confidential.

INTERVIEWER: So what's a doctor's order?

ANSWER: The doctor is going to ... prescribe orders. He's going to say the child needs an IV or needs this kind of drug treatment, or he may need these types of puffers, these X-rays, these tests. We do it all. We transcribe all those orders. We do all the orders into the computer so we've got all the tests, we get all the lab work done, we do it all. The nurses come and look and verify that we have done it, but we are the ones that actually do it all.

INTERVIEWER: And so do you use a computer all the time, or do you also fill out charts by hand?

ANSWER: There's two things we do ... You have a small paper chart which has doctors' order sheets that are in carbon copies, so there's always a copy on the chart of the previous orders. A copy goes down to the pharmacy, but all the orders are transcribed from the chart onto the computer and also onto a cardex. So you also have a cardex that they can flip through quite easily and look at the prescribed medications on.

INTERVIEWER: And you're the person who is responsible for all three?

ANSWER: Yes.

INTERVIEWER: And what happens if you screw up?

ANSWER: Well, that's why the job is so very important that you don't, because you are dealing with medications. All the orders that have been ordered by the doctor, you put into the computer for the meds and what comes out of a printer is called a MAR [an archival] sheet. So you put all the meds ... the orders into the computer. You order what drugs have been ordered, what tests have been ordered, every-thing like that goes into the computer. You have what's called veri-fied orders. That means it goes right on down to pharmacy. It goes right on to the lab and to X-ray. So if you've put a wrong test in and the person gets the wrong test, you're responsible for putting in the wrong test.

INTERVIEWER: Who checks your work, or is it left for you to ...?

ANSWER: The RN will go over the orders and sign them off. But they don't check your work on the computer.

INTERVIEWER: And the work that you've inputted into the computer, does that end up on a piece of paper or does it reside only in the computer?

ANSWER: It resides in the computer ... We put in the medications that are ordered. It goes directly to pharmacy. Pharmacy then produces a [report] that's printed off on a printer on your floor. You put it into a medication binder. So each patient has a separate ... sheet with their medications on it. And they come up every single day. So, and espe-cially sometimes, you will get different [reports] through the day for children. Children are different than adults. Their condition changes very quickly. So let's say it's an asthmatic child. Their puffers may be changed three and four times a day according to how they're doing. And so you might get different [reports] coming up all day long because the medications have been changed throughout the day. Adult patients, usually it's once a day. Doctors come in, write new orders, and the [reports] are printed off each day for each patient. So, some floors don't use cardexes any more. Other floors still feel that they need those cardexes to refer back. And the cardex is simply a cardboard sheet that fits into a ... it looks like a big, giant clipboard. They all have their little pockets with the patient's name on, diagnosis, allergies, and a nurse can flip through very quickly just to make sure ... to see what tests are going to be done, what treatment the patient is on. So everything is in pencil on those because they change so quickly. So we're responsible for doing all of that. Which is a big responsibility ... a liability.

INTERVIEWER: Are there other binders besides the meds binder?

ANSWER: Each patient has their own chart as well, which is in a binder. So they would have their doctor's order sheets in the binder. That's about it for ... well, then you have old records files that come up so if the patient has been admitted previously, the ward clerk is also responsible for ordering their old charts, making sure the old charts are brought up to the floor, and those are stored as well. So they have an old chart [and] a new chart, if they're been a previous patient.

INTERVIEWER: And do you do the storing? Do you do the arrangement of the binders?

ANSWER: We do it. We put everything together. And the binders go in a chronological order. There's a special order for each patient binder. Each patient binder contains doctors' order sheets, history sheets, progress notes. It may have copies, paper copies of their X-rays and lab work that's done. It comes up and into the binders. All that. We have to make sure all that filing is done as well, so we make sure all the things, the binder is kept current, and you make sure you've got the right patient's information in the right binder, in their binder.

The job also has rewards that are specific to care. And it has a downside that creates stress unique to health care work, especially in a ward that deals with children.

INTERVIEWER: What part of the day do you enjoy most?

ANSWER: I love patient contact. I love just working with the staff. I guess I don't know if there's any one part of the day I enjoy more than any other. I guess I just like the whole job. It's a very fast-paced, very busy job. You're always moving.

INTERVIEWER: What's the most difficult part?

ANSWER: The most difficult is when you've got someone dying. You're very involved. If it's an emergency situation where someone has arrested, you're calling family, you're dealing with family members

... Sometimes you're right in there. If there's a code on a child many times I've been in the room because they're calling out to you to get things, to get people there, to get different doctors there.

INTERVIEWER: So who would be the people who would be calling to you?

ANSWER: Nurses and doctors. They would ask for different Ambu bags [a brand of disposable resuscitator], or can you get portable X-rays up here now, can you get me this stat. So they're calling out from the room, or sometimes you're standing right there. Sometimes you're dealing with the families as well. If there's a child that's arrested or even an adult that's arrested, they can't always be in the room when the teams are working on the patient. You're then dealing with the family, getting them into a room where they're comfortable, calling other family members for them. It's sometimes very difficult, a difficult situation. Very emotional. So you deal with families a lot. You're getting the minister or priest to come in for the families in situations like this. It's all a difficult situation.

Like many other ancillary jobs in health care, a ward clerk's skills are acquired through both formal training and on-the-job experience. New technologies, new work organization, and new kinds of health issues all require new knowledge, although much of this knowledge is gained without formal credentials or recognition.

INTERVIEWER: How did you learn how to do all these things? How were you trained?

ANSWER: Basically, I had clerical skills and just started working in the setting and just, I don't know whether it was instinct. Many people can't work in this type of a clerical position. They tried. There's too much patient contact, and they've had to leave because they didn't realize that this isn't just a clerical job like in an office. You're actually dealing with patients, nursing staff, doctors, all forms of hospital staff all day long. And it's not an easy job. It's a high-stress job, and you have to know what's going on all over the floor. There could be a code going on down at the end of the hallway but somebody else needs to go for an X-ray. You have to know everything that's going on so you can direct people where to go, because the nursing staff aren't always at the desk. They're out busy with patients. Well, we're the ones at the desk where everybody is coming and asking the questions, and you really need to know all that information and be able to keep it straight. And with the way that the beds have been cut in hospitals, when a patient leaves you have to be right on getting the bed made for the next patient to come in, because there's a line-up. Emerg is always full. They're always waiting for those beds. You have to be on top of everything all the time. It's a very ... it's a high-stress job.

INTERVIEWER: So are you the person who calls housekeeping when it's time to change a bed?

ANSWER: Yes. There's a system implemented in the hospital right now ... It's a call system that you put in a page for them to come, and that's for portering. You do have the core cleaning people on the floor that you would call... your person assigned to the floor and say, 'Oh, 2005 is empty now. You can clean in there.' And if they need backup because there's too many beds, then you call this system to get backup for them. So basically you're doing a lot of the calling. Besides doing all of that we do have some staffing clerks on some floors, but not all floors have staffing clerks. You may have to call in staff. So in the mix of this, if a psychiatric patient is brought in, let's say, and they need constant care around the clock – which is one-on-one nursing – you may have to find free nurses.

INTERVIEWER: And how do you know who to call?

ANSWER: Well, you have to know your collective agreements as well, because it tells you in there who is the next person. So you would have to know possibly a multitude of collective agreements if you have RNs and RPNs on the floor. Two different collective agreements. You need to know what the collective agreements stipulate about who gets called in next, so that's something else you have to know.

INTERVIEWER: And do you have a binder with a list of the staff to call?

ANSWER: Yes. And you may be doing scheduling as well. I did the scheduling as well. I made up the schedule ...

INTERVIEWER: For which staff?

ANSWER: Well, for everybody. I did RNs, RPNs, and the housekeeping people. Now it's changed a bit, where housekeeping is now having their own staffing person do all of theirs, so that part of it is gone. But someone still has to do all the RN staffing.

INTERVIEWER: Okay. So how do you know what weekends off to give, things like that?

ANSWER: It's all in the collective agreement. You follow the collective agreement and you try and make up master schedules so that they know their master. So that they know what their life is going to be like for the next six months. They can have a mass rotation. They can predict their weekends off and on. They change at vacation. They change at Christmas.

INTERVIEWER: Okay. And if an RN is sick?

ANSWER: You have to replace her.

INTERVIEWER: And it's up to you to replace her?

ANSWER: Yes. They phone me – if they don't have a staffing clerk on the floor. Now as I said, some of the floors are going to staffing clerks where that responsibility has been taken away from the ward clerk, because the ward clerk's responsibilities have just grown so much that staffing is almost impossible to do. So a lot of the areas are going to where they have just one separate person [and] all they do is scheduling of staffing.

The job involves multiple tasks as well as multiple skills. Many of these tasks and skills are hard to see, but are none-the-less critical to the functioning of the system. Like much of women's work, the ward clerk's job is most visible if it is not done or not done well.

ANSWER: There is a multitude of codes. It could be a code orange which is a disaster, which we've had. There's code black for bomb scare. Code brown for chemical ... Well first of all, you need to know all those codes, because if there's a fire on your floor or something like a code red ... I have personally been through two fires on my floor.

INTERVIEWER: And how are people on the floor alerted?

ANSWER: Me. And I phone switchboard. I let them know that there's a code red and where it is. They phone the fire department and get the fire department there. You have to implement a procedure on your floor where someone takes charge, which is usually the charge nurse. She will take charge, put on an orange vest, and she will direct me if we need to start evacuating or moving patients or what-ever. I would call switchboard and say okay, we need to get patients out of here. We need help up here ... Probably the charge nurse and you work hand in hand. The two of you. Everyone is looking to her for direction, her/him. And the two of us work together on a lot of things. What's happening on the floor, we're always updating each other. She needs to know, if she's been off doing something, she needs to know that this is happening on the floor so I'll communicate to her.

There's a lot of other work as well that goes on behind the scenes. There's a lot of just clerical work that needs to be done on the floor as well. All the supplies have to be ordered. We do all that. We do all the payroll for everyone. So all the payroll has to be done. And each day you have to update that because nursing statistics or patient statistics, [it] depends on the number of staffing on the floor. So with all the ways that the government benchmarks hospitals and how efficient they are, you have to make sure you've got the right [number of] staff in the computer that day so that your numbers come out right.

It's up to us to make sure that the right people are put into the computer each day so that ... they get the right budget money to operate the floor. [Our section] manages four different areas so each area that they work in has a different functional code, so if they're working in the intensive care room that day, I have to input their payroll under that function 'cause it comes out of that budget, the same as if they're in pre-op or if they're in day surgery or if they're just on a regular floor ... Everything has a different code. You have to make sure the right codes are inputted, the right shifts. They get shift premium, overtime, weekend premium. All that has to be done.

INTERVIEWER: So you have to keep a lot in your head. Give me an idea what the last half hour of your shift is like.

ANSWER: Well, you're trying to tie up ends ... There could be a lot of admissions because people have been to the doctor, and that's when you're getting your admissions. So starting about noon hour, doctors' offices are phoning and you're admitting patients. And it could be any time. I mean they could come in the morning. There tend to be more between, let's say, eleven and three, you're getting a lot of admissions from doctors' offices. So you're preparing charts. You're getting them all set up. You try and have the chart at least out and ready to go before the patient comes. When the patient comes, you're doing their admission. Every single piece of paper in that chart has to be labelled with the patient's label on. Once you admit them you print a label sheet, so all of this has to be prepared. So if you're getting ready to leave you want to make sure that [for] any patients that are coming, you have charts out ready for them to come. The same with your day surgeries. You want to make sure you discharge them. You want to get ready for the next person coming in, getting a little report ready for them so that they know what's going on themselves to take over.

New technologies mean new skills. They do not, however, necessarily mean less work or less complicated work. And the constant interruptions that result from the nature of clerical work in health care make the job more difficult.

INTERVIEWER: What have computers done to your workload? Have they made it less?

ANSWER: [laughing] You know, with computers they thought it would be paperless. It's not. You're putting it in the computer and you're getting the paper back to file in the chart. I don't think computers have made it easier at all. Charting is much more difficult on a computer than it is handwritten, and it takes longer for everyone to work with a computerized chart than it does with a paper chart. And all of the nursing notes and that have all gone computerized. Even to look into a computerized chart – it's there for anyone to look in. So all the treatment notes. It takes longer to get through those notes to find what you need instead of flipping a page in a binder. You've got to try and find it on a computer screen, and it's much more difficult even to find the blood pressure and temperature on the computerized charts. Like everything is computerized. To me it takes longer to do everything and sometimes it's doubly because you're still doing it on paper. So it just seems ... to me a waste. Every single day there's a new [report] printed for every single patient in the hospital. So every single day you are taking out the [report], printing new [reports] for every single patient every day. And that's just in the last couple years that's happened. Whereas before you would go over, cross out the meds that were on a med sheet, and write it down below. And now it's a new sheet every single day.

INTERVIEWER: It sounds to me like a lot of the work you do requires a lot of focus and concentration. Do you have the space to do that?

ANSWER: Well, we're interrupted constantly. That's another thing. You're right at the nursing desk, right in full view of everybody – patients, nurses, doctors. Everybody is coming at you all day long, so not only are you doing all this work, you're being interrupted continuously. You're answering all the phones on the floor. There's call bells, patient call bells. If there's no nurse at the desk, you're answering the call bell, writing down the message, and making sure the nurse gets the message from the patient. It's constant interruption with your work, but yet you have to know where you've left off and pick up and continue on. It's not a nice, quiet atmosphere. It's very loud. You've got parents at the desk needing information, you know, wanting things for their child; you're taking messages continuously, not only for nurses but some of the doctors. They [the parents] want to leave a message for the doctor so you're making sure that the doctors are getting their messages as well. They might be leaving messages for other family members. You're taking it all. You're doing it all. You're getting all the calls for the new patients and taking the information. You're very, very busy with the phones as well. It's not a quiet ...

INTERVIEWER: Do you have anything to do with the meals being delivered?

ANSWER: The housekeeping people deliver the trays. But if the tray is wrong, then we have to make sure we get the new tray up. So we order all the diets for the patients in the computer. If by chance they sent up the wrong meal or something, the nurse or parent will come out and ask us to re-order. Doctors order what the patient should be on. So you have to follow the directive from the doctor ... During the day, they might run out of a certain supply. They might need a certain type of needle brought up because there's a doctor coming in and doing a lumbar puncture or things like that. We order constantly from a central service area. We order different trays up. Lumbar puncture trays. Just any kind ... it could be a gyne exam; it could be the doctor wants to do a sigmoid on the floor. Any of those things we would order all the trays ... They might simply need a different type of oxygen mask. The nurse will come out and say, 'Can you get me this ...?' So you're ordering it. It could be someone that has a colostomy that needs a different type of applicator. So you again have to know ... and you have to know where to get all these different things. It could be linen that you need.

INTERVIEWER: What's a sigmoid?

ANSWER: A sigmoidostomy is when they scope your bowel and it's not as invasive as going into a day surgery procedure. They do that right on the floor.

INTERVIEWER: Okay. So you have to know quite a bit.

ANSWER: You have to know all your medical terms.

INTERVIEWER: Anything else?

ANSWER: Oh, there's so many jobs that we do that it's hard to list them all.

The hours of the job are nominally seven to three, but this often does not include breaks for coffee or lunch, in part because health care demands are frequently unpredictable. Furthermore, the work may go home with the worker, again as a result of the nature of care.

INTERVIEWER: What do you do during your break?

ANSWER: A lot of times you don't get that break. And the reason is you can't ... You could be in the middle of doctors' orders and if there is some kind of emergency on the floor, you're not leaving the floor. A lot of times, too, the way that pre-op clinic is done, the patients don't always get there on time for their allotted appointment to be registered. Well, you can't just walk away. That backs everything up. So sometimes you're missing your break. No – I shouldn't say sometimes. A lot of times you're missing your break, working through your breaks because the workload is so heavy you're not getting time to have a break.

INTERVIEWER: And can you leave your work behind when you walk out the hospital door at night?

ANSWER: Not always ... I can get teary here. There's some situations that you need counselling for. Which has happened many times, especially working on a pediatric floor. There's the child abuse and that – that's hard to turn off. Even on the adult floor. I worked on an adult floor for many years. Cancer floor. That's difficult. You've got cancer patients there for long periods of time. You become very close to them. It's hard. It's emotional. You try to turn it off. Hopefully, you've got support at home that you can talk it out, and that's what you really need. And there are situations that ... the employer needs to bring in the crisis team to the whole floor, like a post-traumatic stress debriefing, because some situations are very difficult. And that's in any health care, any floor, any hospital has those situations.

Virtually the full transcript of this interview with a ward clerk has been included here because it so clearly sets out the complexity, skill, and commitment involved in the work, as well as the very specific nature of clerical work in heath care. It offers just one indication of the critical role clerical work plays in health services.

In health care, women work as medical and other kinds of secretaries, as ward clerks, as court recorders and medical transcriptionists, as records and file managers, as receptionists and switchboard operators. Not surprisingly, almost all of these clerical workers are women: in all

Figure 2.2 Clerical occupations in health care and social assistance industries by sex, all workers, 2000

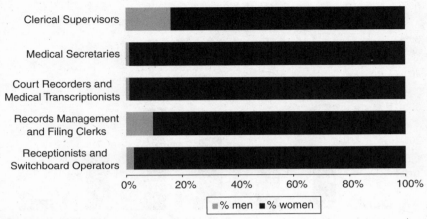

Source: Statistics Canada 2001a.

categories except that of clerical supervisor, women make up over 90 per cent of clerical workers in health care. The men who do this work are more likely to be clerical supervisors rather than clerks (figure 2.2). Although women are still the majority in this supervisory work, they make up only three-quarters of the clerical supervisors in residential care.

It is significant, however, that the men in these occupations tend to have less formal education than the women have. Three-quarters of the male clerical supervisors have high school education or less, while this is the case for less than one-quarter of the women who supervise. Clearly, the greater number of men in supervisory positions does not reflect more formal credentials. Half the women who do clerical work have a community college diploma, and another 9 per cent have one or more university degrees. In other words, the majority have post-sec-ondary credentials. While 6 per cent of women have less than high school, this is the case for 15 per cent of the men in health care clerical work (figure 2.3).

Clerical workers tend to be somewhat younger than the overall labour force and over-representative of visible minority groups. Most of the women are in their 30s or 40s. Unlike many other occupational categories, their numbers drop significantly after age 50. The male cler-

Figure 2.3 Education levels for men and women in secretarial and other clerical occupations (aggregated), 2005

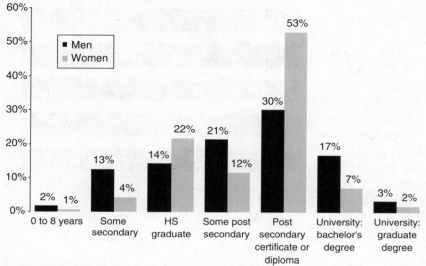

Source: Statistics Canada 2005c.

ical workers are even younger, perhaps reflecting the computerization of the work, the lack of employment opportunities in male-dominated work, and the part-time work available for those who are completing their formal education (figure 2.4).

The proportion of immigrants who do this work is similar to the proportion of immigrants in the general population, but those women self-defining as visible minority are over-represented among medical secretaries, records managers, and filing clerks, and are under-represented in other health care clerical jobs. Males from visible minorities are over-represented in jobs working as receptionists and switchboard operators.

Clerical workers are more likely to have part-time work than are women in the labour force overall. The high proportion of male medical secretaries and receptionists working part-time may reflect their young age. They may take part-time work as a supplement to school. In contrast, all the male supervisors are employed full-time. However, most of the male and female employees, part-time and full-time, have regular – or what is termed permanent – employment. Indeed, they are more likely to have permanent jobs than is the case for the labour force as a whole (see figure 2.5).

Figure 2.4 Ages of men and women in secretarial and clerical occupations (aggregated), 2005

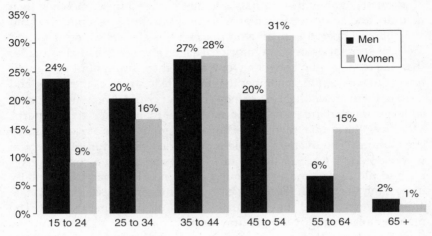

Source: Statistics Canada 2005c.

Figure 2.5 Clerical occupations by full-time/part-time status: health care and social assistance industries and all other industries, 2005

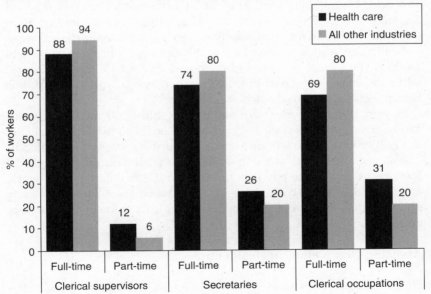

Source: Statistics Canada 2005c.

Wages for clerical workers vary considerably. At first glance, the earnings data on clerical work in health care look relatively good for women. Medical secretaries in hospitals average higher annual incomes than men do, and so do records managers and file clerks, receptionists and switchboard operators in all workplaces. Only clerical supervisors and medical secretaries in ambulatory care face a wage gap that is higher than the average gap between women and men throughout the labour force. But we need to remember that there are few men in these jobs and most of them are young, unless they are supervisors. And when they are supervisors, they frequently earn more than their female counterparts. Moreover, the annual earnings of both men and women are low in these occupations. The average female annual income for full-time clerical workers in 2002 was $25,100, while medical secretaries, records managers and file clerks, and receptionists all earned less than this. Equally important, the men in these jobs earned significantly less than the male annual average. And these figures are for full-time employment. The many who are employed part-time earn even less.

Female-dominated clerical work is low paid everywhere. However, detailed Census data show that the wage gap between the health care sector and other industries is smaller for medical secretaries, records managers, and filing clerks and receptionists (Armstrong, Armstrong, and Scott-Dixon 2006; see figure 2.6). Only supervisors and medical secretaries in ambulatory care fare worse than their counterparts in other industries. In terms of hourly wages, women doing clerical work in health care are paid almost a dollar more than other female clerical workers. Full-time workers in health care average 37 hours a week, while those employed part-time average between 20 hours in the public health sector and 17 in the private one.

In sum, clerical work is women's work, although men are significantly overrepresented as supervisors. Clerical jobs are more likely than other jobs in the labour force to be done by women identified as visible minority. Most of these women are fairly young, although the men are younger. The pay is better than in it is in other clerical work, and the male–female wage gap is smaller. But pay is still low, especially given the fact that over 70 per cent have at least some post-secondary education.

Assisting Occupations in Health Care

Statistics Canada has a category that lumps together nurse aides, orderlies, and patient service associates (often called personal support work-

Figure 2.6 Median hourly wage for women workers in clerical occupations: health care and social assistance industries and other industries, 2005

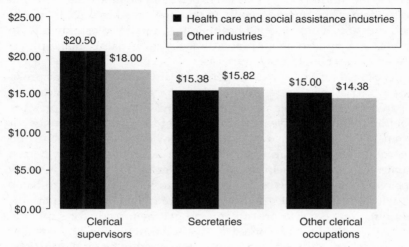

Source: Statistics Canada 2005c.

ers). All these occupations are defined as jobs that involve assisting nurses, hospital staff, and doctors in providing basic patient care. Then there is an additional category for 'other assisting occupations in support of health services,' which Statistics Canada defines as jobs in which workers provide services and assistance to other health care providers. Dental assistants and technicians are included in this large category as well. The boundaries between these groups are blurred not only by Statistics Canada but also in the practice of health care. As a result, it is difficult to separate out those most frequently defined as ancillary from those who are not.

Aides, orderlies, and patient service associates (PSAs or PSWs) can be found in all health care facilities, although they are most commonly employed in long-term care and home care. Their duties vary somewhat from jurisdiction to jurisdiction and from location to location. In Alberta, for example, home support aides provide more than 60 per cent of palliative care, but their share of the work for those with short-term home care needs declined from 55 to 46 per cent between 1991 and 2001 (Wilson et al. 2007, table 4). Nevertheless, there are some common aspects to their work. Most provide personal care, although orderlies mainly transport patients, equipment, and supplies. Wherever it is provided, personal care means bathing, toileting, shaving, and grooming, as well as feeding and offering social support. These providers get people up in the morning and put them to bed at night; they walk them and talk to them. They remind people to take their medications; they take blood pressure, handle mental health issues, and do colostomy care. In home care, they also shop, prepare meals, do banking, make phone calls, and clean people's living spaces.

Interviewed for this book, one personal care worker (who was previously called a health care aide) explained that her college certificate prepared her for a whole range of duties, from taking blood pressure to bathing, and 'every year, we have to retrain on certain things' or learn new skills. She now works the weekday three-to-eleven shift and every other weekend, caring for 17 long-term care residents by herself except when she gets help to use the Hoyer lift for patients who are unable to move themselves. 'So you have to toilet, you have to bathe and you have to change. And if people are in bed, you have to take them out, you've got to dress them and get them ready for supper at five.' Although she has worked in this same home for 20 years, her employment career has been irregular. She 'used to be on days before, then I got bumped and I went on nights, and then somebody got sick and died, God forbid, and then I applied for the afternoon shift.' When she first started working there, residents were younger when they entered and more were simply frail. Current residents are not only older: 'Most people that comes in now have certain type of dementia. Doesn't matter what type, it's a form of dementia now' (LTCb 2006). Out of the 17 residents, 15 are incontinent and half require help eating, some in bed and some in the dining room. These health conditions complicate apparently simple tasks such as bathing. No two baths are the same:

ANSWER: [It] depends on the resident also. There is some resident they are very delightful to give a bath to. There is some that you have to literally beg and sometimes they beat you. And ...
INTERVIEWER: They hit you?
ANSWER: Yeah. You've got to leave. And you've got to return. When you bring them into the shower that's another fight. You have to put on water boots. You have to put on gowns because they'll splash the water. And then when you do give them their bath and they feel the water is very warm and nice they might settle down. And you just give them their ordinary bath. You wash their hair. You finish. You've got to blow-dry their hair. You've got to cream the body,

powder the body. Sometime I use perfume. Depends if they have perfume. And put clean clothes on them. You know, moisturize their face. Sometime we even buy our own stuff to bring in to use on the residents because they need moisturizers for their face.

INTERVIEWER: And for a resident for whom you use the ceiling lift, is there a ceiling lift apparatus in the bath as well or do you ...

ANSWER: Yes, there is.

INTERVIEWER: ... shower in the wheelchair or what?

ANSWER: No, no. We have a Jacuzzi. We have showers. And we have bathtub. And there's a ceiling lift for that which is really good. And then they have the shower chair, which is good also, that you put them on and it goes right in the tub. But with that, you also have to use another lift to put them on that lift.

INTERVIEWER: Okay. So it takes a lot of strength sometimes?

ANSWER: A lot of strength. Most of us that work in the, in this industry develop ...

INTERVIEWER: So you're patting your muscles on your arms.

ANSWER: Yes. We develop arms. Big arms. Because a lot of men would ask if we go to the gym, which we don't.

She goes on to explain that 99.9 per cent of the workers are women because men don't

want to do this job because they don't want the wages we get. They don't want to do what we do ... Most of the wages are not that great. And I don't think men want to look after females that way. And it's not, what should I say, a job that weak of heart can do. There's a lot of feces that you have to wash. I don't think most men want to do that. (LTCb 2006)

Another worker surveyed for our long-term care project wrote the following succinct summary of their work and the views of their work: 'PSWs are the frontline caregivers. We see all and do all but we are treated differently. We are only PSWs. We know nothing to a lot of people, but families, nurses and doctors would know nothing without us' (LTCa 2006).

When they work in private homes, the ancillary workers face not only a wider range of patients and workplaces but also considerable variety in family members and in their forms of participation. A personal support worker, who mainly works 12- to 24-hour shifts in home care, recently provided palliative support for a woman stroke victim who died on her shift. The woman had stopped eating, and the family wanted her to come home. 'I went to the hospital and take her out.' At home she gave sponge baths and skin care while offering comfort and encouragement, as well as doing the cleaning and shopping. This worker had just prepared breakfast, lunch, and supper for the patient's husband, because 'he eat only bread so I said I'd make something good for him,' and had given the patient 'a sponge bath, clean her, clean clothes' and a clean diaper just before she died (LTCb 2006). This worker also regularly does a shift alone with a woman suffering from Alzheimer's disease, working 72 hours straight doing laundry, vacuuming, washing dishes and preparing meals, not only looking after this woman but also her cat. Asked when she sleeps, she replied, 'When she is sleeping, but you have to keep an eye on her,' because she wanders and she also needs a puffer when she coughs. Anther client is a diabetic whose medication and eating must be monitored and who needs some strong encouragement to watch her diet. Summing up, this PSW said, 'They are all demanding.' Sometimes she has to wear gloves and masks, depending on the patient, adding to her stress. Although she has a PSW certificate as well as extra training in Alzheimer's disease and childcare, she is paid only 100 dollars for her 24-hour shift.

These assisting occupations work closely with other providers and perform a wide range of jobs requested by nurses and others defined as direct providers. Optical and pharmaceutical assistants and those who work at benches in medical labs are just some examples of the kinds of workers included here. They collect blood and specimen samples, assist with autopsies and do diagnostic testing, fill prescriptions, conduct clinical trials, mix IV bags and chemotherapy products, to name only some of the varied, complex tasks carried out by technicians. Dental assistants work by themselves cleaning teeth and taking X-rays. They also work alongside dentists, taking charge of the surgical tools and other equipment. As the Hospital Employees' Union in British Columbia points out, many of these technicians are 'dealing with a dramatic expansion in the scope and responsibilities of their work as a direct result of an increasing shortage of technologists and other health care specialists' (*Guardian* 2005a, 11).

Men are most common as orderlies in hospitals, where pay and conditions are often better than they are in other health care settings. The inclusion of orderlies helps explain why, in hospitals, men make up one-quarter of the workforce in assisting occupations. In contrast, 90 per cent of those employed in ambulatory services and residential facilities are women, suggesting most of these are not orderlies. Many will be PSAs. Nine out of ten of those in other assisting occupations and nearly all of the dental assistants are also women.

These workers are not young. The majority are over 40, with most clustered around that age. The youngest group is the dental assistants, many of whom are under 40. And most have considerable formal education, with a majority holding some form of certification. Among the women, 57 per cent have college diplomas while another 6 per cent have a university degree or some form of postgraduate accreditation. By contrast, only 41 per cent of the men have college diplomas, although 15 per cent have university degrees. As is the case with clerical work, the women have more formal education than the men.

This kind of work is disproportionately done by immigrants and people from racialized groups. Compared to the labour force as a whole, women born outside of Canada are significantly over-represented, while foreign-born males are under-represented. At the same time, the proportion of visible minorities is relatively higher than in the overall labour force, especially for men. Both male and female blacks and Filipinos are significantly over-represented in the aides, orderlies, and patient service associates category. Visible minority males are disproportionately found as dental assistants and in the other assisting occupations in support of health services, where they account for one in four of the workers. Most of these men are Asian or south-Asian in origin.

The work is also disproportionately part-time. Only 61 per cent of the women who work as nurse aides, orderlies, and patient services associates have full-time jobs, compared with 74 per cent of women in the overall labour force. Some women take part-time work in order to accommodate their other job at home, like the woman employed in long-term care who reports that she has just returned to work because her daughter is now in school full-time, and she is employed part-time as she waits for full-time jobs to come up (LTCb 2006). But many do so because there is no full-time work. Listen to a worker in our long-term care study: 'I work at two nursing homes part-time to get full-time hours. I am a dietary aide who works very hard. We need more hours at both nursing homes to make my job easier' (LTCb 2006). Fourteen per cent of men in assisting occupations work on temporary contracts, about the same as in the labour force as a whole. Just over two-thirds in the other assisting category have full-time jobs, with men significantly more likely than women to have full-time work. Dental assistants of both sexes are more likely to have full-time work, although nearly one-third of the men have only part-time work.

Because such a significant proportion of those in assisting occupations work part-time or part-year, the data on annual incomes tell only part of the picture. What the data do show is that women earn relatively low salaries, with 2002 annual wages for full-time female nurse aides, orderlies, and personal service associates averaging from $24,972 in ambulatory care to $29,430 in hospitals. There are other rewards, but they cannot make up for the low pay. As one long-term care worker explained,

> I enjoy working with the elderly. It's very rewarding at times but it is physically demanding. I bathe five to six people five days a week (7:30 a.m.–12 p.m.). I am exhausted when I'm done and wish I had more time with each individual. By the time you fill the tub, clean the tub between residents, have a break, there isn't a lot of time to spend with the residents. I wish people in the health care profession would be paid more. We work hard at what we do. (LTCb 2006)

Nevertheless, these workers earn more relative to similar workers outside the health care system, and the male–female wage gap is smaller for those employed in hospitals. While most work a 37-hour week, about 18 per cent of women and 26 per cent of the men work 40 hours or more per week, with 12 per cent of men and 10 per cent of women reporting that they worked overtime hours. What this suggests is both that the work is irregular and that the workers would like more hours of work if given the opportunity.

It is particularly frustrating to base the analysis here on Statistics Canada's category, given the lumping together of those usually defined as health care and those usually defined as ancillary. Greater detail might show particular patterns for personal service associates that distinguish this work from other jobs. From the data available, we can see that immigrants and those identified as visible minorities are significantly over-represented, although the patterns vary somewhat for women and men. Here, too, wages are low and part-time work is common, in spite of the fact that the majority have post-secondary education. But women still fare better relative to men and to women who do similarly defined work in other sectors.

Visiting Homemakers, Housekeepers, and Related Occupations

Like the assisting occupations category, this category lumps together people in a range of jobs, reflecting in part the blurring of the lines between health care and household work. Those who provide home support services such as shopping, cooking, cleaning, and respite to families and individuals who are sick or disabled are here. So are those who keep house in embassies and other similar establishments. Foster parents too are included. The category, then, is broad. With over 80 per cent counted as being in health and social services industries, however, it seems likely that most are care workers. Indeed, half are in long-term care facilities or ambulatory health care services.

As Sheila Neysmith and Jane Aronson (1997) explain in one of their many articles on home care work, those who do it undertake specified tasks such as baths and foot care, meal preparation and housecleaning, shopping and bookkeeping. They also do assessments of health care needs, make medical appointments, and provide emotional support. And they do so on the basis of training and experience. Although often called cleaning ladies by those needing care, they are 'there not for the purpose of cleaning but because of the health and social situation' of those needing care. 'They don't know we have responsibility for everything about them, not just the house. We have to care about them; observe how they are doing; how they are eating; if something is happening' (Neysmith and Aronson 1997, 486).

Again, it is no surprise that 90 per cent of workers in this category are women (figure 2.7). Most of them are middle-aged, with over half between 35 and 54 years old. Perhaps most surprising is their formal certification. Nearly half have a trade or community college diploma. Another 9 per cent of the women and 12 per cent of the men have university or post-graduate education. The proportion that is immigrant is similar to the proportion in the population as a whole, but the women are much more likely than the men to be foreign born. Daiva Stasiulus and Abigail Bakan, in their book on migrant women, document how work in private homes often allows 'relations of continued discrimination' (2005, 87). While the proportion that self-identifies as visible minority is similar to the overall population, male and female blacks and Filipinos are over-represented among these workers.

The rate of part-time work is high for both women and men in these jobs, with the rates for men nearly three times as high as they are in the overall labour force (figure 2.8), although temporary work is less common than in the labour force as a whole. As is the case with other ancillary work, the women who are employed full-time, full-year in these jobs make more than they would in similarly labelled jobs in other sectors. They find their highest pay in hospitals, although women hospital workers face a larger wage gap with men compared to those in ambu-

Figure 2.7 Visiting homemakers, housekeepers, and related occupations in health care and social assistance industries by sex, all workers, 2000

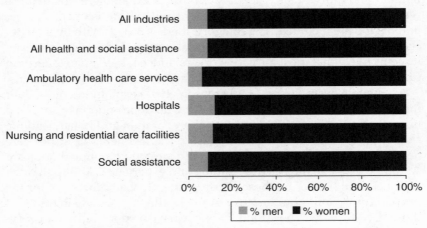

Source: Statistics Canada 2001a.

Figure 2.8 Rates of part-time employment in childcare/home support occupations (aggregate category): health care and social assistance industries and all other industries, by sex, 2005

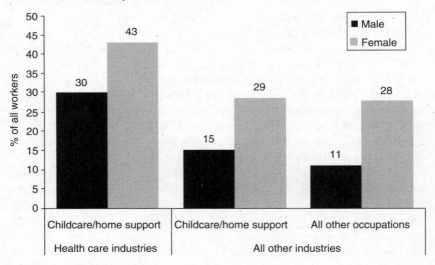

Source: Statistics Canada 2005c.

latory care. However, hourly wages are lower, on average, in health and social services than in all other occupations. The difference both reflects and magnifies the high proportion of part-time work in the health and social service sector.

Unlike clerical and assisting work, then, work in the home is not done disproportionately by immigrants and by those identified as visible minorities, even though a few groups are overrepresented. Like those other two occupations, though, it is disproportionately part-time and low paid. Nevertheless, once again the pay is still better in health care than it is outside it.

Cleaning/Housekeeping, Laundry, and Food Services

Health facilities and homes have to be cleaned, the laundry has to be done, and people have to eat. This is, of course, work that is done in many service industries. However, health facilities are particularly dangerous places for both workers and patients because people are ill, frail, or are facing surgeries that expose them to all kinds of risks from bacteria and other germs. These risks are in the air and ventilation systems, as we have learned from legionnaires' disease. They are carried on equipment, laundry, food trays, and linger in bathrooms, as we have learned with the spread of superbugs such as *C. difficile*. Most of those counted as doing these jobs in health care are working in hospitals or long-term care, but it should be remembered that the 'assisting occupations' and housekeepers described above also do this work, often in private homes.

And for them, it is all health care work. Listen to this cleaner:

> You learn so much from the elderly. They deserve respect. When we have residents move in, we know and they know this is the last place they will be spending the last of their days. Listening, laughter, compassion, and understanding when they strike out at you that you wouldn't take it personal. I have always loved working with people since I was 15 years old. I love the residents in my building, talking to them when I am cleaning their rooms. Some of the stories are great to hear. (LTCb 2006)

The tasks of these workers vary considerably, both from job to job and from hour to hour, in part because it is health care work. A housekeeper (now called a service associate) interviewed for this book talks about how 'we clean; we do floors; we do beds; we do dusting.' They often have to 'double clean,' which means cleaning everything twice. 'So in a patient room, it could take you an hour and a half to do that alone ... because you have to leave at least ten minutes between washes.' There are different cleaners for different areas and a whole range of different things to clean.

> We have to clean up all the instruments that they use. All the equip-
> ment that they use, the nurses pick it up and put it in the hallway. We
> pick up the linen. We pick up the linen. We pick up the garbage that
> they used. If the patient's room is a mess, we have to clean it up. And
> then when we finish all of that, then we go back to our list and see
> how much we can get done out of our four to six, or a four-hour shift
> ... So there's a delivery. You now had the delivery and you have to go
> in and clean the floor because it might be bloody. You have to clean
> the instruments ... And then there's the discharged mother and baby.
> So if they get discharged in the afternoon, there ... could be another
> woman waiting to deliver so the room has to be ... (LTCb 2006)

The worker not only cleans patient rooms and bathrooms. She also transports patients and sets up rooms for meetings, a job once done by a male-dominated maintenance staff.

Like cleaning, the job of feeding patients also varies significantly with the needs of those who are being cared for. A food service worker interviewed for this book talked about the wide range of tasks involved in feeding residents in long-term care. The work begins with filling trolleys to set the table, as it might in any restaurant. But there are also special dietary needs.

> We have papers that we have to follow. There's the name of the peo-
> ple who don't chew any more, so we give mince, or I mean a soft
> diet. And then there's the mince. We have to make that. You don't
> have to toast it. You don't toast those diets. But the regular we have
> to toast. (LTCb 2006)

And there are also special needs in terms of actual eating. Most of the 30 people she feeds are in wheelchairs and many cannot feed themselves. 'We work really hard because, you know, we cannot tell the residents, "Come and eat!" ... They are very old and it's hard for them, you know, to force them to feed.' They take a long time to eat, to chew if they can, and to swallow. Some fall asleep long before they have enough to eat and the time allowed to feed them is over.

Those who do food, laundry, and housekeeping work, as well as those who supervise it, are mainly women. However, there are significant variations within these services. While women account for 85 per cent of the food service supervisors and 72 per cent of the supervisors in health care laundry facilities, they are only 38 per cent of the cleaning supervisors. More detailed data reveal even more segregation. For example, women constitute just over half of those who supervise cleaning in hospitals but just over one-quarter of those who supervise cleaning in long-term care. Because supervisory work usually goes to those with experience, it is not surprising to learn that most of the supervisors are over 45 years old. However, significantly more of the male supervisors are in their thirties, suggesting that gender also plays a role. This variation by gender cannot be explained by formal training. While 77 per cent of the female supervisors have at least some post-secondary certification, this is the case for only 70 per cent of the men. Again, we find a majority of people in occupations often defined as unskilled bringing considerable formal credentials to their work.

It is not possible from Statistics Canada data to determine how representative these food, laundry, and housekeeping supervisors in health services are of the general population in relation to immigration and racialized groups. We know that in terms of the labour force as a whole, male immigrants are over-represented as supervisors in food, laundry, and cleaning services and that this is also the case for females in laundry services. Similar patterns emerge for those identified as visible minority. But we do not know what the patterns look like in health services specifically. As the lines between those in and out of the public health care services become more blurred, we can expect the patterns to become more similar overall.

Work in food, laundry, and cleaning services tends to be precarious for supervisors, with large numbers of them employed part-time or in temporary positions. However, both the women and the men who work as supervisors in health care are more likely than those with similar jobs in other sectors to have permanent positions and to work full-time. Moreover, both women and men have higher incomes as supervisors in health care, and the male–female wage gap is smaller in comparison to the overall labour force. For example, while women employed full-time as food service supervisors average $22,463 a year, those in hospitals average $39,322, earning 87 per cent of the male wage. Nevertheless, it is not all good news for women in health services. The male–female wage gap for cleaning and laundry supervisors is greater than the over-all average, even though these women earn more than their counter-parts outside health care.

According to Statistics Canada, there are three kinds of cleaners. The 'light duty cleaners' clean lobbies, halls, and rooms. This category lumps together those who work in hotels, motels, and resorts with those who work in health care, in spite of the significant differences between health care and hotel service work. About one in five of those counted as light cleaners are employed in health and social services. Nearly three-quarters of them are women, although men make up one-third of those doing light cleaning work in hospitals.

Specialized cleaners, the second category, are those who clean car-pets, chimneys, ventilation systems, and the like. They tend to be self-employed or to work for cleaning service companies. A majority of spe-cialized cleaners counted as working in health care are men, but women are a slight majority in hospitals and do more of this work in long-term care. The third cleaning category, comprising janitors, caretakers, and building superintendents, is male dominated. Indeed, it almost seems that the difference between light cleaners and janitors is gender. More than 70 per cent of janitors and building superintendents in health care are men, whose jobs are described as cleaning and maintaining the inte-rior and exterior of a building. They are distinguished from light clean-ers who 'only clean' and do not do routine maintenance or outside work, or what is described as 'industrial cleaning.'

Like light cleaners, laundry workers in health care are lumped together with those employed in hotels and other, dissimilar organiza-tions. They sort and prepare laundry for washing, operate machinery of varying sizes, and handle the clean laundry for distribution. Even though this is usually heavy work involving a great deal of lifting, four out of five laundry workers in health care are women. Men are most commonly found in hospitals, where the loads may be heavy, but they still make up less than one-third of the workers. In long-term care, there are very few men doing laundry. There is a second category of laundry workers, consisting of those who iron, press, or otherwise finish gar-ments. These too are mostly women who work in hospitals.

In food services there are cooks, food counter attendants, and kitchen helpers. Given the association of women with food preparation, the fact

Figure 2.9 Highest educational attainment in the chefs-and-cooks occupational group, health care and social assistance industries, by sex, 2005

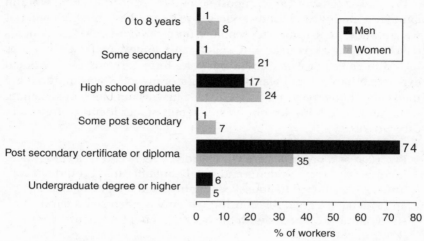

Source: Statistics Canada 2005c.

that women make up more than four in five kitchen workers in health care seems obvious. Where health care differs significantly from other sectors is in the proportion of women who are cooks. While men are the majority of cooks in the labour force, women represent nearly 70 per cent of those in health care. Men are more common in hospitals, where they account for one-third of the cooks and where they operate in huge kitchens. But in other health services, it is women who do most of the cooking. They make up almost all the cashiers in health care as well.

Most of the women who do this work in health care are over age 35, although there are more women in the younger age categories than is the case for other jobs in this sector. Male cooks in particular seem to be clustered in younger age groups. This is the only ancillary group where the men have more higher education than the women (figure 2.9). Eighty per cent of the men, compared to 40 per cent of the women, have university, college, or trade certification, while 29 per cent of the female cooks (and only 2 per cent of the men) have less than high school education. Almost all male cashiers have some post-secondary education, compared to about half of female cashiers. It seems likely that the young men working as cashiers and cooks more than account for the education difference. In the rest of the jobs in this category, women appear to have more formal education than the men.

Who are these women with post-secondary educations who work in laundry, cleaning, and food services? We do not have much detail, but we do know that some are people whose foreign-earned credentials have not been recognized in Canada, and some have lost other jobs in health care. For example, in our long-term care survey, a woman explained that 'before I was bumped out of my job, I was in nursing. I then chose housekeeping' (LTCa 2006). She was not alone in switching from nursing to housekeeping, while retaining her identity as a health care worker.

> I worked as a personal care worker for 14 years and was very much involved with my residents and family but after that I could not continue, so I switched to housekeeping to lessen the personal strain and still have a good relationship with my residents and family. I still volunteer off hours with the residents about ten hours a week. (LTCa 2006)

Most of those employed in food services are Canadian born, with immigrants under-represented in these jobs. It is not possible to calculate the distribution of visible minorities from the data available. We do know, however, that those men and women identified as visible minority are significantly over-represented in light cleaning, laundry, and food services in general, suggesting that this would be the case in health services as well.

In the overall labour force, cleaning, laundry, and food services jobs tend to be disproportionately part-time, especially for women. The status of these jobs in health care is no exception, with only 63 per cent of the women and 77 per cent of the men employed full-time (figure 2.10). Nevertheless, these workers still fare better than their counterparts outside health care in terms of full-time work. Cooks do significantly better in terms of full-time jobs compared to those in other sectors. Nearly three-quarters of the women and over 80 per cent of the men who are cooks have full-time work, compared to just over 60 per cent in the workforce as a whole. Maybe this is why we find more young men in these jobs.

Both women and men in health care industries are also likely to have higher wages than those in other sales and service jobs. Women in health care sales and services average $3.51 more an hour and men

Figure 2.10 Rates of part-time employment in the food services and cleaning services occupations, 2005

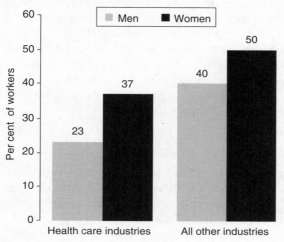

Source: Statistics Canada 2005c.

$3.78 more. In food services, while women average $3.30 more per hour than in food services jobs outside health care, the advantage is even greater for men: $6.67 more an hour. This does mean that the male–female wage gap is higher in health care, however.

Once again, the practice of lumping together workers from health with those in other sectors makes it difficult to develop a full portrait of these ancillary workers. Many of the patterns we can see are similar to those in other ancillary jobs, with few exceptions. As is the case in the occupations already described, the overwhelming majority of cleaning, laundry, and food services workers are women. Indeed, women's share of the cooking jobs is greater here than it is in the labour force as a whole. Men, however, are disproportionately supervisors throughout cleaning, laundry, and food services. Men are also more likely to be found in heavy cleaning, even though women do more than their share of the 'heavy' work. The only ancillary job in which men are the majority is specialized cleaning.

In these jobs, too, women on average have more formal education than the men. The exception is in food services, where the higher proportion of men with post-secondary education may be explained by the young men who cook and those who work as part-time cashiers. It is difficult to determine the proportion of immigrants and those identified as visible minorities. The data indicate over-representation among these jobs in the labour force as a whole, and this suggests there would be over-representation in these health service jobs as well.

As with other ancillary jobs, the wages are low and part-time, and temporary work is common. Nevertheless, the pay and the male–female wage gap is lower than for similar jobs in the rest of the labour market. The exception is in supervisory jobs, where the male–female wage gap is greater than it is elsewhere.

Security Work

Security in hospitals is there to protect both buildings and people; both patients and providers. Unlike many of the places where security personnel work, the overwhelming majority of health care organizations operate 24 hours a day throughout the year. Moreover, many of the people these workers encounter are under severe stress, and security personnel need to handle incidents as health issues rather than primarily as control ones. Not infrequently, the security guard is the only one available to ask for directions or other forms of assistance. Security personnel deal with codes that are complex, requiring an understanding of what these codes mean in health as well as security terms. This why the British Columbia Nurses' Union, for example, wants 'all health authorities to provide 24/7 security staff who are trained to protect nurses, other health care workers and patients in all ERs around the province' (*BC Nurses' Union Update* 2007, 22).

Three-quarters of those providing security are men, as is the case in the rest of the labour force. However, women make up over one-third of those who do security work in long-term care facilities. Among the men employed in security work across industries, blacks and South Asians are over-represented as compared to their presence in the overall labour force. Both men and women employed in the health sector are more likely to have full-time work compared to those who work elsewhere.

Managers

If health care workers are defined as those who provide clinical or direct care, then those who manage in health care should be defined as ancillary. According to Statistics Canada, managers are those responsible for planning, directing, controlling, and evaluating services, but not for delivering them. As a result of their research on European health services, Ann Mahon and Ruth Young (2006) conclude that there are now three kinds of managers in health services. Historically, and still commonly in many places, medical professionals work their way into senior managerial roles and may continue do some doctoring or nursing. In recent years, it has become more common for those involved in clinical practices to take special training in administration and management. Many of these individuals are nurses who, in various circumstances, can still take up care work. Finally, and increasingly, there are the managers with a distinct professional role resulting from specialization in management rather than in the provision of health care. While many of these professionals have focused on health services in their formal education, it is becoming common to assume that any kind of managerial training is relevant to health services. Indeed, experience in other sectors may be highly valued.

As is the case with other ancillary workers, the line between care and other work is often hard to draw. According to Mahon and Young (2006), some managers are focused primarily on strategic management, developing the overall goals of the organization and providing a broad view for organizational direction. Others are more directly involved in daily activities, ensuring these are carried out through the oversight of tasks and people. For the first kind of managers, the distinction between delivering care and managing it may be clear. Such managers are most common in large hospitals. But the lower the level of management, the smaller the facility, and the more managers with clinical backgrounds, the more difficult the lines between care delivery and management are to draw. In organizations that are attempting to flatten hierarchies, some may work as managers today and directly deliver services tomorrow (Wotherspoon 2002).

Most of those classified as managers in health care work in hospitals, long-term care, and ambulatory services, in that order. Women make up just over half of the senior managers, with their numbers particularly high in long-term care (59 per cent) and social assistance (67 per cent). Women are more common than men among those defined as lower-level health care managers within institutions, where they account for 73 per cent of those employed. Women are more likely to be managers in health care than in other sectors but, given that more than four out of five workers in care are women, they do not have a proportionate share of management jobs. Moreover, they are more likely to manage the smaller organizations and at lower levels. For example, 30 per cent of

Figure 2.11 Age in management occupations, by sex, 2005

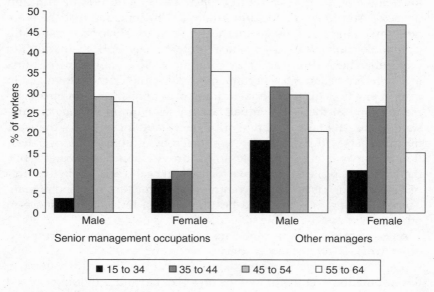

Source: Statistics Canada 2005c.

the hospital managers are men, with women's shares increasing as the size of the organization decreases.

Among senior managers in health care, the women tend to be older than the men (figure 2.11). This perhaps reflects different career paths, with women emerging from the ranks and men directly from management in other organizations. It may also reflect gender bias in promotion. The pattern is less marked among middle managers, where there is only a slight preference for younger males.

Senior managers are more likely than middle managers to have university degrees rather than college diplomas, suggesting many middle managers emerge from clinical practice. This pattern may reflect the fact that most of the older nurses were educated in colleges or hospitals, rather than in universities, while all doctors have university degrees. It is not surprising, then, that men in both senior and middle management are also more likely than women to have university degrees. However, even here, detailed Census data reveal that more of the female senior managers have post-graduate or professional degrees (Armstrong, Armstrong, and Scott-Dixon 2006).

Figure 2.12 Highest educational attainment in management occupations, health care and social services industries, by sex, 2005

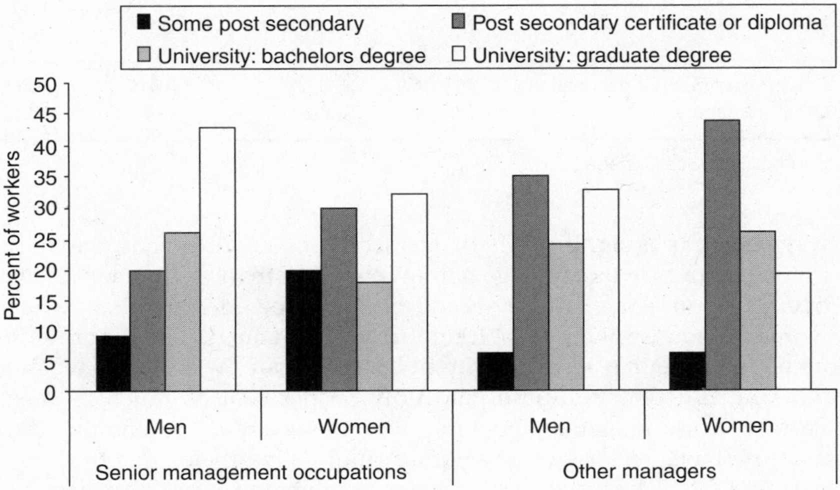

Source: Statistics Canada 2005c.

Compared to management positions in other sectors, senior manage-ment positions in health care are somewhat more likely to be held by those born outside Canada. However, immigrants are somewhat under-represented in relation to their share of the overall labour force. Fourteen per cent of senior managers and 16 per cent of other managers are immigrants, while those born outside of Canada make up almost 20 per cent of the labour force as a whole. Visible minority men and women are not as well represented in management positions. Visible minority women and men each make up only 3 per cent of those in senior management. Visible minority women fare better than men in middle management, accounting for 5 per cent of this occupation. But this is still a far cry from the 13 per cent they represent in the labour force.

Managers in health care are more likely than other managers to hold full-time permanent jobs, regardless of sex. Nevertheless, 18 per cent of the women in senior management still have only part-time jobs, while men are slightly more likely than women to have contract positions. Both sexes also do better than managers outside of health care in terms of pay on both a yearly and hourly basis, although the male–female

Table 2.1 Median hourly wage for men and women in management occupations, 2005

	Median hourly wage		Gender wage gap	
	Men	Women	$	%
Senior management occupations	$49.74	$29.81	–$19.93	59.9
Other managers	$32.00	$26.44	–$5.56	82.6

Source: Statistics Canada 2005c.

wage gap varies significantly by facility. Women working as managers in long-term care face a wage gap much larger than women face in the overall labour force, and it should be remembered that this is where women are most likely to be found in senior management. For middle managers, the gap is largest in ambulatory care, with those women working full-year, full-time paid only 56 per cent as much as men. Women working as managers in government fare better compared to men, perhaps because of pay equity rules. Nevertheless, as the wage data in table 2.1 show, hourly wages for female senior managers are considerably below those of men. Women and men in the public sector also have shorter hours than those in the private sector and, unlike in the private sector, there is little difference between the hours women and men work.

Although women account for four out of five people employed in health and social services, their numbers decrease as the level of management position and the size of facility increase. Some of this disparity can be explained by the presence of physicians in senior management and the legacy of male dominance in that profession. However, the extent of the disparity suggests continuing discrimination. Immigrants fare better in health services management than they do in the labour market as a whole, but this is not the case for those identified as visible minorities. And like other ancillary jobs, hours and pay for women managers are generally better in health care than in other sectors, although this is not the case in long-term care.

Unpaid Ancillary Work

If we define health workers as 'all people engaged in actions whose primary intent is to enhance health ... this means that mothers looking after their sick children and other unpaid carers are in the health workforce' (WHO 2006, 1). Yet paid work is what makes it into most discussions of the health care labour force. There are, however, a growing number of references to women's unpaid care work and its economic contribution, in large measure as a result of feminist efforts (Bakker 1998; Stone 2000). This unpaid work not only includes that done by mothers, daughters, sons, husbands, neighbours, and friends in the home, but also includes work done without pay in health care facilities (Baines 2006; Coleman 2003). Some of this work is unpaid overtime put in by those usually paid for the work.

The Canadian Institute for Health Information (CIHI 2002, ix) notes that the 'largest groups of unregulated health care providers are family members, friends and community volunteers' but provides no further elaboration. A special issue of its *Health Policy Research Bulletin* on health human resources recognizes that 'historically, the family has been key in providing care' (Hawley 2004, 9). It goes on to say that 'today, however, most women participate in the paid labour force and have less time to meet the needs of family members who are ill, especially when they care for their own children as well,' thus acknowledging that this is primarily women's work. It is women who take the main responsibility for cooking, cleaning, feeding, and caring for the frail, the disabled, and the ill, combining all these jobs into one.

Research by Decima reported that nearly 80 per cent of family caregivers are women (2002, 1). Other data suggest men do more than 20 per cent of care for seniors, in part because of the way this caregiving is counted. Statistics Canada includes in caregiving work inside activities such as housekeeping, meal preparation, and personal care, and outside activities such as house maintenance, lawn mowing, bill paying, and transportation. In 2002, women providing unpaid care were recorded as averaging 20 hours a week in housekeeping activities related to caregiving for seniors and nearly five hours providing personal care. Men, by contrast, average only six and a half hours a week doing inside house work and a little over one hour in personal caregiving. Most of men's contribution is outside the house, doing maintenance (five hours a week) and providing transportation (three hours a week) (Stobert and Cranswick 2004, 3).

And even these data may underestimate the total time women spend in tasks with the primary purpose of enhancing health, because the blurred boundaries make it difficult to differentiate the kinds and amounts of care work women do in the home. Women are more likely than men to see what they do in the home as simply part of being a

Figure 2.13. Participation in unpaid ancillary-type tasks, by sex, 2005

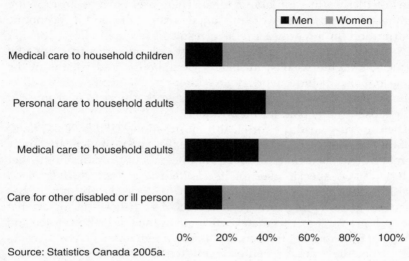

Source: Statistics Canada 2005a.

woman rather than as care work to be reported. In 2005, more men were regularly doing such work than they were in 1986 (Marshall 2006, 7). But it is still the case that 90 per cent of women between the ages of 25 and 54 do housework daily, compared to 79 per cent of the men in this age range. What Statistics Canada defines as core housework – meal preparation, meal clean-up, indoor cleaning, and laundry – is done daily by 85 per cent of the women in this age group, compared to 59 per cent of the men. Women do much more of the unpaid personal and medical care (figure 2.13) and generally spend more hours doing these jobs (table 2.2).

Moreover, it is women who carry the heavy loads. In 2002, 44 per cent of employed women between the ages of 45 and 64 were classified as providing high-intensity care involving four or more hours a week, while this was the case for only 27 per cent of the employed men (Pyper 2006, 38). Although women in Canada and United States have reduced the time they spend doing housework during this period, they still average almost two hours more a day doing such work (Marshall 2006, table 1). It is important to note here that Statistics Canada data suggest men do more care work around the home because work dismissed as ancillary when it is paid is counted as caregiving when it is unpaid.

Table 2.2 Time spent on unpaid ancillary-type tasks by participating adults, by sex, 2005*

	Median duration	
	Male	Female
	Minutes per day	
Medical care to household children	50	60
Personal care to household adults	40	30
Medical care to household adults	60	75
Care for disabled or ill person (non-household)	90	120

Source: Statistics Canada 2005a.
*Note that the universe of this table is people who reported one or more occurrence of this activity on the reference day.

   Women of all ages, stages, and cultural backgrounds do unpaid ancillary work to enhance health (Guberman 1999; Morris 2004). However, high-income women are the least likely to do such work and the most likely to put in hours similar to those of men (Statistics Canada 2006a, 3). Married women provide more hours of care work than do single women (Pyper 2006). Men are most likely to do the unpaid work when they are single and young, although they are increasingly providing more of this work when their elderly spouses are sent home for care. And for both women and men, the unpaid care work is increasing. As an Alberta study, for example, puts it, 'the relatively small amount of home care provided to dying persons raises concerns about informal caregiver burden' (Wilson et al. 2007, 59).

The Composite Picture

These data tell only part of the story, mainly because there are only limited data available at this level of occupational detail. We have, for example, not included the male-dominated trades and maintenance group, primarily because this work in health care is so hard to track in detail using Statistics Canada data. If we look at ancillary workers as a group, however, it is possible to reveal other patterns (Armstrong and Laxer 2006). For example, one in ten ancillary workers has an income that is below Statistics Canada's poverty line. The majority do not have benefits. Two-thirds do not have pensions; less than half have extended health or dental coverage. Comparisons between ancillary workers and those the Romanow Report describes as direct providers reveal significant disparities, not only in relation to the incomes, which are often justified in terms of educational attainment, but also in relation to unionization and benefit coverage.

In sum, ancillary work is women's work. Some occupations that are female dominated in the labour force are even more female dominated in health care. Significant numbers of men are found in senior management, in supervisory ancillary work, in security and cleaning, although their share of these jobs is smaller than their share in the overall labour force. Ancillary work is low paid, often part-time and/or temporary. But women do better in health care than they do in similar job categories in the rest of the labour force. While similar jobs are low paid throughout the labour force, they are in general better paid in health care. This is especially the case for men. The wage gap between women and men also tends to be smaller in health care, but this is not always the case. Moreover, health care jobs are also more likely to be full-time and permanent, with more benefits and much higher rates of unionization, than similar jobs in other sectors (Armstrong and Laxer 2006). Most individuals work as employees, with the exception of some managers, researchers, consultants, sonographers, dental technicians, and medical transcriptionists, who tend to be self-employed and relatively well paid. Self-employment is also more common among homemakers and housekeepers, where it is most likely to mean precarious work and pay.

The profile of those who do jobs labelled ancillary in health care differs to some extent from that of those employed outside health and social services. Compared to the labour force as a whole, immigrants and those identified as visible minorities hold a higher proportion of ancillary jobs. Visible minorities are over-represented in most clerical jobs, other assisting occupations, food, laundry, and cleaning work. They are, however, under-represented as managers, especially in senior positions. Immigrants are over-represented in other assisting occupations, in food, laundry, and cleaning jobs. Greater detail reveals greater differences both between women and men and among women. For example, women who work as visiting homemakers are more likely than men who do this work to be foreign born. While the number of people identifying as visible minority in these homemaking jobs is similar to the proportion in the larger labour force, male and female blacks and Filipinos have a larger share of jobs here than they do overall. The women tend to have more formal education and training than the men, except in the most senior management jobs and in the cooking jobs. Indeed, many women have much more formal education than the label of unskilled would suggest. The men who cook often work part-time, while those who work as cashiers and clerks are younger than the women who do this work. Meanwhile, most of the women who work in the laundry and kitchens are middle-aged or older.

This portrait needs more work to fill in the depth and range of the work and the workers in ancillary health care. It does, however, provide at least an outline that allows us to further investigate the structures and processes that help explain these patterns. Like this portrait, our explanations are based on feminist political economy, which we discuss in the next chapter.

3 Determining Who Counts

The very term 'ancillary' implies a particular understanding of health care. It invokes a notion of clearly defined activities with definite boundaries between work that is central and work that is peripheral or not even part of health care. The notion of ancillary work fits best with a medical model of health care focused on the scientifically based treatment of body parts, with doctors as the central authority. Diagnosis and cure are directed by a physician whose expertise and authority are based on a command of scientific research that establishes causes and corrective treatments. Thus the physician is at the centre, directing the treatment that is understood to be the purpose of health care. In such a model, health care workers are those who have acquired formal, advanced training and who are focused primarily on interventions, treatment, and cure, or on carrying out the directions of those who have such a focus. It is not surprising, then, that it is doctors and nurses who are the subjects of research and statistics on health care work, given the dominance of allopathic medicine that puts them at the centre of diagnosis and cure.

Our alternative model grows out of feminist political economy and what is usually called a determinants of health approach. This model leads to a much broader definition of both health care and health care workers, a definition that sees those termed ancillary as critical to care. Our model also suggests that in addition to a medical model and medical dominance, there are other interests that benefit from defining these workers as being outside health care, and other ideas that play a powerful role (Kelleher, Gabe, and Williams 2006). This chapter sets out the theory that underpins our argument and guides us to identify health care workers in the way we did in chapter 2. This theory helps us identify the distinct features of health care work that separate it from other forms of paid labour, as well as recognize the ways ancillary workers contribute to care.

Feminist Political Economy

Political economy has a long and varied history, and it continues to evolve as an approach to understanding the forces, structures, and relations that shape our worlds. The constant change results in part because political economy is usually understood as a method of analysis rather than as a set of fixed texts setting out answers. It therefore changes along with historical developments, with emerging evidence, and with debates among its practitioners (Vosko 2003). Nevertheless, there are some assumptions that unite those taking a political economy approach.

The name 'political economy' comes from the central assumption that the political and the economic are integrally related. This unity of the political and the economic is not primarily understood in the sense of institutions and people, but rather in the more abstract sense of a fundamental link between power and economic control. Together, these two elements set the context for understanding developments such as health care services. Equally important, a political economy approach does not consider states, markets, ideas, discourses, and civil society as independent variables that can be examined as individual entities. Instead, they are analysed as interrelated parts of the same whole.

This assumption leads us to ask in whose interests and for whose benefit are structures and relations developed. It draws our attention to the ways inequities in power pervade our relations both with others and with institutions, as well as the ways in which these inequities are created and recreated on multiple, interconnected scales. Dorothy Smith argues that a political economy approach helps us see what she calls the complex 'relations and apparatus of ruling' (1992, 4). At the same time, taking a political economy approach allows us to make the link between private troubles and public issues, as C. Wright Mills (1961) put it in *The Sociological Imagination*. Or as second-wave feminism would have it, the personal is political and the political is personal. This notion leads us to examine health care and those working within it in relation to the political economy – broadly defined – and as a component of the political economy.

Analysis begins with how people provide for their basic, socially determined needs; that is, with how goods, services, and people are produced and reproduced on both a daily and generational basis and with our ideas about what is necessary for survival. How we work together to communicate and to obtain food, shelter, jobs, joy, and babies shapes our limits and possibilities. A particular form of capitalism sets the stage without determining the outcome. This mode of production, like the markets and structures that are key components of it, is understood as being socially constructed, and thus open to change. Indeed, the analysis of how and why change occurs is central for political economy. Within this capitalist mode of production, the search for profit plays a critical role.

This leads to another central assumption about change. According to political economists, we make our own history, albeit under conditions not of our own choosing. We are born into particular existing conditions and relations. Yet we are the subjects of history, working collectively and individually to make change or support the status quo. Because we are active in creating our places and spaces, analysis must be historically specific in searching for the forces at work and the properties of the structures and relations that result. These forces include cultural and ideological ones; that is, the ideas, discourses, and practices that dominate and those that subvert existing relations. These ideas and subjectivities are not seen as free floating or as unrelated to our experience. Nor are they understood as entirely independent of the political economy. Rather, subjectivities and ideas are perceived as emerging with our experience and being shaped by the relations of ruling, as Dorothy Smith (1992) outlines. Some of these relations of ruling are more powerful than others in shaping our subjectivities, in large measure because they control what Smith calls the means of mental production, of which the most obvious examples are the media and the education system. Investigating developments in health care, then, means exploring both the most powerful forces at work and those that resist them. It means locating developments in health care not only within specific political economies, geographical locations, and time frames, but also relating these developments to people in particular social locations. It means analysing how health care and ideas about health care are actively created in specific places, thereby recognizing the importance of experience.

Perhaps the most complex assumption in a political economy approach is that related to dialectics or contradictions. Far from understanding history as a process that unfolds in an orderly way, according to some widespread consensus, political economists see history as being built out of multiple sources of tensions and contradictory tendencies. The search for profit provides one example. Some of those searching for profit look to health care, seeking to make it a source of surplus value by charging prices well over what the companies pay for labour, equipment, and materials. These companies seek to pay as little as possible for what they buy and to sell as much as they can at the highest prices possible. Drug companies are only one type among many such organizations. Their search for profit often puts them in conflict with both those who actually make the drugs for the drug companies and with those who need the drugs or pay for them. At the same time, those searching for profit in car manufacturing may well support a public, non-profit drug plan in order to lower the prices they pay to provide drug coverage for their employees. In other words, the car manufacturers and drug companies hold contradictory positions in relation to for-profit health care, just as those with drug needs and the actual producers of the drugs do. Within health care, employers searching for profit by reducing labour costs may create conditions that raise injury rates to such a level that labour becomes scarce and workers more expensive, creating an internal contradiction. Such contradictions are important to identify because they are often a source of change. Moreover, specific locations can be inherently contradictory. For instance, citizens experience critical tensions between wanting to control the amount of money spent from the public purse and wanting to have a public health care system cover everything quickly. Or there may be contradictions between taking time to ensure new drugs are safe and bringing new drugs quickly to the market for those needing them. Most political economists would agree that these kinds of contradictions are also important to identify, because they should be recognized and handled in ways that promote equity.

Initially, political economists tended to focus on inequities related to class and on relations found in the formal economy. Largely in response to feminist critiques, political economists are increasingly including households, communities, and unpaid work in their analyses. Equally important, the concept of relations of ruling is no longer restricted to considerations of class but has expanded to an examination of how gender inequities pervade societies (Andrew et al. 2003; Armstrong and Connelly 1999; Connelly and Armstrong 1992). Other social locations, especially those associated with racialization, immigration, geography, sexuality, and age, are now understood to intersect with those of gender and class. And feminists have been central in emphasizing the importance of ideas, experience, and culture. Understanding health care in this way means not only including and linking paid and unpaid work, but also relating health care work to various social locations and especially to the gender divisions that penetrate it.

Guided by this framework, we locate formal health care services within a global and local political economy, relating them to forces inside and outside their usual boundaries. We link households, communities, and formal economies, stressing the divisions and inequities related to various social locations, placing a particular emphasis on gender. We explore the pressures that promote an increasing division of labour, pressures that come from the search for profit, from efforts by health care workers to shape their labour, and from patients as well as policy makers who are seeking better care. These pressures include the ideas produced inside and outside formal institutions, as well as those arising from experience. We draw on both official statistics and reported experiences to develop a picture of the work, because we understand both statistics and experience as evidence. We include in that work all those involved in care, because we see the work as a whole rather than its separate parts creating a health care service. And we emphasize contradictory tendencies and developments in health services, as well as in efforts to improve care. In addition, we recognize the aspects of care that reflect an understanding of health care as a set of relationships' rather than simply as measurable tasks (Armstrong and Armstrong 2004b).

Like other theorists, we grapple with the problem of separating out the parts for analysis while trying to integrate them into the whole, and with the problem of capturing complexity and differences while highlighting more general patterns. For the purposes of this book, there are chapters on different aspects of the whole. But the guiding thread of our framework directs us to see them as necessarily not only linked but occurring together.

The Determinants of Health

A political economy framework fits with many of the assumptions of a determinants of health approach. Indeed, political economists such as Ivan Illich (1976), John McKinlay (1984), and Lesley Doyal and Imogen Pennell (1979) have played an important role in the development of this approach. Its focus is on a range of factors that influence people's health, with health rather than illness the central concern. From this perspective, health results primarily from favourable economic, social, and physical conditions and relations, as distinct from the effects of most health care interventions, which are undertaken after someone becomes diseased or injured. This approach thus locates biology and health care in a broader context, one that focuses on the root causes of health and ill health. Here we outline the more popular forms of the determinants of health approach, then discuss our political economy application to ancillary health care work.

The Lalonde Report, produced under the direction of the then Canadian Minister of Health and Welfare (Canada 1974), was one of the first public policy papers to set out a determinants of health approach. This perspective also sees health as socially constructed rather than simply biologically determined or technically produced. According to the 1986 Ottawa Charter, a statement produced by the First International Conference on Health Promotion, 'Health is created where people live, love, work and play.' The Ottawa Charter defined health promotion as 'the process of enabling people to increase control over and to improve their health' (Canada 1986, 1). Creating health means building healthy public policy; creating supportive work, home, and community environments; strengthening community action; developing personal skills; and reorienting health services to promote health rather than simply focus on treatment. The subsequent Adelaide Conference in 1988 defined health as a fundamental human right and stressed the importance of equity, identifying improvement of women's health as a priority not only because women suffer from inequality but also because they are critical in the daily promotion of health, especially as mothers and unpaid care providers. Three years later, the Sundsvall Conference (WHO 1991) highlighted the spiritual, social, cultural, economic, political, and ideological dimensions of workplace and other environments.

A determinants of health approach is increasingly promoted in Canadian health care reforms. For example, in its October 2005 report, *Improving the Health of Young Canadians*, the Canadian Institute for Health Information begins by stating that 'the health and well-being of Canadians is linked to a number of factors, including health services; social, economic, cultural and physical environments; and interactions between individual biology and behaviour' (CIHI 2005c, unpaginated). Health Canada recognizes 12 determinants: biological and genetic endowments; gender; income and social status; employment; education; physical and social environments; social support networks; healthy child development; personal health practices and coping skills; culture; and health services.

And these Canadian organizations are not alone. The 2005 Organization for Economic Cooperation and Development's publication *Health at a Glance* considers health determinants, 'reflecting growing policy interest in striking a better balance between spending on prevention and care' (OECD 2005, i). Closer to home, the introduction to the Romanow Report talks about the many presentations made to the Commission on the Future of Health Care in Canada that 'focused on the need to improve our understanding of the determinants of health,' arguing, for example, that 'the food we eat directly affects our health and our health care system' (Commission 2002, xix).

There is more than one list of determinants, in part because the definitions of categories and boundaries vary. However, most assume, as Robert Evans, Morris Barer, and Theodore Marmor put it in their influential book *Why Are Some People Healthy and Others Not?*, that 'medical care is but one of many socio-economic "institutions" (e.g., income maintenance, social security, education) that affect health' (1994, xiii). Through a brief exploration of the 12 determinants listed by Health Canada, we seek to reveal their role in health without claiming that they constitute a definitive list.

We begin with biology and genetic endowments, mainly because it is often assumed that these are the critical factors in health and illness. Undoubtedly, our bodies and the genetic makeup we inherit play a role in health. However, biology is frequently understood as unchangeable even though it is profoundly influenced by social contexts. These contexts are unequally structured for women and men, as well as for different groups of women and men and for different individuals. The age of puberty, for example, varies significantly among economic groups, and women employed in some jobs cease to menstruate (Messing et al. 2000). Even genes are influenced by the physical, social, and economic environment, as are our definitions of what is genetic (Basen, Eichler, and Lippman 1993). Equally important, the meaning and consequences of genetic factors are structured by such environments (see for example Mitchinson 1991).

Gender, understood as a term emphasizing the social construction of differences linked to sex, is also on the Health Canada list of determinants. Feminists throughout the world have emphasized the centrality of gender in the creation of health and care. Recognizing gender means recognizing the gendered consequences of subordinate relations and conditions. In these relations, women participate on unequal terms with men. This inequality has consequences for the health of both women and men. As Richard Wilkinson shows, in 'societies where women's status is closer to men's, both men and women [have] better health' (2005, 217).

The Fourth World Conference on Women agreed that 'women's health involves women's emotional, social, cultural, spiritual and physical well-being and is determined by the social, political and economic contexts of women's lives as well as by biology' (United Nations 1995). A gendered approach thus means much more than analysing data by sex. It means recognizing what women share socially as well as biologically. And it means understanding differences among women as well, differences related to their various social, cultural, sexual, physical, and economic locations and abilities. The claim is not that gender is primary but rather that it always must be taken into account, considering the ways it intersects with other factors.

Canadian women have been active participants in the global efforts to include gender in discussions of the determinants of health. They have been active as well in pointing out that the ways in which health services are organized and delivered have a profound impact on women's health. As the authors of *The Politics of Women's Health* put it, medicine has played 'an active role in perpetuating some aspects of women's oppression while helping to reduce other dimensions' (Sherwin et al. 1998, 3). Gender matters not only in how women are treated as patients in the health care system but also in how they are treated as workers in and outside that system. With women accounting for four out of five health care workers, gender is clearly a factor in care work. Canadians have contributed to a broad literature establishing the invisibility and undervaluing of women's health at work and women's health care work, both paid and unpaid (Armstrong et al. 2002; Grant et al. 2004). What Karen Messing (1998b) calls one-eyed science has both used men as the standard in research and ignored the particular hazards in women's work. Armed with such research, women in Canada have been successful in having both sex and gender recognized as health determinants. Moreover, they have convinced the federal government to require all policy to include a gender analysis (Status of Women Canada 1995; Women's Health Bureau 2003), although the statement is more relevant as theory than as practice.

Women in Canada and elsewhere have also highlighted the importance of racialization as a health determinant and as a factor in care work (Das Gupta 1996; Doyal, Payne, and Cameron 2003; Guruge, Donner, and Morrison 2000). Racialization is not identified as a determinant of health by Health Canada, but culture is, suggesting some differences related to the social relations of racialization. The absence of racialization from Health Canada's list could be understood as a failure to recognize the importance of racism, although it may also be meant to emphasize how other differences that result in poor health may be linked to discrimination, stigmatization, and exclusion. However, as Richard Wilkinson explains, it is easier to remove cultural markers than it is to remove those linked to racialization (2005, 229).

The federal government and some provincial governments have some policies on employment equity that acknowledge inequities resulting from racism. And the Canadian Charter of Rights and Freedoms can be understood to acknowledge racism. There is still, however, a long way to go before a determinants of health approach makes racism central and recognizes the ways in which it interacts with other determinants of health.

Income and social status also have a profound impact on health. The poor live shorter lives than the rich, and their lives are marked by more frequent bouts of ill health and disability (Wilkinson 1992). It is not only absolute income that matters to health, however. Relative income is also very important. Indeed, overall inequality in a society is a critical indicator of overall health, with greater inequality leading to poorer health (Wilkinson 2005). And we know both that inequality is increasing globally and nationally (Spiers 2000), and that women continue to be paid less than men (Hennessy 2006). Moreover, the 'quality of social relations and low social status are among the most powerful influences on health' (Wilkinson 2005, 101). Low social status is often linked to income, although it is also linked to jobs such as cleaning and laundry, regardless of pay. And sometimes low pay is justified in terms of the high value attached to the job. As Anthony Heyes (2004) argues in an article on the economics of pay in the health sector, low wages may be taken as a sign of the moral commitment of those providing care.

Social relations and social status are often related to employment. Paid work can promote health by providing material and psychological rewards as well as social contacts (Carver and Ponée 1995), and unemployment can destroy health (Avison 1998). For many, however, the formal workplace is dangerous to their health (Stellman and Daum 1973; Stellman 1977). And the risk does not come only from obvious dangers such as chemicals and guns, falls and fumes. Research in the United Kingdom shows that there is a strong relationship between health and location in the workplace hierarchy, with mortality rates near the bottom of the hierarchy three times higher than the rates for those near the top (Marmot 1986). Lack of control over tasks and over the ordering of tasks can produce more dangerous stress than does running the plant (Karasek and Theorell 1990), and low co-worker support can undermine mental health (Shields 2006b). A summary prepared for the National Forum on Health (1998), a group appointed a decade ago by the prime minister to look at the future of health care, sets out a range of factors, starting with the global, national, and sectoral contexts, through to organizational structure and environment, task requirements, and individual practices that shape health at paid work and that need to be addressed in promoting health. Households, too, can be workplaces that promote health or undermine it. Both violence and accidents are common consequences of relations and conditions in the household (Lakeman 2006; Rosenberg 1990). Moreover, stress caused by the conflicting demands of paid and unpaid work can be a particular health hazard for women (Shields 2006b).

Paid workplaces and households are often more than just working environments, they constitute our most important physical and social environments as well. Like the work that goes on within them, they can either promote or undermine health, or even do both at the same time. The nineteenth-century public health movement was built on evidence demonstrating the importance of clean air and water, on the critical nature of housing and crowding, and on the significance of safe, nutritious food (Copp 1981). The identification of bacteria emphasized the importance of washed hands, clean surfaces, and sterile equipment while more recently, legionnaire's disease made us recognize that ventilation systems play an important role in the transmission of illness. And we have all become increasingly aware of air, water, and soil pollution (Zayed and Lefebvre 1998). Health services constitute the physical and social environments not only for workers but for patients and residents as well.

Employment, in turn, can either provide us with the sort of social networks that promote good health or do the reverse by undermining our ability to form social networks. Although we most often associate social networks with households and communities, our work may not only be the place where we meet people but also where our health is influenced in ways that threaten social relations at home. As Jeanette Cochrane succinctly put it, the 'stressors we encounter in one area of our lives are certain to have an impact on other areas of our lives' (1995, 131). Sexual or other harassment at paid work, for example, can undermine relations at home. In a special issue of *Health Policy Research Bulletin*, the Director of the Public Health Agency of Canada pointed out that 'the association between social networks or social support is not new' (2006, 3). He reported that in recent consultations, 'Canadians highlighted the importance of a sense of belonging, as well as the need to have supportive families, friendships and diverse communities.' Such relationships are beneficial in themselves, and they promote access to other resources that contribute to health.

Education is linked to employment, influencing the kinds of jobs and income available. Education can also mean that we know about the kinds of personal practices, like eating our vegetables and cooking them appropriately, that can contribute to good health. Literacy is particularly significant, determining access to a wide range of resources (Breen 1998). Equally important, education can provide skills that allow people to gain satisfaction in both their paid and unpaid work. Doing a job well can promote health. It is an ongoing process, requiring continual attention to new learning from others and with others. While formal education is the most obvious form, the informal acquisition of skills and knowledge that happens through work can be as important as the ones recognized through certification. In what has become a classic in nursing literature, Patricia Benner (1984) shows how nurses move from novice to expert more through providing care than through formal education. The possibilities for learning on the job, however, are shaped by the organization of work as well as by the nature of the workplace relations.

The National Forum on Health (1998) devoted an entire volume of research findings to another of Health Canada's determinants; namely, healthy child development. It seems obvious that our early years have a profound impact, not only on our well-being as a child but also on our adult health. What may be less obvious are the ways that the work of adults, and especially of mothers, influence the environments in which children grow up. Mothers who are stressed at their paid jobs take home their stress, and may take that stress out on their children. In one long-term care research project, every group of workers we interviewed talked about finding themselves yelling at their children more as the pace of their work increased and the number of staff declined (Armstrong and Jansen 2003). Women can also bring home other health hazards at work, as we learned with SARS.

Lifestyle behaviour, or what Health Canada calls personal health practices and coping skills, are perhaps the most talked-about health determinant. It is difficult to pick up a magazine or newspaper without seeing a story about eating your spinach or joining a gym. Governments, too, have made fitness and eating well a central theme in their health promotion strategies. The federal government is now offering tax credits for parents whose children participate in certain sports the revenue department understands as contributing to health. Undoubtedly, practising yoga and eating spinach in appropriate measures can improve health. However, in order to participate in such activities, people have to have the time, the energy, and the resources. The will is often not good enough. With multiple paid jobs, for example, a long commute, and no access to childcare, it is difficult for a woman to find the time for yoga. And in any case, yoga may not be sufficient to overcome the stress caused by such work demands. Moreover, workers may know about workplace health and safety strategies but be unable to follow them because the equipment and/or the pace of their work is unsafe. Similarly, workers may have the money to buy spinach and even the time to cook it, but if the available spinach carries harmful bacteria, health is not promoted by the practice. Workplaces shape the possibilities for coping and for staying healthy. In health care, they do this not only for workers but for patients as well.

Finally, health services are recognized as a determinant of health. This too seems obvious. Indeed, a determinants of health approach emphasizes how health is determined by more than medical interventions, assuming that health services play a critical role. The interaction between health services and other factors tends to be less obvious, however. For example, in her paper for the National Forum on Health, Kimberly Scott (1998, 153) talks about how a new wave of hope for health in indigenous peoples results from their increasing 'control over human services,' including those relating to health care. In other words, racialization, or culture, as Health Canada would have it, is related to power over and relations within health services. Similarly, conditions for work and pay of workers not only influence those providing care but also the care they provide.

In short, a determinants of health approach tells us that health is critically influenced by social, economic, and physical environments, by relations as well as by structures and technologies. Health is not only determined by genes and care; it is not only about cuts and chemicals. Health is created everywhere. And it is created in classed, racialized, and gendered ways.

Although our political economy approach builds on the increasingly popular determinants of health literature, it differs from the most common applications in at least two important ways. First, instead of treating these determinants as largely independent variables, we understand them as interpenetrating ones. This means that we stress the importance of these variables within health care, in terms of both patient and worker health. This not only implies a broader notion of health care work and of who counts as a health care worker, but also an emphasis on the particular characteristics of health care work. This is the subject of the next chapter. Our focus here is on paid health care work, but it is based on the understanding that most health care work is unpaid and done primarily by women. This unpaid women's work has a significant impact on the value attached to women's paid work, an issue discussed further in chapter 5.

The second way our approach to the determinants of health differs from the more standard version concerns the importance we attach to the ways these determinants are shaped by global as well as by national, regional, and local forces in interconnected and often contradictory ways. In spite of the emphasis on the social, much of the current determinants literature ignores power inequalities at various levels and the ways in which political economies influence health and care. The most popular determinants of health approaches provide no context for the social determinants of health (Poland et al. 1998). And there is little explanation for changes over time or among groups, except for those explanations that look to individual practices or values. In an effort to identify some of the pressures leading to transformations in ancillary work, chapter 7 focuses on the global context for health reforms and the ways these play out at the national level in Canada. However, the entire analysis presented here is understood within this context.

4 Identifying Contributions to Care

In this chapter, we begin by setting out what distinguishes health care from other industries. In arguing for the specificity of health care, we are laying the groundwork for the way we count the skills of health care workers and the way we assess current reforms strategies. Our understanding of the distinctive nature of health care work grows out of our feminist political economy and determinants of health approach. This understanding leads to the analysis of nursing work that follows, an analysis that is intended to show both the integral relationship between nursing and ancillary work and the critical role ancillary work plays in care.

The Specificity of Health Care

Providing health care is not the same as being employed in any other industry. The work differs significantly from making a car on a Toyota assembly line, from offering a greeting at Walmart, from answering the phone for Rogers, and from cleaning a room in a Hilton Hotel. Understanding the specificity of care is a critical starting point in any analysis of health care and of the people who are health care workers (Armstrong and Armstrong 2004a, 119–25)

Perhaps most significantly, health care is a human right. Collectively, we have a responsibility to provide care for those who need it, and individually, we have the right to receive it. While we can argue about what exactly is included in the range of necessary services, there is global agreement that a minimum of health care must be available to all as a matter of right. Because health care is about human life, its risks and consequences cannot be assessed exclusively or even primarily in economic terms. This right distinguishes health care from most other services, as do the risks.

Health care is also a social relationship. This has a number of implications. First, it involves what Arlie Hochschild (1985) calls emotional labour. But care work differs from other work that can be considered emotional labour, such as that of flight attendants, in that it is provided to people who are at least in some ways particularly dependent and vulnerable for variable lengths of time. Moreover, both provider and patient are emotionally involved in the care process, and providers frequently identify with those needing care (Aronson and Neysmith 1996b; Baines 2004a). Listen to this woman, interviewed for this book, who provides personal care in a long-term facility:

> I like my residents. [laughs] Because you know what? My mom is 70-something and she has heart problems. She has arthritis. She has the works. And I've been in the hospital twice being sick. And I have a son with sickle cell anemia. So in a way I think of myself and I think of my mom and I think of my son, and what I do for these residents I want somebody to do for my mom, for me, and my son. So in a way I walk in all the residents' shoes 'cause I went to bed one night and I wake up sick. I have to go to the hospital. I didn't know what was wrong with me. I had to have surgery 'cause a cyst broke. And it was so bad that they said it was leaking toxin poison inside. And I was sick. So they treat me well in the hospital. (LTCb 2006)

She acts on this concern. One of the residents is a young woman.

> We do our talking when I'm giving her a bath. That's when we talk. And when I'm putting her to bed at night, we'll do our talk. Even now, I'm off for three months, I go back once in a while to see her 'cause she's pretty young. (LTCb 2006)

The second implication arising from the social dimension of health care work is that those seeking care are frequently vulnerable and limited in power because of a significant knowledge and/or capacity gap between themselves and the health care workers. As Nancy Folbre puts it, those who need care are not like other consumers. 'Those receiving care often lack the information or experience required to assess the quality of what they are receiving, and seldom have the flexibility to engage in "comparison shopping"' (2006, 18).

Third, those needing care are active participants in the process, with needs and demands that vary considerably from person to person and in the same person over time. A British study concluded that good care is 'individualized, patient-focused, and related to need; it is provided humanistically, through the presence of a caring relationship by staff who demonstrated involvement, commitment and concern' (Attree 2001, 456). In a Canadian study of how women define quality care (Armstrong et al. 2006), the most common answer was 'time,' by which they meant all of the above, plus time to listen, to hear, to know the individual, to respond to that individual within the context of her life. The personal support worker interviewed for this book offered the example of residents with special needs:

The resident need to have somebody that they know. They need to feel comfortable. And when agency staff come in also, there's things that they can't do for those residents, because basically things that we would do that we know this person like, they don't know. So they're going to do the basic care and that's all that patient is going to get for that day is the basic care. But I'll know. You know what? If Mary doesn't eat, [I'll say,] 'Can you give me an Ensure [a brand of nutritional drink] for Mary? She didn't have anything today and she needs something.' So I'll go get her Ensure. Or I'll sit and say to Mary, 'You know what Mary? If you don't eat you're going to get sick and weak, so come on. Please. Eat something for me, or for your daughter.' And she would say, 'Okay, I'll drink or eat something.' Agency won't do that because they don't know that. (LTCb 2006)

Partly as a consequence of care being a social relationship, health care needs are also usually unpredictable for both the patients and providers, often generating high costs that are well beyond the means of most people. Equally important, care frequently requires quick, context-specific action. Without such action, permanent injury and even death may result. And this is not an occasional issue, as it may be in construction work, for example, but rather a constant one. This makes standardization difficult, not only from person to person but also from day to day (Aronson and Neysmith 1996b). This variability also makes it difficult to monitor providers, who often must consider the context and the particular, current needs of the patient.

This variability additionally means that health care usually involves a host of people with specialist training. A coordinated team inside and outside facilities is required to cover the range of skills involved in care. This team extends beyond the specialized knowledge of paid professionals to the entire range of ancillary workers and also to family, friends, and neighbours. So for example, a personal support worker interviewed for this book explained that although she sometimes calls 911 when a particular patient with Alzheimer's disease has a crisis, she sometimes calls the neighbours. 'We could call them and they would assist us' (LTCb 2006).

The specificity of health care work means that the determinants of health take on a particular importance within health care. Social, physical, and psychological environments are even more critical for those who are ill, frail, or who suffer from chronic conditions that make them particularly vulnerable. The importance of these determinants is intensified within the health care workplace. Health care is about vulnerable individuals whose body parts cannot easily be divorced from their environments.

Moreover, the environments for health care are much more likely than other environments to constitute risks that are particularly dangerous to those requiring care. Indeed, the environments for care are part of care and can be as critical to health as clinical interventions. Environments can influence whether such interventions succeed or fail. For example, as a report from the United Kingdom Department of Health explains, 'MRSA [methicillin-resistant *Staphylococcus aureus*; an infection] in fit healthy people is not a particular problem' (2004, 4), but it has become a major problem in health services. Research in British Columbia suggests that homemaking services may be even more important than nursing ones in maintaining care in the home and in preventing a move to facility care, precisely because the frail and ill have lower immune systems (Hollander and Tessaro 2001). The influence of environments is in part why there is a term for illnesses that result from being treated in the system: 'iatrogenesis' refers to illness or death caused by health care.

Take food, for example. The National Health Service in the United Kingdom describes health care food as 'a token of exchange between hospital and patient, and it matters tremendously how it is made available to patients, how it is prepared and how it is served' (NHSEstates 2003). Steven Gelber (2005) reminds us of the healing potential of food for hospital patients. While the healing aspects of food matter to us all, they have a particular importance when patients need to be tempted to eat. But food is more critical than this in care. Food not eaten, the wrong food eaten, or food eaten at the wrong time in the wrong way can be especially dangerous to the ill, frail, or disabled. So can food that is not correctly prepared. Michael Rachlis points to a Saskatchewan study showing that over half of those long-term care residents studied suffered from a form of malnutrition, which in turn made them particularly susceptible to disease and less likely to be protected by a flu shot. 'If you're frail to begin with, it's crucial to eat very, very well' (Rachlis 2004, 153).

Yet while the Romanow Report identifies food as a critical factor, it dismisses those who prepare and serve the food for the ill and disabled as non-health care workers. In her 1982 study of U.S. hospital workers, Patricia Cayo Sexton suggested that 'medicine's indifference to diet and nutrition is perhaps associated with both profits and prejudices.' Profit features prominently because it is more advantageous economically to quickly treat or cure with pills and surgery than it is to do so through nutritional approaches and through making dietary workers integral to care. Prejudice also features prominently because this is traditional female work. 'Since food, diet, nutrition are the basic products of that historic female enterprise, they may be seen as essentially marginal to hospital operations, along with the dietary workers associated with them' (Sexton 1982, 38).

A similar point could be made about laundry and housekeeping work, where indifference may be compounded by the preponderance of immigrants and people from racialized groups in such work. Because those needing care tend to be particularly vulnerable, they have special needs for clean physical environments and require special protection against the heightened risks posed by others who are ill. For example, research in the United Kingdom demonstrated that high cleaning standards play an integral role in controlling infection (Wilcox et al. 2005). Similarly, Canadian research has concluded that a reduction in resources assigned to housekeeping has been an important factor in the spread of *C. difficile* in hospitals (Valiquette et al. 2004). Beds, bathrooms, and toilets all pose health risks. Health care laundry that has not been appropriately handled can become life threatening for patients (Orr et al. 2002). Recent concern over patient safety and SARS has begun to shift attention to the determinants of health within hospitals (*Healthcare Quarterly* 2005). However, very little research has been done on the safety of care in homes, communities, or even in long-term care institutions (Hassen 2005, 9).

Infections are far from the only risks particular to health care. Bed sores provide just one further example. A systematic review of research on pressure ulcers (Reddy, Gill, and Rochon 2006, 974) concluded that these common, painful, and costly problems in patients can be prevented by using better supports such as specialized foam and sheepskin overlays, ensuring good nutrition with dietary supplements, and moisturizing skin regularly. In other words, they are problems specific to those needing care and they require care of the sort provided by ancillary workers.

Those who use the health care system also have particular needs in terms of social supports. When someone is ill, facing surgery, or struggling with a chronic illness or disability, the need for social support seems obvious. With the amalgamation of hospitals and other facilities in locations that may be far from friends and families, and with most women working in paid jobs, there is more pressure on paid providers to offer support. Doctors spend little time with patients, and increasingly this is the case for nurses as well. Thus, ancillary workers are frequently the only people available to chat with and respond to calls for help. For example, patients talk to those cleaning around their beds, and often influence that cleaning in the process. 'Cleaning staff play an important role in handing people blankets and out-of-reach items, opening drink containers, getting personal items, notifying a nurse of problems and conversing with patients' (Cohen 2001, 8). Because health care is an interactive process, the people who need care are constantly defining new needs in ways that may pay little attention to the titles and credentials of workers. They want and need support now. By way of illustration, a clerical worker interviewed in an Ontario study told a story about a woman who had been informed she had cancer by a doctor and nurse who then were immediately called away. 'She had just been told and she broke down crying and the housekeeper that was cleaning up went over and she said, "Do you want a hug?"' (Armstrong et al. 1994, 59). There is often no time to call a person with formal training for working with cancer patients.

Health care also requires interaction among those who provide care, because care itself must be integrated through the complementary skills of a range of providers. Health care necessarily involves a team that includes those who perform surgery and those who make sure the surgery is clean; those who determine whether patients eat and those who help them eat; those who determine what records should be kept and those who keep them. Team members are interdependent in ways that blur distinctions between ancillary and direct care. Although the division of labour has become more clearly defined in recent years, as we shall see later, coordination across job titles is critical to care and often means different categories of workers take on tasks assigned to others when a health crisis demands it. The British House of Commons Health Select Committee warned in 1999 that 'the often spurious division of staff into clinical or non-clinical groups can create an institutional apartheid which might be detrimental to staff morale and to patients' (quoted in Sachdev 2001, 33).

The specific nature of health care work is also underscored by a consideration of the determinants of health approach, with its lessons concerning employment, working conditions, gender, culture, and social support within jobs. In other words, it leads to a concern for the health of health care workers. As Jennifer Stone, vice-president of the Canadian Institute for Health Information explained, the 'challenge, at a systemic level, is to keep health-care workers employed, satisfied, in good health, on the job, motivated and effective' (Conference Board of Canada 2005, 13). Nevertheless, most of the research on these issues has focused on the regulated professions and especially on nurses (Canadian Nurses Association 2004), and very little of it takes gender or culture into account. In one of the few studies that not only links patient safety and worker safety but also includes a range of providers in a variety of settings, Annalee Yassi and Tina Hancock conclude that 'looking after the well-being of healthcare workers results in safer and better quality patient care' (2005, 32). However, here too the focus is still on nursing staff, albeit a broadly defined nursing staff.

Ancillary workers often have part-time, temporary, or casual work, which means they often do not have sick pay or medical benefits (Armstrong and Laxer 2006). As a result, they frequently go to work sick, increasing the risk both for other workers and for those in care. New managerial practices and contracting out too frequently mean ancillary workers are unfamiliar with the physical workplace, with the patients, and with other workers. This too can harm workers and place those with care needs at risk (Baines 2006).

In sum, a determinants of health approach may be the dominant discourse in policy circles but it is not dominant in research and practice within health care. The role of ancillary workers in determining health within facilities and households is seldom considered, and reforms are seldom assessed with the role of the determinants of health within care in mind. Health care differs from other work in significant ways, creating demands and expectations not found in other work. At the same time, the health of ancillary workers is often ignored, as is the role gender and race plays in their health. Those who do the work do not need the research to tell them health work has special demands and that ancillary work plays a critical role in care. 'Whether it be clean rooms, laundry, bathing, dietary, they are all essential parts in their well-being' (Armstrong, Armstrong, and Daly 2007), as one worker succinctly explained. This book seeks to address these gaps by considering ancillary workers as part of a health care team.

The Origins of Ancillary Work

Almost all the work currently done by ancillary workers was once done by nurses. And one of the first people to emphasize what we would now call the determinants of health within health care was Florence Nightingale, the woman often recognized as the founder of nursing training. Tracing the history of ancillary work through nursing allows us to see both the central role this work has played in care and the part it continues to play in determining health. By tracing developments within nursing work, we can see that work currently defined as ancillary was once part of nursing precisely because it is essential in care. Indeed, ancillary work is still required of nurses if it is not done by others because it is so critical to care. The lines between direct and non-direct care work are difficult to draw because both are integral to care and because there is constant overlap in the work of a team that includes those defined as core and ancillary. A consistent application of a determinants of health approach leads to such a conclusion.

There are old and new debates about how the occupation of 'nurse' should be defined. Should it include, as Veronica Strong-Boag argues, the entire range of 'women's longstanding responsibility for maintaining family and community' (quoted in Bates, Dodd, and Rousseau 2005, 8)? Or should 'nurse' be used as a more restricted term, applied to those paid for care work in the regulated nursing professions? The debate arises from the fact that women have, throughout recorded history, done care work and that care work has involved a wide range of activities, regardless of whether or not the work is paid and labelled as nursing, and regardless of where it is done. The debate also arises from the overlap both between paid and unpaid nursing work and between more restricted definitions of nursing tasks and those of domestic labour. Indeed, as Christina Bates, Dianne Dodd, and Nicole Rousseau make clear in their introduction to *On All Frontiers: Four Centuries of Canadian Nursing*, nurses' struggle for professional recognition 'had as its starting point a determination to banish the taint of domestic labour' (2005, 9). It is a struggle that continues today, because domestic work remains central to care work, because domestic work is denigrated, and because care work is not always easy to divide into discrete tasks that separate the clinical from the domestic, and direct care from non-direct care.

Paid nursing work was primarily done in private homes until well into the twentieth century, although some nurses worked in hospitals and some may have worked in other kinds of residential care facilities. In French Canada, the first formal health care was provided mainly by nuns, who trained each other and worked without pay (Coburn 1987). Some midwives had trained in France's formal system, and Aboriginal women continued their traditional practices (Benoit and Carroll 2005). In English Canada, the public hospitals for the military were initially staffed by male nurses. But this practice of hiring men for nursing work was and is the exception outside military and mental hospitals (McPherson 2003, 10). In response to epidemics of cholera, typhoid, and smallpox that swept eastern Canada in the second quarter of the nineteenth century, hospitals recruited female lay nurses and paid them a wage (Coburn 1987, 443).

The label 'nurse' was applied to a wide range of women who provided a wide range of services. Most were immigrants from servant classes and acquired their skills on the job. Their tasks included 'cleaning and changing patients' clothes when they were admitted, monitoring symptoms until the doctor stepped in, restraining delirious patients, changing patients' soiled bedding and bedshirts, distributing medications and meals, and cleaning the patients and the rooms' (Bates, Dodd, and Rousseau 2005, 15). According to a Montreal doctor writing in the nineteenth century, these nurses were 'ill-educated,' although he may have been referring to formal training and reflecting his own class position (Gibbon and Mathewson, quoted in Coburn 1987, 443). Other evidence suggests that nurses had diverse levels of education and skills (Bates, Dodd, and Rousseau 2005, 25).

'Cleanliness was not a feature, either of the nurse, ward or the patient,' in part because germ theory had not yet been propagated and in part because both the patients and the nurses had few resources (Gibbon and Mathewson, quoted in Coburn 1987, 443). Hospitals in

general were often dangerous as a result, dangerous to both the providers and the patients, although Kathryn McPherson (2005) argues that
there was a wide range of care that included high quality care.

Nurses in Canada helped improve hospital safety following Florence
Nightingale and others in establishing training schools for nursing that
articulated the skills and duties of nurses. Nightingale emphasized
'nurses' nurturing work, their management of sanitary conditions and
their "ability to make the hospital a home"' (McPherson 2005, 79). In the
process, she and other reformers simultaneously enhanced the prestige
of nursing and formalized training while firmly tying it to women's
work. The combination of trained nurses, germ theory, cleaner environments, better funding, better techniques and richer patients all contributed to making the hospital a safer place for care.

At the beginning of the twentieth century, there were only two categories of women listed in the Canadian Census as working in health
care: graduate nurses and students. According to George Torrance
(1987, 481), even during the time between the two world wars hospitals
were characterized by very little division of labour. Graduate nurses
supervised student nurses, 'who not only provided most of the bedside
care but also did many of the domestic chores as well.' Some cooks,
kitchen helpers, and cleaners could be found, but many of them, like
the nurses, lived in the hospital residences. Wages were low for all these
women, with little difference perceived between general duty nurses
and maids. Nurses in private duty, who made up the majority of graduates, faced 'pressure to blur the distinction between nursing and
domestic work' (Keddy and Dodd 2005, 47).

All this started to change in the period after World War II. Hospitals
grew rapidly, prompted by the development of new technologies and
antibiotics, by returning soldiers' need for care, and by new approaches
to health care such as the medicalization of childbirth. Public financing
of hospitals and then hospital insurance gave an enormous boost to
hospital expansion. Between 1946 and 1971, the number of hospital
workers grew four-fold to over 270,000 people, accounting for 6.1 per
cent of the total employment growth in Canada during the postwar
quarter century (Armstrong 1977, 300). Work in public health and residential care also expanded along with the welfare state. With enormous
labour force growth came both managerial and labour strategies that
contributed to increasing specialization within health care work (Armstrong and Armstrong 2003). This division is more common in Canada
than it is in many other countries, where fewer distinctions among

nurses are made. As the WHO (2006, 4) points out, 'health management and support workers slightly outnumber health service providers in high income countries, while the opposite is the case in low and middle income settings where health service providers typically constitute over 70 per cent of the total health workforce.'

Until the 1960s, nursing students provided a significant proportion of the health care labour force. Nurses-in-training lived in residence and worked as apprentices in the hospital. Most were Canadian born and white, and were usually women who did not have the resources to pay for their own education (Kirkwood 2005). These unpaid apprentices provided direct care, but they also did the whole range of tasks usually called domestic. However, the changing demands of increasingly technical nursing work, new ideas about the organization of both care and nurses' education, and pressure from nurses' organizations combined to transform nursing education. Beginning in the 1960s, students left the residences and their unpaid work. They entered formal educational institutions, in the process leaving the nursing labour force until graduation and also leaving much of what we now call ancillary jobs to others who had to be paid for the work. It is during this period as well that more foreign-trained nurses were recruited in order to increase the supply and reduce the power of nurses that the shortages had created. But the work remained highly female-dominated, with women accounting for well over nine out of ten registered nurses.

Meanwhile, as we shall see later in greater detail, these formally educated nurses had been forming professional associations and unions that became increasingly successful in demanding not only decent wages and working conditions but also the right to leave some of those domestic tasks to others. It was, in part, an attempt to distance themselves from the association with women's household work and to gain status by means of that distance. Faced with rising labour costs and armed with new managerial strategies, health care organizations introduced new occupational categories. The new division of labour developed gradually, but the trend was consistent, carving pieces out of nursing work to be done by those who had less formal training and less power. What we now call ancillary work emerged. And it was mainly the result of women handing over some of women's work to other women.

While the new division of labour was intended to define boundaries and leave nurses free to focus on the clinical aspects of care, the boundaries remain blurred. As one nurse interviewed by Riva Soucie for her thesis on nurses' learning explained, 'We have fewer clerks too, so a third of my day is spent answering phones. If there's a cutback it always falls back on nurses. If a cleaner calls in sick, guess who's putting new sheets on the burn stretcher? The only people that are there all the time are nurses' (2005, 57). A nurse surveyed about conditions in long-term care wrote that

> too much nursing time taken up doing work in dietary, passing juice, cleaning tables, passing snack cart. Nursing on evening shift in my facility get 3.5 hours per shift for nursing care. The rest is kitchen work, supper breaks, paper work. Tic sheets are four pages long and it takes 4–5 minutes per shift to do. When floor is in quarantine because of illness outbreak, no extra help is offered. My floor is working three staff for 48 people. (Armstrong and Daly 2004, 20)

The boundaries remain porous not only because the nurses are always there, but also because the work must be done. It is critical to care.

Equally important, the boundaries between cleaning, dietary, clerical, and other workers are not always clear either. Celia Davies draws our attention to the 'often unacknowledged therapeutic role that such workers play as they build close relations with patients and clients' (1995, 20). So does Jerry White in his study of Canadian hospitals. 'The bond of caregiving work, loyalty to patients, and service orientation' (1990, 70) united these workers in their opposition to changes that threatened their role in patient care, a point Robin Badgley (1975) had made more than a decade earlier.

The reason for this brief rehearsal of history is not simply to emphasize the legacy of Florence Nightingale or the significance of ideas about women's work. Both are clearly important in making nurses feel responsible and in holding them responsible for the entire range of care work. These factors are also important in establishing the value attached to the various aspects of nursing work, as is the historical division of labour itself. But this section is intended to make an additional and equally important point. Cooking, cleaning, feeding, recording, and laundry are critical, even integral, components of care work. Although the work can be divided among many different people, the work itself is part of a whole and requires intricate orchestration through teamwork. When such work is not done by others in a timely and efficient fashion, nurses must do it precisely because it is essential to care. It is these other people, the ones now doing work previously done by nurses and still often done by them, whom we include as health care workers and focus on here.

Conclusions

Based on our feminist political economy take on the determinants of health, this chapter argues that health care has to be understood as different from other industries. The nature of health care shapes the work, making it different from employment in other sectors. We cannot equate work in health care with work in the rest of the service sector. Cleaning, laundry, record keeping, and feeding take on a specific form in health care, where people who do this essential work form part of the health care team. At the same time, the conditions for employment in care have an impact on care itself, as well as on the health of the workers. This in turn can have implications for overall costs. And as we shall see in the next chapter, the fact that this is primarily women's work has important implications for the structure of the work and value attached to it.

5 Making Gender Matters Visible

A determinants of health framework leads to the definition of ancillary jobs as health care jobs and of those who do the work as health care workers. Feminist political economy helps us understand how such low value can be ascribed to this work and these workers. Combining these approaches helps us understand both the invisibility and the undervaluing of this traditional women's work, and women's efforts to shape their own labour.

We begin this chapter by exploring the nature of women's care work, with the intent of showing how the blurred boundaries between paid and unpaid health care work as well as those among different kinds of care contribute to the low value attached to such work. In order to challenge this low valuation, we examine some of the skills, effort, responsibilities, and conditions involved in this work. But women have not simply accepted these definitions, conditions, and valuing of their work. The chapter concludes with a brief analysis of women's resistance through unions, professional organizations, legislation, and individual action.

Women's Care Work

Health care work is women's work. This statement refers to what women do, what we say they do, and what we think they should do. In other words, it has material and ideological roots as well as discursive ones. The boundaries between male and female labour vary historically and with class, physical location, racialization, immigration status, and age, among other social locations. Although the boundaries change, what persists is a division of labour between women and men. This division is not simply about difference but also about power and assigned worth. In general, to call something 'women's work' means it is less valued work, in terms of both prestige and pay. It also usually means fewer resources of the kind that would provide the basis for allowing women's views to prevail, or at least to have a significant influence.

Health care work is perhaps the best example of what is meant by the notion of women's work. Throughout history, across social and physical locations, women provide the overwhelming majority of paid and unpaid care work. Feminist historians have demonstrated that there has been considerable variation in the extent to which women have worked for pay in Canada over the last three hundred years, leaving some with little time to do work in their own households and others with no households or only minimal ones (Arat-Koc 1995; Bradbury 1997; Hamilton 1978; Strong-Boag and Fellman 1997). And they have demonstrated that there has been considerable variation in the extent to which women could and did undertake care work for their own household members and friends. But it is clear that when cooking, cleaning, laundry, and basic personal care were provided, they were mainly provided by women.

It is also clear that although there were significant variations in expectations about women's care work, there was still considerable consensus that this was women's work. In nineteenth-century Nova Scotia, a Reverend Sedgewick obviously had a particular class of women in mind when he preached that 'when sickness seizes on the household and chiefly on the heads of households, how timorous and tender her influence then. She is the ministering angel, whose presence and sympathy extracts more than half the evil from the disease and mitigates and soothes where she cannot deliver' (quoted in Cook and Mitchinson 1976, 25). But in order for such women to be ministering angels, other women were cleaning, cooking, doing laundry, and handling much of the heavier aspects of care work. When such work in the home was paid, it was usually done by women who had recently immigrated (Arat-Koc 1995; Strong-Boag and Fellman 1997). Even with paid assistance, however, all but the very wealthiest women in Canada worked side by side with the women who were paid to help (Langton 1950; Mitchell 1981; Parr Traill 1969).

Boundaries between unpaid domestic work and paid work were blurred within the household. So were the boundaries between care work and other forms of labour. Indeed, paid nurses most frequently worked in private homes until World War II. Cleaning up after a sick husband, parent, or child, washing their laundry and serving them food, organizing for their care and keeping their records were tasks difficult to separate definitively into care work or housework for both paid and unpaid workers. Such tasks were difficult to sort in part because they were usually done by the same women in the same place or at least by most women some of the time. Boundaries were similarly blurred between care work inside and outside the home, since the overwhelming majority of women working in the labour force cooked, cleaned, did laundry, served food, nursed, taught, and recorded (Ramkhalawansingh 1974) – just as they did in the home.

Attitudes about what women can and should do have changed significantly over the last three hundreds years. When surveyed, most Canadians now agree that men as well as women should do work in the home. However, a majority still think children will suffer if women are employed while their children are young, and see caregiving as mainly women's work (Zukewich Ghalam 1997). The 2006 decision by the federal government to pay families $100 a month per preschool child rather than provide day care services suggests that there is still considerable support for having the mother look after children at home. Moreover, as we have seen in chapter 2, women continue to do most of the care work in the home, 'both in terms of the likelihood of providing care and [in] performing the most intensive tasks such as bathing, dressing and cooking' (Williams 2004, 10). This notion of care work being women's work extends far beyond the care for children, however. Our search turned up no similar surveys regarding opinions about who should care for the sick and the elderly at home and in the labour force, but here too we know that women are more likely than men to provide the care. Despite significant changes in attitudes, care is still primarily understood as women's work, and it is still the case in practice.

Women now work in virtually every job in the labour force, and the majority of Canadians see this as appropriate (Zukewich Ghalam 1997, 15). However, most women remain heavily segregated into work that is similar to work in the home. One in five women in the labour force work in health and social services, where they account for four out of five workers (Statistics Canada 2006d). Outside the health sector, women are also disproportionately represented in service work closely related to their work in the home. In his research on hospital workers in Ontario, Jerry White (1990, 40) reports that many of those he interviewed commented on how similar their work was to what they did at home.

Women interviewed about their work in long-term care noted that they went home at night to start some of the same work again, although they also recognized that there were critical differences between their work at home and in health care (Armstrong and Jansen 2003).

Feminists have for a long time argued that the association in ideas and practices between women's care work in the private household and their similar work in public workplaces contributes to the low value attached to this labour when it is paid a wage, although it is not the only factor (Armstrong 1987). Other factors include the association of care work with servants and especially with racialized and immigrant groups (Baines 2004c). Boundaries between women's different kinds of care work have been blurred throughout history, and they are blurred on a daily basis today. Indeed, as more paid and unpaid health care work moves into the home and more unpaid care work is provided in care institutions, the blurring has increased (Armstrong and Armstrong 2005). Women paid to provide personal care often work along with unpaid female relatives and friends in private homes and in public care facilities. In both places, the tasks undertaken by women often overlap, regardless of title or pay. One advantage of this overlapping is that it reflects the integration of care work – the combination of the full range of care tasks. But there are also disadvantages. The blurring of boundaries makes it harder to see the work as skilled, as valued, and as care. It is also difficult to see the effort the workers must exert and the responsibility they carry. Ancillary work can suffer as a result.

Skills and Care

Our notions of skill play a significant role in the construction of ancillary work. The Nova Scotia minister (quoted in Cook and Mitchinson) who lectured on women's place made a strong plea for the education of women, arguing that that they required a curriculum that included 'the sublime science of washology and its sister bakeology. There is darnology and scrubology. There is mendology, and cookology in its wide comprehensiveness and untellable utility, a science that the more profoundly it is studied it becomes the more palatable, and the more skillfully its principles are applied' (1976, 21). While this may sound like a parody, it is clear from the rest of his speech that the minister saw this work as similar to other work that required a formal education, like being a biologist. He went on to say that 'knowledge of housekeeping ... is essentially necessary' (22). As dated as his views of women may seem, at least he recognized that such work involved skills. Contrast this to a recent Statistics Canada publication that described work such as cooking, cleaning, laundry, and personal care work as 'support occupations requiring few skills' (Galarneau 2003, 15).

Defining Skills

What do we mean by skills? Academics, policy makers, and managers often talk about skills but seldom define with any precision what they mean by the term. Skills are frequently used as a justification for pay, prestige, and power without any clear explanation of how they are understood or measured. As Attewell shows in his examination of the concept, skill is 'a complex and ambiguous idea' (1990, 422).

At a minimum, there is some agreement that skills refer to learned capacities. However, what constitutes learning and capacities remains a subject for debate. Most frequently, skills learned in a formal setting and resulting in some form of accreditation are more visible and valued. Statistics Canada, for example, typically measures skills in terms of credentials. According to a 2001 report, skill levels reflect 'the level of education normally required in the labour market for a particular occupation' (Statistics Canada 2001b, 6). Here, 'highly skilled' means the job normally requires a university education and 'skilled' means a college credential or an apprenticeship, while 'low-skilled' jobs require high school or less. Skill thus becomes equated with the education level set as a job requirement. It is about the job rather than the individual holding the job, although it may be the case that jobs held by those with university degrees become defined as requiring degrees – a process that equates the skill of the work with the skills of the worker.

This approach tells us only what signifies a skill rather than what skill is. It does not tell us what capacities people require to do the job. It also assumes that what is specified in a formal job description reflects the capacities that are required, and that these are acquired in formal education resulting in a credential. It thus ignores the learning acquired through other means, including what is learned informally on the job or in other places. A chef is someone in a job that requires a chef's certificate. This approach also ignores the skills people use that may be acquired through their formal education but are not formally required in the job. Home care workers who have nursing education provide just one example.

Most commonly, then, formal certification becomes a proxy for skilled work and skilled people. However, skill may also be defined and measured more directly. Literacy skills, numeracy skills, computer skills, interpersonal skills, technical skills, and clinical skills are just some of those aspects of work or workers that have been identified. But these too are open to interpretation and are not simple to assess. There is often disagreement about which of them are required in a job, about how they can be measured, and about the level of capacity required within each skill. Moreover, these skills too may be reduced to what is learned through formal training rather than learned on the job. For example, many clerical workers simply teach themselves the new computer programs that they use continually, but there may be no explicit requirement for this in the job description. What is required in the job is negotiated, as is the recognition of the skills this negotiation represents.

A review of the literature leads to the conclusion that skill is both a measurable capacity and a socially defined one. Whether it is recognized and measured, how it is recognized and measured, and what value is attached to the recognized skills is about social process rather than about objective measurement (Fudge and Owens 2006). We cannot simply say a job is skilled or unskilled on the basis of credentials alone or on the basis of recognized skills. Rather, we have to examine the work of a particular job and the social relations that surround it, including the power and gender relations.

Gender Skills

What counts as skill is profoundly gendered. As Jane Gaskell explains, when we look at the skills of any job, 'we come face to face with basic questions of value, of power, of women's place in the world. When people overlook women's skills, devalue them, give them low ratings, it is not a technical glitch, but a reflection of the status and power women have not had in the world' (1991, 142). Gender plays a critical role in both the visibility and value of skills. And so, often, does racialization for similar reasons (Baines 2004c).

If we understand skills as learned capacities, then it is important to establish that the skills are learned. Many of the skills women have are assumed to be part of being female, to be natural rather than learned capacities (Steinberg and Haignere 1987, 163), in part because women begin learning them at a very early age. As Mary Corley and Hans Mauksch (1988, 136) explain, a 'set of characteristics which would otherwise earn applause and prestige can be neutralized, if not trivialized, when identified with the presumed natural consequences of low status attributes.' The very association of certain skills with women may mean low status for those skills. The Ontario Pay Equity Tribunal, after listening to extensive expert testimony, concluded that 'the sex of the job incumbent has been a factor contributing to the traditional placement of the job within the hierarchy of the workplace in both wages and status' (Ontario Pay Equity Hearings Tribunal 1991, 7). As the quote from the Nova Scotia minister illustrates, there have been periods when the skills traditionally associated with women have been thought of as skills that have to be carefully taught. Veronica Strong-Boag (1985) has documented how domestic science emerged as a discipline and a practice in homes in the first half of the twentieth century. In Ontario, domestic science was introduced as the 'feminine of manual training,' (quoted in Danylewycz 1991, 127), offering women 'an array of household science and related sex-typed courses' (129), including instruction in sewing, laundry, food preparation, general housework, and home nursing.

But for the most part, the skills involved in cooking, cleaning, doing laundry, and providing personal care are associated with women in ways that leave their acquisition obscured and their value degraded. Even clerical work tends to get lumped in with assumed natural characteristics. Indeed, we are increasingly sending care work home to be done by women there, without providing much training or many supports, based on the assumption they can do what any woman can do. As a dietary aide in long-term care put it, 'We feel we are not appreciated and undervalued. We are known as uneducated and low on the totem pole' (Armstrong, Armstrong, and Daly 2007). Managers in the paid labour force assume women will not only know how to provide the extra support we call care but also assume they will take on the care work in addition to their assigned jobs, and will usually do so without being paid for this care (Baines 2004a; Rasmussen 2004).

Where skills are learned and who teaches them are also critical to their recognition. And those who do ancillary work tend to learn their skills primarily either at home and/or on the job. In both cases, they usually learn them from other women also thought of as unskilled. As the housekeepers interviewed for this book put it, they were taught 'by the girl that had already been working it' (LTCb 2006). In neither case do these skills result in a piece of paper that testifies to the workers' accomplishments. Indeed, the association of skills with the home itself tends to both obscure them and denigrate them, given that household work is much less valuable than labour market work in our society. Moreover, women often do similar work both in the labour force and in the home. The similarity in the skills employed contributes to their invisibility in both places.

Formal skills learned in educational institutions are much more likely to be recognized. Few places of higher learning teach cleaning and laundry skills, although there is such a program for hospital cleaners in British Columbia (Cohen 2001), and a British university has a Cleaning Science Training School (Herod and Aguiar 2006). Both clerical and personal care skills are taught in post-secondary institutions, but such female-dominated programs themselves are assigned lower value than many male-dominated ones requiring the same length of training. Equally important, many employers do not require people to have these credentials in order to do the work and thus lower the value of the certification for those who have it. Moreover, the large number of women with these skills tends to lower their value, confirming the assumption that they are only doing what any woman can do (Armstrong and Armstrong 1983). So does the large number of women who are immigrants or are from racialized groups, both groups often possessing little power.

This leads to the issues of status and power raised by Gaskell. The visibility and value of skills are negotiated. Women have limited power in these negotiations. Skills in clerical and personal care jobs are assumed to require generic women's skills – therefore any woman can be hired to do the job. Sonja Sinclair titled her book *I Presume You Can Type* (1969) as a way of emphasizing the assumption that women's innate skills extend to clerical work. In the case of cooking, cleaning, laundry, and personal care work, the question is not even asked because the assumption is implicitly made. Women's power is limited by the segregation of the labour force itself, a segregation that pits so many women against each other for this women's work. Women's power is also limited by their responsibilities or assumed responsibilities in the home, and it is limited by the men who still dominate decision making in many arenas.

The Ontario Pay Equity Commission (1988, 2) begins its explanation of why pay equity legislation is necessary with the following statement: 'Historically, men and women have tended to do different kinds of work. Work that has traditionally been performed by women, however, has generally been undervalued.' Care work is gendered work, and work done by women is less likely to be seen as skilled or rewarded as skilled. This is particularly the case with those skills mainly learned at home by large numbers of women, the kinds of skills required in ancillary work.

It is not only the skills used in ancillary work but also the effort and responsibilities, along with the working conditions, that are undervalued. Housekeepers often manage by themselves, moving heavy equipment and taking responsibility for ensuring a bed is safely cleaned. When they porter, they push heavy beds around 'people in chairs, and garbage cans, and there's lots of IV poles. There's lots of stuff in the dialysis area, equipment' (housekeeper/porter, LTCb 2006). Personal support workers must determine when to call the doctor or the neighbour, supervise the taking of medications, and 'give her her puffer when she is coughing' (LTCb 2006). Ward clerks must keep information confidential, decide when to call in codes and even handle wheelchairs (LTCb 2006). Dietary workers lift heavy trays of dishes, push trolleys, and make sure people needing care eat. Many of these skills, efforts, responsibilities, and working conditions are specific to health care work, as we argue in the next section.

Health Care Skills

Just as health care work is assumed to require women's generic skills, many of the skills required in health care are assumed to be generic to service work. When managers and government started to talk about 'hotel services' in hospitals, the claim was being made that the work and the skills involved in cooking, cleaning, laundry, feeding, and clerical work in health care are generic and the same as those required in hotels. It was further claimed that the work required no more than the skills any women has by virtue of her gender. Yet there is considerable evidence to suggest both that the work is skilled and that it is specific to care. In chapter 4, we argued that health care is a particular kind of work. Here we expand on the specific nature of health care work in order to expose the link between the specificity of health care work and the skills, effort, and responsibilities it requires.

Most importantly, health care work is about people who are ill, injured, disabled, or frail. As one long-term care worker so succinctly put it, 'We're in charge of people's lives on a daily basis' (Armstrong, Armstrong, and Daly 2007). This makes the job demanding in particular ways. An 18-year veteran in long-term care explained, 'Although it is very challenging and stressful, it is the most rewarding job I have ever had. To be able to help someone who can't help themselves and share their good times and bad is the reason I go to work every day' (LTCa 2006). Patients and residents are more vulnerable than the rest of the population, less able to help themselves, and often emotionally fragile as well. Remember the interview in chapter 2 with the ward clerk, who talked about how difficult it is when a child is dying: 'You've got cancer patients there for long periods of time. You become very close to them. It's hard. It's emotional.'

Because it is about people in such states, 'uncertainty is a feature of caring and flexibility of response is required' (Davies 1995, 19). Much is unpredictable in advance, and irregularity is a constant. Asked how many baths she gives each day in her long-term care facility, a personal care provider can only answer, '[It] depends on if the person has a lot of mess on themselves, you have to give them a bath. You can't just wash it off. You have to bathe them' (LTCb 2006). Irregularity requires workers who can respond to the irregularity, making judgments about what is to be done. When a patient's blood pressure suddenly drops, for example, and several nurses rush in to surround the bed, the dietary staff needs to stop putting down the tray and alter her work schedule. A personal support worker has to drop everything when a patient goes missing: 'So you start your building search' (LTCb 2006). When one resident takes too long to eat or falls out of bed, the food service workers have to adjust the times for everyone else (LTCb 2006). The doctor runs out of supplies, or wants a different oxygen mask, or a patient waiting for tests has a cardiac arrest. As the ward clerk explained, this means 'we're interrupted constantly.' If a patient with a micro-organism resistant to antibiotics (MRSA) is admitted in the middle of the night, 'the ward clerk will page housekeeping and tell them the room has to be double cleaned.' Or 'we have an emergency surgery so that means that I would have to go in and wash the OR floor. And then something else would happen and they had a delivery. Then I would have to go to the new life centre and clean' (LTCb 2006).

In health care, personal contact is critical. This makes boundaries among tasks difficult to maintain. What should a cleaner do, for example, when a patient asks them to pick up their dropped glasses or simply wants a chat when the cleaner is the only one in the room? As a housekeeper explained,

There's the families that are so happy to see you because they know that you chat with the patient in the bed and you help them and, you know, they become part of your day. So you set up the tray and you talk to them and you make sure everything is within reach. And you know people will help themselves if you set them up. So that was part of my job to set them up. The family is always the nice family that says, 'I know you're really busy but could you get mom some ice for her jug?' No problem. (LTCb 2006)

Because care is about whole people with varied needs and preferences and about active subjects, there are often significant differences from patient to patient. Those needing care seldom know who is assigned to what and simply want care now. Ancillary workers often fill in the gaps for a range of other workers. 'In the face of escalating bed and staff shortages, these workers are the "eyes and ears" for other health care professionals' (*Guardian* 2005a, 11). A housekeeper in chronic care explained that helping patients is 'not on the task sheet. But if you don't take the lids off, they don't get their food ... You open up the food. You open up the cartons. You take the plastic off or she'll eat the plastic' (LTCb 2006). Clerical workers often become involved in patient care as well. A study of medical receptionists (Patterson, Del Mar, et al. 2000) found that although their job descriptions focused on clerical tasks, their work often involved patient assessment, monitoring, and even therapy.

Many of the hazards to patients and providers are specific to health care, and so are many of the ways of responding to them.

You have to wear gowns and gloves when you go into isolation rooms to clean them after people have left or even in the course of the day. Every time you go into a room that has been put on isolation, there is a chart on the wall or on the door. And some rooms have masks, gowns, and gloves that you have to wear every time you go in that room. Or there's other rooms that you have to wear a gown and gloves, double gloves. So when you go in that room you have to wear this attire, and when you come out of that room, before you step out, you have to discard your gown and gloves and the rest of it into the garbage and wash your hands before you leave the room. (Housekeeper interview, LTCb 2006)

Not your average hotel cleaning job! The consequences of mistakes, of poor quality and poor timing can literally be deadly.

You know what? I think people need to know that we deal with germs that are superbugs, And that ... as a housekeeper, you have the potential to infect the whole building if you don't do something right. If you don't take your gown and your gloves off and leave them in the appropriate spot, if you run from the emerg department to an isolation room because that room needs to be double cleaned now, because there's another patient to come into it and that person is not there any more, if you don't take your stuff off properly, you could possibly infect the whole place. (Housekeeper interview, LTCb 2006)

Concern over the spread of infections has highlighted a significant difference between health care work and other industries, leading to a growing awareness of the skills involved in the work (United Kingdom, Comptroller and Auditor General 2004). Research across the globe has demonstrated that a high standard of cleaning is central to ensuring a safe environment in health care (La Duca 1987; Wilcox et al. 2005).

According to Health Canada (2005, 19), nosocomial infections, 'which are acquired while in a health care setting or as a result of medical procedure, affect approximately 250,000 Canadians per year, with anywhere from 8,000 to 12,000 estimated deaths per year.' And these data do not take into account those who are receiving care in the home. The British government now recognizes that 'cleanliness is of paramount importance to patients and the public and has a role to play in the prevention and control of healthcare associated infections' (Davies 2005, 4). A housekeeper interviewed for this book explained not only how she single cleans for pneumonia and double cleans for MRSA, but also about the different kinds of cleaners used for each room and for each health issue, and a different cloth for every bathroom. These differences from hotel cleaning means the skills required are different as well.

In her research into the work of hospital cleaners, Karen Messing found that the skills, the complexity, and the demands of work were often invisible to patients, other health care workers, and managers. Indeed, the women doing the work were themselves often invisible, as keeping out of the way in a manner that made them hard to see was one of the job requirements. Cleaners are required to adapt 'chemicals, methods and tools to different situations,' reflecting the constantly changing environment in health care work (Messing 1998a, 174). Both the equipment and patients' belongings cover a broad range of configurations that do not match the computer description of the job (Messing, Chatigney, and Courville 1998, 453). Moreover, workers have to take particular care to ensure they do not disrupt delicate equipment as they clean around it. Knocking over intravenous equipment could cause major havoc, for example. Their work is often interrupted by patients and providers, and they frequently have to respond to changes caused by emergencies or by the non-routine nature of much of health care work.

Although cleaning in health care has received some research attention, it is hard to find research on those who do clerical, laundry, and dietary work. Yet is it clear that each requires particular skills. In clerical work, records must be meticulously kept in ways that require considerable knowledge about health issues, as we saw in the interview with the ward clerk in chapter 2. Indeed, much of their work requires specialized knowledge and a specialized vocabulary related to health care organizations and health issues. Accuracy is particularly important, because errors can have life-and-death consequences. Almost all of the clerical work deals with confidential information. Much of it also involves contact with people who are ill or are distraught about those who are ill. It takes skills and effort to get accurate information and to get people to understand the information they need.

The food service worker interviewed for this book (LTCb 2006) talks about how she has to check the reports each day to know when to prepare separate food for someone who has something like diarrhea. For those who cannot swallow easily, 'you have to give that thickening juice. You have to mince that,' with the mincer designed for that purpose, before stirring to make the food palatable.

> It's too many things. You have to write it down who take this, who take that, and who take this. And you make a mistake ... you might end up, for example, for the person who is diabetic ... with sugar. So you have to make sure that, you know, what you're giving is the right diet for the residents.

Food preparation too requires such knowledge, with special care taken to ensure that foods meet the specific dietary needs of the ill, frail, and disabled. Getting people to eat takes both skill and effort, especially when eating is painful or uncomfortable.

Laundry workers in health care must carefully separate laundry, not in terms of colours and materials as we do at home, but rather in terms of diseases and patients. Laundry from isolation wards has to be washed in manually loaded machines and specially treated (Cohen

2001, 12). Uniforms are separated from bed linens, and all of them have to have approached with caution to ensure they contain no biohazardous wastes or dangerous articles such as needles. Both the machines and the garments and linens that are washed are significantly different from what is seen in most commercial laundries.

As a result of quite recent research, we do know more about some of the skills involved in personal care work. Based on his experience of working in a nursing home, Tim Diamond found that personal care jobs were much more complex than a label of 'unskilled' would imply.

> The social relations involved in holding someone as they gasp for breath fearing that it might be their last, or cleaning someone, or laughing with them so as to keep them alive, feeding them or brushing their teeth, helping them to hold on to memories of the past while they try to maintain sanity in the present. They are unskilled and menial practices only if nursing assistants are presumed to be subordinates in the medical world. (Diamond 1988, 48)

Working with the ill also means constant communication among workers as well as with patients or residents. A personal support worker explained:

> We talk with each other. If I'm leaving and Susan, who is my replacement at night, I will say ... 'Keep an eye on Mrs. White for me please. She is not feeling well. And make sure you report anything, because she's a bit feverish and stuff, so could you keep an eye on her?' And that's how we do it. The staff do that. Or we'd say ... 'Sam came out of bed twice, so could you watch him? Keep an eye on that so he doesn't fall. Make sure the wheelchair brake is on so he doesn't fall.' But we still tell each other, you know. We don't depend on whatever. We still tell each other ... 'Oh by the way, Ben has shingles.' (LTCb 2006, using fictional names)

As Cynthia Cranford (2005, 101) points out, personal care work is 'intimate and intermittent,' usually involving women and often involving women from racialized groups. But it is not only those designated as doing personal care who are engaged in this way. For example, a food service worker 'talks to the residents when I finish my job because, you know, when you are on the job, especially when short, there is really no time to talk to them' (LTCb 2006).

Those who deal directly with patients, such as attendants and personal support workers, also have to use considerable skill in lifting patients. Often lifting involves a mechanical device that requires training and judgment to operate, as well as the personal skills necessary to get the patient to cooperate and the assessment skills involved in knowing which device to use in which space. Moreover, lifting often involves teamwork and the ability to not only know when you need help but also to work with others to do the job (Messing and Elabidi 2003). It also means knowing how to work with the patient.

Jane Aronson and Sheila Neysmith's research with home care workers reveals the wide variety of skills they employ in carrying out their personal care and housekeeping tasks. They have to listen, to talk and negotiate a plan with the person who needs care. They have to take individual preferences, attributes, abilities, and health issues into account while keeping communications open. And they often teach clients how to cope. This complex process is 'accomplished by means of observation, particular knowledge of the individual, a careful according of self-determination to the clients and a large degree of flexibility on the part of the home care workers' (Aronson and Neysmith 1996a, 8). The workers have to juggle tasks and demands from patients as well as from employers, often changing their approach with each person and over time. In addition, they have to deal with family and friends, as well as with other paid providers.

Although still often defined as unskilled, these providers are increasingly adding tasks that are recognized as skilled and even regulated in many provinces. According to the New Brunswick Advisory Council on the Status of Women (Smith 2004, 4), personal care providers are delegated basic nursing duties 'such as catheter care, dressing changes and giving medications.' And they are taking on more and more of these kinds of jobs, in part because they are the ones who are there when the need arises and in part because employers want more done by those who are paid less.

In sum, health care requires particular skills, and ancillary workers bring skills to their jobs that are critical to care. We focus on skills here because the work is so often defined as unskilled. We have included in this discussion of skills the kinds of responsibilities these workers take within the health care system, but we have paid less attention to the effort and the working conditions involved in the work. For example, we have not considered the physical strength involved in lifting trays of food, in pushing wheelchairs and beds, or the conditions involved in visiting homes that are operating as drug dealerships. However, it is the effort, responsibilities, and working conditions that are central to understanding the health hazards at work, and thus we describe some of them in the next chapter.

Regulation and Training

The notion of skill is central to the regulatory framework governing health care workers. For well over a century, multiple regulations have been developed to establish in law who can do what to whom in Canadian health care. Such regulations have a long history, reflecting the efforts of both providers and governments to control who could call themselves a practitioner, and to establish standards as well as education and training requirements. Viewed by some as primarily a means to establish a monopoly and limit competition (Naylor 1986; Johnson 1972; Witz 1992), such regulations have been defended by others as a means of ensuring quality care and protecting the interests of the public based on expert knowledge (Manitoba Law Reform Commission 1994). In short, they are about who is formally defined as skilled.

'Regulation of occupations can be in the form of certification, licensure, or registration' (CIHI 2002, 24). Some providers, like doctors and dentists, are required to have a licence to practise, and these licences are governed by a body composed primarily of those considered to be experts in the field. Only those with a licence can legally do certain types of work or tasks. Initially, those required to have a licence had a defined scope of practice that established what they had the right to do and how to do it. Increasingly, however, there has been a move towards narrowing the scope of practice to specific tasks considered high risk, some of which may be delegated to others (CIHI 2002, 24). In effect, some deregulation is happening across Canada and more workers are encouraged to do a broader range of tasks.

Certification allows those who have met the established requirements to use a title such as massage therapist, although others may be able to do similar work without using the name. Some occupations require members to register and may require specific tests to grant registration. Registered nurses are an obvious example. As of 2003, more than 30 health care professions were regulated in at least one jurisdiction, but the nature of the regulation varies significantly across Canada (CIHI 2005a,14), suggesting the significant role negotiation plays in defining skills.

Licensing, certification, and registration are primarily about formal education in post-secondary institutions but also usually involve some on-the-job apprenticeship. Regulations in health care are thus focused on the individual worker. Regulations recognize the skills acquired through the education system and acknowledge, through the application of standards, the quality of those skills. What gets recognized and who gets to do the recognizing is a profoundly political process, albeit one presented as reflecting technical measurements. Patricia O'Reilly (2000) has documented some of the power struggles that were evident in recent consultations over the development of a new regulatory framework in Ontario. Some groups were successful in gaining recognition and others gained new rights. But many groups seeking legal status were excluded or marginalized, reflecting the political nature of the process.

Ancillary workers remain among the excluded and marginalized. Indeed, they do not even appear in O'Reilly's book or in other discussions of regulation. Ancillary workers are largely unregulated as individuals under provincial or territorial legislation. Some of the male-dominated work in trades and stationary engineering is regulated, and some provinces are moving to regulate training for security guards. But most of the female-dominated jobs are not regulated. There are post-secondary courses in health care clerical work, housekeeping, management, and in personal care work. There are a number of private organizations offering training courses in these fields as well. However, there is significant variation in the extent to which these credentials are required for employment in health care, and there is little if any legal regulation of this work in health care. Occupational health and safety regulations may be the exception, with all jurisdictions requiring some training in this regard.

To say that there are no regulations applying to the individuals working in ancillary jobs is not to say that they have no training. Many have taken post-secondary courses specific to their jobs, and large numbers have formal education beyond high school, as we saw in chapter 2. Many also have on-the-job training that does not lead to credentials but does increase their capacity to do the work (Armstrong and Daly 2004). Almost all hospitals report providing some on-the-job training, although it is difficult to tell how much of this training is provided to ancillary workers. Long-term care facilities are less likely to provide such training and less than half of the ambulatory health care services report doing so (CIHI 2005a,15). In other words, those services that employ a significant proportion of ancillary workers provide the least on-the-job training.

The World Health Organization's report *Preparing a Healthcare Workforce for the 21st Century* (WHO 2005a) focuses on the skills needed to care for people with chronic conditions, arguing that reforms in training are necessary. This 'requires a fundamental change in perspective from the familiar approach,' one that pays particular attention to a longitudinal perspective and prevention (WHO 2005a, 18). Five core competencies are listed: patient-centred care, partnering, quality improvement, information and communication technology, and a public health perspective (20). However, the report talks only about professionals. There is no discussion of the ancillary workers who play a critical role in public health and prevention, not to mention in the provision of long-term care.

So unlike the regulated professions, ancillary jobs lack the recognition, control, and standards that go along with regulation. And the public lacks the protection regulation is said to bring. The lack of regulation suggests a lack of skill requirements, reinforcing the undervaluing of the work while failing to ensure that the workers have the skills required. Women in Canada receive less employer-supported training than men, in part because there is little recognition that skills are required and in part because many women have already acquired skills through informal means (Kapsalis 1998). The failure to regulate and recognize the skills can be understood only through a lens that acknowledges the roles played by gender, racialization, economics, and power.

Skills can be recognized without regulation, and regulation can mean a form of gatekeeping that excludes workers in ways that emphasize gender, race, and class divisions. So regulation must be approached with caution, and other strategies should be considered to protect workers and those needing care. What is needed is supported, certified training, and recognition of previously acquired skills, however learned.

Resistance

Moving into the Labour Force

Many factors have contributed to changes in women's health care work. One of the most important has been the massive movement of women into paid work. As women have entered the labour force in

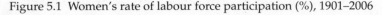

Figure 5.1 Women's rate of labour force participation (%), 1901–2006

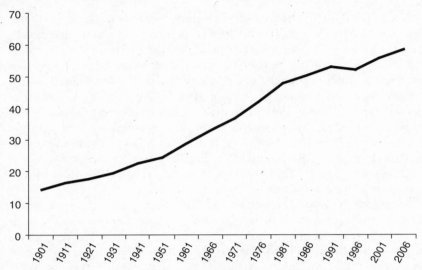

Data for 1901–61 from Statistics Canada, *Labour Force Historical Review*, Series
D107–122 (Statistics Canada 2005a). It includes women aged 14 and older (although it
includes ages 10–13 in 1921 and 1931) and excludes Newfoundland in all years.
Data for 1962–75 from Statistics Canada, *Labour Force Historical Review*, Series
D431–448 (Statistics Canada 2005a). It includes women aged 14 and older, excluding
the Yukon Territory, the Northwest Territories, and Aboriginal population on reserves.
Data for 1976–2006 from Statistics Canada, CANSIM table 2820002, Vector Series
V2461686. It includes women aged 15 years and older (Statistics Canada 2006b).

large numbers, they have increasingly resisted both their segregation
into traditional women's jobs and the conditions in those jobs.
Although this movement is familiar to us all, it is worth briefly review-
ing here because it sets the stage for the discussion of resistance within
health care work that follows.

Although Canadian women's labour force participation rates
dropped somewhat after the Second World War, they have been rising
steadily since the 1950s (figure 5.1). In 1951, just over 20 per cent of
women were in the formal labour force (Armstrong and Armstrong
1994, 16). By 2006, three-quarters of women were counted as part of the
paid workforce (Statistics Canada 2006d). Most of these women are
married and a significant proportion have children, representing a dra-

matic shift from the pre-war workforce of single women who worked beside a few married ones who seldom had children (Statistics Canada 2006d). It should be noted, however, that between 2004 and 2006 labour force participation rates for both women and men declined slightly (Luffman 2006), but that in 2007 they began to edge back up.

As a result of this steady increase, women's labour force participation has become similar to that of men. Like men, women now remain in the paid workforce for most of their adult lives. The primary difference is that women are much more likely than men to work part-time. In 2005, 26 per cent of employed women, compared to 11 per cent of employed men, did part-time work (Statistics Canada 2005c). It should not be assumed, however, that this part-time work is a matter of choice for most women. Although 23 per cent of women between the ages of 25 and 54 took part-time work because they were caring for children and another 8 per cent did so because they had family or other personal responsibilities, 32 per cent said they took part-time work only because they could not find full-time employment (Statistics Canada 2005c). In other words, more women worked part-time because that was all the work they could find than did so in order to provide unpaid care and do domestic work. And even when women give family responsibility as the reason for working part-time, we cannot assume this is a choice, especially given the lack of childcare and home care. This is important to remember when we look at the large numbers of ancillary workers who have part-time jobs.

The data on reasons for working also help us see why women take and stay in ancillary work, in spite of the poor pay and conditions. Women seek and take paid work for the same reasons as men: they need the money. Women's income is what helped maintain the income levels of husband-wife families before 1979. However, even with the majority of married women in the labour force, real family incomes have frequently failed to keep up with cost of living increases since 1979. Median family income declined between 1993 and 2004, while the number of low income families grew (*Perspectives on Labour and Income* 2005a, 64). In an increasing number of cases, it has been a wife's earnings that kept poverty at bay. According to Statistics Canada data, 'The contribution of wives' earnings to dual-earner families' ability to stay above the low-income cut-offs (LICOs) was overwhelming where the wife was the primary earner: 7% of such families fell below the LICOs in 1993, whereas almost half (45%) would have done so without her earnings' (Statistics Canada 1998, 4). Even in households with a man as primary earner, 9 per cent would have fallen below the poverty line without women's pay (Statistics Canada 1998). 1997 data show a continuing decline in family income, with more families in the bottom 30 per cent of income earners. More recent data show inequality among households continues to increase. 'While the poorest 10 per cent of families in most cities saw their income fall during the 1990s, those in the top 10 per cent saw increases of between 5 and 10 per cent' (Galloway, quoted in Jackson 2005, 27). Now, at the height of the increase in married women's labour force participation, data indicate that the majority of dual-earner families have mortgages to pay and that there are only small differences between dual-earner and single-earner households in terms of possessions such as dishwashers, freezers, and microwave ovens (Statistics Canada 1992). For the women without partners or without employed partners, the economic need is even more obvious.

This growing participation has been accompanied by continued segregation. Women still remain concentrated in teaching, nursing and other health occupations, and in clerical and service work (Statistics Canada 2004, 8). And women still, on average, earn less than men. The combination of rising participation and continuing segregation was an important impetus for the growth of feminism. Women increasingly had little choice about working for pay but in the process, they became increasingly aware of the inequalities in both pay and employment conditions. Feminists in and out of the labour force fought successfully for a range of legal and social protections.

Women gained the right to stay in employment after marriage and after pregnancy, with maternity benefits provided for those who qualified under unemployment insurance. They won the right to equal pay for work of equal value in many jurisdictions, and protection against sexual harassment. Birth control and divorce became easier to obtain and abortion is no longer illegal. The Charter of Rights and Freedoms includes provisions to protect women from discrimination from governments, and human rights legislation is intended to ensure equality between women and men as well as among women. Labour standards legislation also helped ensure holidays, overtime pay, protection against unfair dismissal, and minimum wages at the same rates for women and men. It should be noted, however, that such legislation is most likely to apply to those with full-time employment who are not self-employed and who are not on temporary work permits or similar arrangements. Moreover, new employment practices such as contracting out often remove workers from these minimal protections, and many people with insecure employment fear they will put their tenuous hold on jobs at risk if they demand their rights (Cranford et al. 2005; Vosko 2006).

It seems safe to say, then, that most women have responded to the growing demand for ancillary workers because they need the money and because these are the jobs available to them. Of course, they may get other rewards from the work, but this does not mean they have many choices about whether to take the employment. The women's movement worked hard to win legal and social protections for women that would improve their conditions of work. Many ancillary workers participated in these efforts and benefited from their success, as they did from their participation in unions. But too many remain unprotected, and some victories have turned into losses, as we shall see in the next sections.

Unions and Professions

Workers have been organizing to protect themselves and the public for well over a century. Health care is no exception, but the biggest growth happened in the post-war period. Indeed, professionalization and unionization after World War II provide a major explanation for the better pay and smaller wage gap of ancillary workers compared to others with similar work in the private sector.

The men who worked as doctors also had a long history of organizing to ensure and protect their work (Naylor 1986). Most of them remained self-employed, and they used their professional organizations to establish shared practices and fees, to determine who could become a member and what they needed to know, to negotiate with those who paid or attempted to regulate them, and to develop collective benefits and services. They organized on the basis of what they defined as their profession, distinguishing themselves from unions. Like craft unions, doctors' organizations are based on their members' skills rather than their workplaces, as is the case with industrial unions. Unlike craft unions, however, professional organizations see themselves as united by particular intellectual disciplines that are taught in universities, based on theory, and motivated by altruism. There is a great deal of debate both about what particular traits characterize a profession and whether such characteristics are the primary reason for their members' power or a justification for their power (Freidson 1970; Johnson 1972). And there are issues to be raised about the gendered nature of both professions and the analysis of professions, about the failure to protect women, about the exclusion of women, and about the relegation of some female-dominated professions to the category of semi-professions, such as nursing and teaching (Armstrong 1993; Witz 1992). What is clear is that the medical profession's success in requiring a university education and in controlling entry has meant that it was long dominated by white men with access to economic resources. And they have used their power to influence the power of others within health care.

Women who worked for pay in health care took longer to organize, in part because of the demands of their other, domestic jobs and in part because they were often forced out of their paid health care jobs when they married or became pregnant. Almost all of them were called nurses and they were outnumbered by doctors a century ago, although official counts probably left out the many women who worked as lay nurses (Coburn 1987). Most nurses worked in private homes, unless they were members of the religious orders that provided most of the institutional care. The combination of scattered workplaces, religious commitments, and ideas about women's place made it difficult for them to organize. So did employer practices that often required women to leave paid work once they married. The Nightingale tradition also played a role. Nightingale schools established in Canada in the late nineteenth century embraced notions of female obedience and military order. As Judi Coburn has made clear, these nursing schools sought 'the instilment of strict authoritarian values,' a stance evident in the motto 'chosen for the first school of nursing: "I see and am silent"' (Coburn 1987, 447–8).

Nevertheless, nurses did start to organize. It is not surprising that nurses sought to follow the male lead and look for recognition as a profession. Not only were doctors the model in health care, but doctors also had considerable power, authority, and income, all of which were attributed to their professional status. Following the doctors' lead, nursing graduates formed the Canadian National Association of Trained Nurses in 1908. This professional organization sought to encourage 'mutual understanding and unity among nurses in Canada' (Mussallem 1988, 401), and to elevate 'the standards of education and promotion of a high standard of professional honor and establish a code of ethics' (Jensen 1988, 560). Like doctors, nurses struggled to ensure the legislative regulation of their profession. However, the first mandatory regulation was not introduced until 1953. And like doctors, they worked to make university education a requirement for recognition as registered nurses. This too has taken much longer than it did for doctors and only recently have most provinces adopted policies that move in this direction. Not all nurses are happy with this development, in part because it follows the doctors' pattern rather than stressing the unique approach of nursing work, and in part because it requires more economic resources and therefore limits the entry of marginalized groups.

By the 1940s, the registered nurses were represented at the national level by the Canadian Nurses Association (CNA). Although the CNA supported collective bargaining for nurses, it insisted that it remain a professional organization and that there be no strikes. But this changed when a 1970 ruling in Saskatchewan argued that the provincial branch of the CNA could not act as a union because it included nurse-managers on its board. From this point on, nurses' unions began to emerge and act much more like other unions. Today, over 80 per cent of employed nurses belong to unions (*Perspectives on Labour and Income* 2006a, table 2). However, not all nurses have the right to strike, and some are restricted by legislation on essential services (Haiven 1995).

Union organizing was facilitated by federal funding, first of hospital construction and then of hospital care. Nurses were brought together in large workplaces where their shared time and experiences made organizing easier. The movement of nursing education out of hospitals also helped, because nurses were less subject to the daily discipline and cultural traditions of nursing at the same time as they were more exposed to the challenging critiques developing in post-secondary institutions. The women's movement helped as well, especially in terms of its successful demands to allow women to stay in their paid jobs after marriage and childbirth.

The combination of the growth in hospital size and the success of nurses' unions in demanding better pay and conditions contributed to the increasing fragmentation of nursing work. So did the development of technology and science, not only in medicine but also in management. More of the work previously done by nurses came to be done by others. Some, like the therapists and technicians, defined themselves as professionals and have organized on that basis. But most, like nursing assistants, personal care providers, cleaners, dietary aides, and launderers, defined themselves as workers and started to organize their own unions. The biggest growth in female union membership took place between 1965 and 1975; most of this growth was in the public sector and much of it was among ancillary workers (White 1993, 55). Data

Figure 5.2   Union coverage in ancillary occupations in health care, Canada, 2005

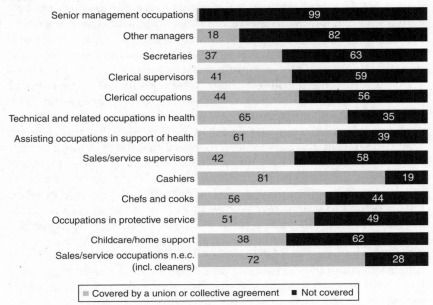

Source: Statistics Canada 2005c.
Note: 'union member' has been aggregated with 'not a union member, but covered by a collective agreement,' since the number of observations in the latter category is quite small for most occupations (although between 4 and 6 per cent of supervisory and managerial positions may fall into this category).

suggest that by the 1980s, a majority of the ancillary workers belonged to unions. Although education and public administration have higher rates of unionization, health and social services remain among the most unionized sectors for women workers (*Perspectives on Labour and Income* 2005b, 62), with 54 per cent of those defined as support staff belonging to a union. As figure 5.2 indicates, however, there are significant variations among ancillary occupations in terms of the proportions covered by collective agreements. Only a minority of clerical workers in health services have such protection, and this is the case for less than 40 per cent of those doing home support or childcare. The shift to home care, then, means a shift to a less unionized labour force.

Unionization gave many women negotiated pay and working conditions, a legally binding contract, third party arbitration, and some job
security (White 1993, 62). As a result, wages improved significantly.
Benefits such as vacations, pensions, and extended health insurance
were introduced and expanded. Hours of employment became regular-
ized. The wage differential alone demonstrates the advantage women
have with a union. In 2005, women without union coverage who were
employed full-time averaged $21.81 an hour compared to $16.94 for
non-union members. The difference was even greater for women working part time: $19.59 compared to $11.81 an hour (*Perspectives on Labour
and Income* 2006a, table 3). Moreover, unionized women employed full-
time worked fewer hours than those without union coverage, while
those unionized workers employed part-time had more weekly hours
than their non-unionized counterparts. And unions made a much bigger difference in women's wages than they did for those of men (*Perspectives on Labour and Income* 2006a, table 3). While the difference for
male full-time employees was $2.47 an hour, it was $4.87 for women.

Unions have also helped reduce the wage gap between women and
men. In Manitoba, for example, the union local in the Winnipeg Health
Sciences Centre won a pay equity settlement in 1973 that not only
increased the wages of laundry, dietary, nursing aides, and housekeeping staff by amounts ranging from $29 to $109 a month, but also demonstrated to women and men the value of their work (White 1980, 103–
6; McPherson 2003, 255). In Ontario, five unions representing 100,000
women employed in nursing homes, shelters, home care and other
community agencies won a $414 million pay equity settlement in 2003,
which significantly raised wages for some of the lowest paid ancillary
workers (Perry 2003).

Unions in health care are not solely focused on benefits for the workers. In his book *Hospital Strike*, Jerry White (1990) documents a strike
primarily motivated by what workers defined as bad care. In an interview for our book, a personal support worker spoke of going to arbitration to ensure that sick workers were replaced. Without the full staff
complement, she explained, the residents 'cannot be changed the way
they're supposed. There is not going to be any bath because I cannot
give bath because you've given me four or five or six extra residents to
look after. So those residents going to suffer' (LTCb 2006). The arbitrator agreed.

However, cutbacks in health care, reorganization, and new managerial strategies have taken their toll. Many of the ancillary jobs have

been contracted out to private companies in a manner that undermines collective agreements and unionization. In British Columbia, the government simply tore up existing union contracts (Cohen and Cohen 2004). 'The impact on wages and working conditions was immediate and stunning: wages for the privatized housekeepers were cut almost in half, benefits were eliminated or drastically reduced, and union protections abolished' (Cohen 2006, 195). The union fought the government all the way to the Supreme Court, using the Charter of Rights and Freedoms. In a landmark decision (*Health Services and Support – Facilities Subsector Bargaining Association v. British Columbia*, 2007, 6), the Court determined that the provisions in the provincial government's legislation dealing with contracting out, layoffs, and bumping 'infringe the right to bargain collectively protected' by section s.2(d) of the Charter. In the process, the union and its various supporters won an important victory, at least against the process the government used, and established the right to both bargain and have collective agreements in force.

In some other jurisdictions, the collective agreements have simply not been protected and new workers not unionized. Between the first half of 2004 and the first half of 2006, the proportion of support staff in health care that was unionized declined from 56.3 per cent to 53.8 per cent, and the proportion covered by collective agreements dropped from 57.7 per cent to 56.4 per cent in just two years (*Perspectives on Labour and Income* 2005b, 64; 2006a, 67). Gradually, unions are making a comeback. In 2005, the Canadian Union of Public Employees in British Columbia signed a collective agreement for ancillary workers employed by Sodexho, a Paris-based company, and with ARAMARK, for cleaning staff working in hospitals and other care facilities (*Guardian* 2005b), although neither contract restored previous gains. The Supreme Court decision described above, which came after these organizing activities, should provide further support for their efforts.

Even those workers who have remained employed in the public sector and have remained union members have experienced a deterioration in their employment relations and conditions of work. The number of full-time, full-year nursing jobs has declined. Wages and benefits have failed to keep up with inflation. Unions representing registered nurses have enjoyed some recent success in demanding better wages and conditions as well as a strategy to address future demands as a result of the perceived shortages. But other workers in health care have been less successful. This is especially the case in the areas where it is assumed that any woman knows how to do the work and where visible minority and immigrant women are found in significant numbers.

In Calgary, regionalization of health care services led to privatization of laundry services in two major hospitals in 1996 (Harder 2003, 134). The unionized laundry workers, most of whom were immigrants and earning low wages, initially agreed to pay cuts averaging 28 per cent as a way of saving their jobs. But when the Calgary Regional Health Authority contracted the work out to a for-profit firm, these workers lost their jobs. The Authority claimed it would save $2 million over five years and put priority on surgical services rather than on laundry services, pitting patients against providers.

Both the Canadian Union of Public Employees (CUPE) and the Alberta Union of Public Employees (AUPE) became involved, initially by advancing their own bid to operate a laundry in Calgary. When this was rejected and the firings announced, these unions and others supported the illegal walkout of laundry workers from the Bow Valley Centre. Public support was strong as a result of questions concerning politicians personally benefiting from the contracting out of the services, the overall cutbacks in health care financing, and the unfair treatment of a particularly vulnerable workforce. 'The rising level of public support for laundry workers and the growing sense of scandal led to a softening of the planned cuts' (Harder 2003, 136). The Authority promised not to contract services out for a year and to pay severance if later contracting out resulted in job loss.

In the end, the Calgary Regional Health Authority did contract services out to non-unionized employers, and a significant number of the laundry workers took the retraining option offered by the government. Lois Harder (2003, 137) argues that the union's initial success was due in part to making visible the valuable service provided by laundry workers, in part to social justice claims, and in part to strategies related to local issues. However, she links the ultimate failure to protect these laundry workers to the political and economic environment in Alberta as well as to the absence of a strong gender analysis and women's movement. She concludes that in this kind of environment, 'the possible range of legitimate political action is increasingly circumscribed' (Harder 2003, 137).

In Ottawa, the Montfort Hospital privatized the cooking, cleaning, laundry, and maintenance work in its long-term care facility in 2006. Workers were paid between $8.25 and $14.00 an hour. Since 2003, the Canadian Union of Public Employees had been seeking wage parity with workers in publicly run home care, asking for wages between $16.63 and $18.93 an hour, rates that were not only higher but also more equitable. In December 2006, an arbitrator agreed and ordered significant wage increases. The company responded by terminating their contract with the hospital. According to a CBC News (2006) report, 'The Compass Group – a food-service company that claims on its corporate website it earns annual revenues of more than $27.2 billion and employees 400,000 people worldwide – said it can't afford the pay increases.' Both workers and patients were abandoned. According to its website, this company won the 2005 Canadian Council National Award for Public–Private Partnerships on the basis of their Milton Cook Chill facility, which provides food to Canada's largest prison 'and additional institutions' (Compass Group Canada 2006), suggesting factors other than conditions for workers are the criteria for this award.

Although the majority of those defined as working in the health care sector are still covered by collective agreements, there is no guarantee that this will continue to be the case. Indeed, reforms seem to be designed to undermine union protection. The farther care moves away from hospitals and direct providers, the less likely workers are to have union coverage. While three-quarters of those employed in large health care workplaces are unionized, only a minority are unionized in smaller ones (McMullen and Brisbois 2003, vii). Meanwhile, reforms are intended to shift care outside hospitals as much as possible, where unions are less likely. Moreover, unions are increasingly unable to protect workers from layoffs, pay cuts, and other losses. Jane Aronson and Sheila Neysmith (2006) report that the home care workers in their study thought their unions were irrelevant or actually harmful in preventing job losses in the wake of the Ontario government's move to contract out their services. And unions are not always responsive to the concerns workers have for patients and residents, or for the skills workers want to protect in their jobs. Equally important, the gains one union makes may mean losses for other unions, as has sometimes been the case when one union gains the right to do work previously done exclusively by another.

Women's Individual Responses

The most visible forms of resistance are those undertaken by unions, professional organizations, by the women's movement or other groups. But women also act on their own in multiple ways to resist negative developments in health care and health care work. As is the case with actions by groups, the consequences may be contradictory for women.

Women feel responsible for those to whom they provide paid care and often put in unpaid work hours to ensure that the care they see as necessary is provided. Yet women are also held responsible by their employers for adequate care, regardless of paid work hours and work-loads during those hours (Armstrong and Armstrong 2003). Donna Baines (2004a, 269) talks about this extra work in the labour market as both an exploitation of female caring and a 'form of worker resistance to uncaring social agendas.' As Baines puts it, there is pressure from employers to do extra work, especially on younger workers (2004a; 2004c). At the same time, older workers in particular feel compelled by their own gender identity to complete the work. Similarly, in their study of home care workers, Jane Aronson and Sheila Neysmith found that the women were committed to the well-being of those in their care and that this commitment 'was, for many, a central feature of their per-sonal and work identities' (2006, 37–8). Research from Norway suggests that managers expect this willingness to take on extra work, while at the same time attributing it to women's inability to set limits (Rasmussen 2004). Not surprisingly, not all women fit this pattern. According to British research, some women respond to the expectation by doing only the minimal amount of work, thus demonstrating that the form of resistance is not about innate female characteristics (Lee-Treweek 1997).

More recently, Baines (2006) identifies significant differences between women and men in undertaking the additional work in their labour force jobs. Men are more accustomed to and more practised at setting boundaries, not only within their workplaces but also outside them. And their employers do not have the same expectations that men will voluntarily add extra work to their workload. In Baines's research, it is the men who are more likely to respond by working to rule through meeting the minimum requirements.

This extra work takes multiple forms. Women work through their mandated breaks; they come in early and stay late without additional pay. They also take on tasks beyond those prescribed by the employer. For example, the personal care provider interviewed for this book pre-pared meals for the husband of her patient, even though the patient could not eat anything and such meals are not part of her workload. He was eating 'only bread. So I said I'd make something good for him. So I made a good breakfast. I made a good lunch and I made a good supper.

I bake chicken and some rice' (LTCb 2006). A dietary worker came in to visit a resident when she was on disability leave, because she knew the woman had no relatives who came to see her (LTCb 2006). In the Aronson and Neysmith study, a woman moved to a new agency so she could continue with her patient, taking a pay cut in the process (2006, 37). Women even spend their own money on things they see patients and residents need but which the system no longer provides (Baines 2006). While these forms of resistance often bring personal rewards to the worker and help ensure better care for those who need it, they may cost the worker her own health in the long run. Equally important, such actions may obscure the care deficit created by restructuring and current work organization. The workers may become 'shock absorbers' that cushion the effects of restructuring (Aronson and Neysmith 2006), and at a minimum, fail to encourage more collective and structural reforms.

Not all the forms of individual resistance at paid work involve personal sacrifice or volunteerism. One form of resistance came out in our interviews with workers in long-term care. Workers reported being restricted in terms of how many diapers they could use on residents each day and were told they could only replace the diaper when the urine reached the line on the diaper intended to indicate saturation. In our interviews, the workers indicated that they individually found ways around the rules. Consider this exchange among women from several workplaces:

They have diaper police.

There's only so many that are sent to each unit. It's one per shift. It's unbelievable.

And management will go round and they will look in all the closets and all the drawers and they will pull all the hidden stuff out. I mean the girls hide it all over.

We have to steal them. [laughter]

Seriously. You want to take care of your residents properly. If they're wet, you want to change them. If I've got a baby sitting in front of me, that baby I feel dampness, we're likely to change them. With our elderly we say, 'At 75 per cent, we change them.'

It's absolutely true what they're saying 'cause we have the same ...
There's not the nursing staff to toilet every hour like they want and
what they need.

... We do the best we can do in the time that we're given ...

And the products that we're given to do it with.

It's not that we feel good about it either.

No.

(Armstrong, Armstrong, and Daly 2007)

In another interview for the same study, the workers talked about how
their actions encouraged family members to successfully demand a new
diaper policy. Individual actions thus resulted in structural change.

Resistance is not limited to paid work. Indeed, some women may
take paid employment in order to escape unpaid care work or at least to
get enough money to pay for support. Women who provide unpaid
care are also active in community organizations such as the Caregiver's
Association, working to change government policies and support other
providers. Many also lobby governments on their own to change rules
and programs that have a direct impact on those for whom they provide care. These individual actions too can produce real change. At the
same time, the increasing burden on women as unpaid care providers
may limit the energy they have to give to making change that works for
them.

Conclusions

In sum, care work is traditional women's work. This material and ideological designation has influenced the development of nursing work
and the value attached to ancillary work. Distinctions among various
kinds of health care work are blurred by the female domination of the
sector, as well as by the nature of the work itself. This chapter links the
specifics of health care work to the gender of jobs in an effort to show
that the skills involved are hidden and undervalued, in large measure
because the work is done by women. The problem does not simply lie
in ideas about what constitutes women's work or even exclusively in

their responsibility for domestic work. It is also the result of a segregated labour force and the limits on women's power. Racism also plays a role, compounding the problems for women and some men in the most marginalized jobs.

The rise in female participation rates in the paid labour force has contributed to the demands for more women's rights, for care programs, and for unionization, as well as for greater recognition of the skills involved in the work. Individually and collectively, women have struggled to change their work and the care people receive. Women in all health care jobs made significant gains until the late 1980s, when cutbacks and new managerial strategies combined to challenge these gains and their health. Unlike workers in officially designated health care jobs, ancillary workers are not protected by fear of shortages or by working in the public sector. Increasingly, they are not protected by unions either, as work is contracted out to non-union firms. At the same time, demands for unpaid caregiving are rising, complicating their struggles at home and in the labour force. Women have been successful in making more of the skills used in care work visible and in winning better conditions, although these gains are constantly being undermined by both government policies and private-sector employer actions. But some of their efforts to resist the care deficit have negative consequences, both for the women who provide care and for the system as a whole, by hiding the growing care deficit. Other efforts lead to government resistance in forms that can also undermine workers health and the system as a whole. The invisibility of the skills involved in this women's work contributes to these contradictory developments and is linked in turn to the invisibility of the hazards they face in this work, the subject of the next chapter.

6 Exposing Health Hazards at Work

Health care work is dangerous to women's health. A gender analysis helps us understand both what the hazards are and why they have been largely ignored. The segregation of women into jobs defined as requiring little effort helps render many of the hazards invisible. So does the focus on male work and the tendency to use male-dominated work as the standard for safe practices (Messing 1998b; 2004). Attention to patterns along lines of racialization is also required (Waehrer, Leigh, and Miller 2005), although we have even less research to inform such an investigation.

The Canadian Institute for Health Information reports that health sector workers are over 50 per cent more likely than other workers to miss work due to illness or injury (CIHI 2002, 87), with weekly absentee rates of 7.2 per cent for health care workers, compared to 4.8 per cent for all workers. Moreover, health care workers are absent for longer periods of time, 11.8 days per year on average compared to 6.7 for all workers. In 2005, health care and social assistance workers lost 14.4 days overall due to their own illness or injury, up from 10.7 days in 2003. But those defined as support staff lost 18.1 days in 2005, while nurses lost 13.9 (*Perspectives on Labour and Income* 2006b, table 4). And the increase in lost working days was greater for support staff. As Annalee Yassi and Tina Hancock observe, it is 'well documented that the healthcare sector is plagued by high rates of work injuries and illnesses, absences from work and related costs' (2005, 32). But even the high recorded rates may understate the problem. In a survey of workers in Ontario long-term care facilities, 97 per cent reported they had been ill or injured as a result of work at some time over the last five years, with over half saying they had suffered illness or injury from work more than 11 times during that five-year period (Armstrong and Daly 2004, 28).

Not all illness or injury is reported, however, usually because it does not result in work absences. Under Canada's various labour codes, workers are not guaranteed payment while they are away sick. Thus workers with the lowest pay and without union protection are the most likely to work sick or injured. This is more likely the case for ancillary workers than for others in health care, and is especially the case for home care workers. Moreover, women are less likely than men to make claims for workplace injury under workers' compensation plans and are even less likely to receive compensation when they do, in part because they have difficulty countering perceptions that their work is safe. They thus remain invisible in these injury data, as well as uncompensated (Chung, Cole, and Clarke 2000; Lippel 1995).

Given the much higher rates of illness and injury in this sector, it is logical to assume that it is the nature of health care work itself that causes the problem. And undoubtedly, there are aspects of work in care that create specific kinds of risks. Indeed, this is one of the factors that differentiates care work from other forms of labour. Part of the problem is also the aging labour force. With a majority of workers over 40 years old doing the work, it is not surprising that injury rates are high, especially given the nature of the work. However, the dangers inherent in health care work can be mitigated by strategies to protect workers. Similarly, the aging of the workforce can be countered with strategies to accommodate workers in the workplace. But instead of addressing the health issues raised by these two factors, new methods for work organization are exacerbating them (Baines 2006; Cloutier et al. 2007; Seifert and Messing 2004).

In spite of the high rates of illness and injury, and in spite of their high cost not only to employees but also to employers, there has been very little research done on the health hazards faced by the full range of health care workers, and even less done from a gender perspective. As early as 1977, Jeanne Mager Stellman exposed the health hazards women face in clerical, laundry, cleaning, and care work. She argued that women were hesitant to expose the hazards they faced, in part because they feared the consequence would be an assumption that they were too weak for the work and that this, in turn, could lead to job loss. At the same time, employers were blinded by assumptions about the safety of women's work and by their search for profit. Instead of addressing health hazards, employers demanded evidence of direct causal links that were difficult if not impossible to establish, especially given assumptions about women's health and about the truth of scientific claims. In the introduction to Karen Messing's book on women's occupational health, Stellman points out that 'even the most straightforward measures are susceptible to inherent bias' (1998, ix). Messing exposes the science that mainly assumes what applies to men applies to women, ignores women, or bases research on stereotypes about women and their work. '[Women's] differences from men can be emphasized or ignored by scientists, but the result of both procedures is the neglect of problems experienced by women workers' (Messing 1998b, xviii). In his more recent book on the gender dimensions of occupational health, Laurent Vogel (2003, 75) makes a similar point about the bias in European occupational research. He explains that there has been investigation of nurses' workplace health issues, primarily because there is a significant recruitment problem. With fewer recruitment problems in ancillary work, however, there is less incentive to do research on the hazards they face.

In spite of this bias and the limited nature of research on the health of ancillary workers, it is possible to draw on a range of international and national research to provide a partial picture of the hazards they face. The following sections explore some of these hazards while identifying areas in need of additional research.

Infection and Respiratory Diseases

The greatest risk health care workers face, and perhaps the most obvious one that distinguishes their work, is the risk of infection and respiratory diseases (Ducki 2003, 217). Hepatitis B and AIDS, teratogenic viruses, and tuberculosis are particularly dangerous hazards but not the only ones (Cesana et al. 1998). It is perhaps not surprising that those who provide personal care are at risk of infection or that women are more likely to get work-related infections than men, given the high proportion of women in health care work (European Agency for Safety and Health at Work 2003, 66). But the risk is not restricted to those providing personal care. 'Support service staff, regardless of their specific work assignment, frequently come into contact with infected patients and contaminated surfaces' (Otero 1997a, 1). A U.S. study found tuberculosis infection was significantly linked to occupation and that not only nurses but also housekeeping, laundry, and security personnel were at high risk (Louther et al. 1997). Cleaners and dietary staff often have personal contact with patients on a daily basis, as do many clerical staff. And no people need be there for infection to spread. Beds, equipment, and bathrooms are prime locations for some of the most dangerous and difficult-to-control infections (Valiquette et al. 2004). Health care laundry that has not been appropriately handled can be a threat to those doing the work, with the risk of acquiring hepatitis A or B only one example (Borg and Portelli 1999; Otero 1997b; Wa 1995). It is not only facilities that create such risks. Working in a variety of private households, with a variety of patients, can also expose providers to a range of infections and environmental hazards.

Equally important, as the outbreak of SARS (severe acute respiratory syndrome) demonstrated to the world, ancillary workers also face the risk of carrying infections out of the facility. According to one housekeeper, the worry is 'always in the back of your mind – it's probably not in the forefront – but in the back of your mind that you could bring this home or you could get it yourself' (LTCb 2006). Unpaid providers face the risk of infection being brought home along with the patient.

Although health care inevitably involves exposure to people with infections and to equipment or materials that carry diseases, the high infection rates are not inevitable. They can be controlled with good management and staff training that includes the entire health care workforce (WHO 2002). The Campbell Commission investigating the SARS outbreak used the evidence from contrasting experiences in Vancouver and Toronto to argue that applying the highest level of precaution when there is an undiagnosed respiratory disease can successfully contain such diseases and protect both workers and patients (Merck Frosst Canada 2007, 1). Cleaning, laundry, dietary, and clerical work are all part of that high level of precaution. The Commission also concluded that not only were workers left unprotected, but that those managing the crisis did not understand the important difference between infection control and occupational safety (Abraham 2007, A1). Both the precautionary principle and an emphasis on workplace safety are possible to implement, as the Commission suggests.

Lifting, Bending, Twisting, and Musculoskeletal Injuries

Back injuries have always been a problem in health care, but their numbers are increasing as workers age, work intensifies, and staff numbers are reduced. Also increasing are other forms of musculoskeletal injuries, such as problems with neck, shoulders, arms, elbows, and knees (Shannon et al. 2001). 'Limb disorders include a wide range of inflammatory and degenerative diseases and disorders that can affect tendons, ligaments, nerves, muscles, circulation and joint cartilage and result in pain and functional impairment' (European Agency for Safety at Work 2003, 41).

Many of these injuries come from lifting. And the problem is not simply that women's upper arm strength is often more limited than men's. As a French study notes, the 'loads to be handled in hospitals very often exceed men's as much as women's capacities' (Davezies 2003, 264). There are fewer people trying to lift sicker ones, and they often have no time or opportunity to get help from others or from a mechanical lift. Those who work alone in private homes are particularly likely to lift people alone, without mechanical aids or, too often, even without training. According to a British Columbia study, in one four-year period in the late 1990s, nearly 40 per cent of accepted Workers' Compensation Board claims from home support workers were for over-exertion injuries involving persons. 'These claims amounted to 4.5 million dollars and more than 65,000 days lost' (Paris-Seeley, Heacock, and Watzke 2004, 1). And that only calculates the costs to the employers. The average per-patient costs for hospitalization are highest for those with musculoskeletal and connective tissue injury, and such injuries are among the top five in overall hospitals costs (CIHI 2005b, 46). Equally important, actual costs to women are underestimated because many of their compensation claims for musculoskeletal injuries are rejected (Lippel, 2003).

But the problems of back injuries and lifting are not restricted to those providing personal care. Fact sheets provided for dietary workers in Ontario make it clear that heavy lifting is one of their work hazards, as are long periods standing that can lead to back pain (HCHSA 2004, 1). A dietary worker interviewed for this book is on workers' compensation from back injuries resulting from pulling and lifting heavy loads out of the commercial dishwasher and then twisting in a confined space. The 'bending that is there all the time' when serving food from heavy pots and sorting dishes only made it worse (LTCb 2006). Housekeepers also lift heavy machinery and garbage; laundry workers hoist heavy bags of soiled linen. If you are a housekeeper, 'when you work on a ward, when you're working in patients' rooms, it's a lot of bending and stretching.' In chronic care, 'they throw stuff' or drop their Ensure on the floor.

It's really sticky. So they would spill it on the floor ... The nurses or whomever happened to knock it off the table top. Often it's in a cor-

ner that it leaks because it's tipped off the table. And you can't just
mop that up. You have to get back there. The rooms are crowded ... a
four-bed room is more crowded. By the time you get over bed tables,
side tables, a bed, a favourite chair, the stuff that people collect, especially in a chronic care setting ... you have to move all that and then
you have to scrape the floor and the wash the floor. (LTCb 2006)

A Scandinavian study of hospital kitchen and laundry workers found
that workers 'had various aches in the muscular-skeletal system, which
they suspected were the consequences of prolonged standing and lifting of heavy objects' (Gunnarsdóttir and Björnsdóttir 2003, 70). Here
too, lack of equipment, reduced workforces, little training, and pressure
to work at high speeds can increase the risks. Being on their feet all day,
whether in the laundry, the kitchen, or on the ward can also put strain
on the back as well as on other parts of the body (Laperrière et al. 2005).
    The good news is that some initiatives are helping to reduce these
injuries while improving patient safety and clinical outcomes (Yassi
and Hancock 2005, 34). Patient lifts installed in British Columbia have
reduced injury and increased patient satisfaction. Adaptive clothing
has made dressing patients easier, and training in handling stroke
patients has helped improve care and limit worker risk. However, such
strategies do little for those who lift non-patient loads. But there is
every reason to believe that in laundries and kitchens, in cleaning and
clerical work there are ways to organize work and workers in order to
reduce the risks.

Chemicals, Needles, and Cuts

The chemicals handled in health care are dangerous and varied. Those
who provide personal care are exposed to chemicals in treatments and
even in the breath of patients (Fuller and Bloom 2005). Among the
chemical hazards are antineoplastic and antiviral agents, sterilants,
and formaldyhyde (Cesana 1998, 23). All cleaning and laundry work
involves chemicals (Zock 2005), but particular chemicals are required in
health care to ensure that dangerous bugs are kept under control. Contact dermatitis, for example, can result from specialized cleaning agents
(Haj-Younes, Sanchez-Politta, et al. 2006). Indeed, health care cleaners
have three times the injury rate of other cleaners, often as a result of
chemicals (Workers' Compensation Board, quoted in Cohen 2001, 9). A
California study reported that home care workers found the hazards of

common housekeeping tasks as serious as those related to lifting (Stock 2005). Cleaning chemicals are part of those household risks. Similarly, health care laundries use toxic substances to ensure that germs are destroyed, with chlorine bleach just one of many (Belkin 1998). Indeed, there are chemicals used throughout the hospital that can pose a risk to anyone who works there.

Needles are another risk specific to health care. They carry all kinds of risks, not only for those who give them but also for those who clean up afterwards. Research reported in *Executive Housekeeping Today* (1991) found that housekeepers, not nurses, were at the highest risk of sharp-object injury. Laundry workers too face injury from needles when they find them in the linen. Dietary workers face other kinds of risks in terms of punctures from knives, cuts from carts, and burns from hot dishes (Beaupré 1991). Also exposed to such risks are those who provide unpaid care, usually without much training and often without any means of disposing of the needles and other dangerous paraphernalia.

Here too it is possible to develop alternative approaches that would at least reduce the risk. Alternative chemicals are available, as are different approaches to cleaning. More time to dispose of needles can also help limit needle stick injuries. Better equipment, such as appropriate gloves, can protect workers. A Toronto hospital (Visser 2006) was able to reduce needle injuries by changing equipment, changing managerial strategies, and through training, suggesting such a three-pronged approach could work in other areas as well.

Lack of Employment Security and Control

Along with recent changes in the health care work environment such as contracting out and the implementation of new managerial practices has come insecurity about employment. As we have seen, ancillary workers have high rates of part-time work and many are without union or benefit protection. All of these factors can contribute to concerns about employment security and have an impact on health. Equally important, those with ancillary jobs have never had much control over their work processes, and lack of control can be hazardous to health (Karasek and Theorell 1990). New work organization strategies, together with for-profit managerial practices, have made it even less likely that these workers have control over their work or their pay.

A variety of studies have shown how lack of employment security can lead to stress-related health symptoms and damage to mental health

(Hammerstrom 1994; Lisle 1994). Moreover, 'stress can alter immune response and influence the onset and progression of physical illness' (Shields 2006b, 6). And it is not only the workers who suffer. Research in India demonstrated that 'accident frequency and severity rates were found to be significantly higher in temporary workers,' leading to the conclusion that both inexperience and insecurity contribute to greater injury and to accidents that have an impact on patients as well (Saha et al. 2005, 375). Similarly, a survey of research on the increase of precarious employment shows the significant health consequences of employment insecurity (Quinlan et al. 2001), not the least of which is low or irregular wages of the sort becoming common in health care.

Research initially done in the 1970s (Karasek 1979) demonstrated that low levels of control over a job combined with high demand can lead to physical illness. Later research has confirmed this relationship (see Marmot et al. 1999) and showed that women face more of this 'job strain' than men do (Hall 1989). The strain is a particular problem in jobs defined as unskilled, jobs like ancillary work. And the strain is increasing. Research on long-term care in Ontario and British Columbia, for example, reveals the increasing workloads for ancillary workers that have been combined with more managerial control and less decision-making latitude (Armstrong and Jansen 2003).

At the same time, jobs have become more precarious for these workers, creating employment strain. Employment strain, like job strain, is about lack of control, but in this case the question is control over hours of work, over pay and benefits, and over when you are employed (Vosko 2006). In Ontario, for example, the Minister of Health and Long-term Care has argued that 'just because it is a public health-care system doesn't mean ... that we should expect to pay more to sweep the floor in a hospital' (*Toronto Star* 2004, A1), implying wages should be cut in these jobs. In our long-term care study (LTCa 2006), a worker said she 'chose this because of a genuine concern to provide good care to the elderly. Sadly, it takes years to get a permanent position, so your life is given over to taking whatever shift you can get. You become exhausted working back-to-back shifts, then getting no shifts at all.' As another explained, insecurity is not only unhealthy for the worker but also for the organization.

All positions as a HCA I held part-time. In order to make ends meet, I held two to three part-time jobs at a time. This is difficult doing double shifts or sometimes working 30 days without a day off. This is stressful for home life. Also on a regular basis my job would either be eliminated, hours cut, [there would be a] heavier workload or bumping out of position. No job security is very stressful, hard to feel loyal to the company. (LTCa 2006)

Stress also makes people sick, as does dissatisfaction with the job. Workers are more likely to suffer burnout, low self-esteem, depression, and anxiety (Faragher, Cass, and Cooper 2005). Research shows that such symptoms have begun to show up in unpaid caregivers as well (Morris 2004).

Even for those with relatively permanent employment, irregular shifts scheduled without consultation can be equally stressful, especially for women trying to juggle childcare and elder care responsibilities. A personal support worker (LTCb 2006) reports that 'in a two-week period, I'm on four shifts.' She also works Saturday and Sunday every other weekend. Split shifts, with workers scheduled an hour or two early in the day and then another couple of hours later in the day, have become increasingly common in home care and cause particular stress for women with other care demands (Baines 2006, 140).

Moreover, the stress, along with constant exposure to people who are ill, makes it more likely that workers precarious employment will get sick, even though they are less likely to get sick pay. Another worker in long-term care (Armstrong, Armstrong, and Daly 2007) reported that 'this past year, I've been ill two times – illness from residents – and have no paid sick days. Very unfair. Lost nine days of pay.' Without sick pay, there is considerable pressure to return to work before full recovery, putting both residents and workers at further risk.

Job strain and employment strain are clearly women's issues. Women report more stress than men, and those with the most stress are those with lower levels of income and formal education (Shields 2006b). In an Ontario study of women in female-dominated occupations, nearly half of the women indicated that stress was their major health issue resulting from work (Feldberg et al. 1996). It is not surprising that women report more stress, given their segregation into the lowest paid work, their low pay, and their other unpaid work in the household and community. And their responsibility for unpaid care is rising just as their stress at work is increasing. This is also not surprising, given that women often have little control over their work in either sphere.

One job spills over into the other. According to a long-term care worker, 'When I am stressed out, my family feels the brunt of it; I complain, I'm tired, [I get] a lot of demands. [I] get told what to do all day [and] do not want to have demands on me when I get home' (LTCa 2006). Ancillary work is a prime example of stress creating strained relations in and out of the paid workplace. In this case, the costs of the strain are borne by those needing care and by the system as a whole, as well as by the workers. Listen to another long-term care worker:

I come home exhausted mentally and physically and wonder if I have actually helped anyone and what I have missed or forgotten. My spouse, who is not well, is left long hours on his own and I would dearly love to have more time with my grandchildren. I understand these problems are widespread in all aspects of home care, causing burnout. (LTCa 2006)

Here, too, there are some solutions at hand. Employment security, which means a guarantee of a job with pay and conditions that are comparable to the one currently held (as distinct from job security, or a guarantee to the current job) allows employers some flexibility while providing workers with some stability. Several provinces once had such provisions, so this is hardly a radical or untried approach. More full-time jobs would also help and could save money in training and admin-istration in the long term, because full-time employment could mean more highly skilled workers, fewer injuries, and more continuity in care (Piercy 2000), in addition to healthier workers who are better able to organize their unpaid care work. A national childcare and home care program would relieve some of the burden of unpaid work, giving women some control over their work in both spheres. And greater worker control over the ordering of tasks and over decision making about care could improve the health of both patients and providers, as research on those providing home care has demonstrated (McWilliam et al. 2001).

Workplace Organization

Employment strain and job strain are integrally related to work organi-zation. Social scientists have long maintained that workplace relations, especially those related to the possibilities for social support and partic-ipation in decision making, have an important impact on health (Doyal 1995).

The speed of change, combined with the speed-up in work, has reduced both worker decision making and the possibilities for making social connections at work. The president of the Canadian Safety Institute argues that 'part of what has created compromises in patient safety is the fact that we are asking staff to master new technologies, processes, drugs, equipment, knowledge, etc. at an alarming rate, and asking them to be increasingly efficient and effective' (Hassen 2005, 9). But is it also the case that the same factors that threaten patient safety can threaten worker safety as well (Cohen et al. 2004).

As researchers for the Canadian Policy Research Networks explain, 'restructuring typically had a short-term, bottom-line focus that did not consider the longer-term consequences for health human resources' (Koehoorn et al. 2002, 4). As their report points out, 'workload and other pressures, work schedules, job control, role stressors, and job insecurity' all influence employee health (5). But there has been little research linking these conditions to patient outcomes, especially in relation to ancillary work.

There is more than enough evidence to suggest that restructuring has a negative impact on the health of ancillary workers, however (Polanyi, Eakin, Frank et al. 1997). A Quebec study (Cloutier et al. 2007) found that restructuring undermined the kinds of relational and emotional rewards home care workers gained from their relationships with clients. This in turn contributed to a rise in both musculoskeletal and psychological health problems. The health consequences are not restricted to care in the home. A housekeeper in a hospital (LTCb 2006), for example, often works from six to ten o'clock, leaving her only four hours to complete the assigned cleaning and other tasks now part of her work. 'You have a list of jobs that you have to do and you start right off and you're not going to be able to finish it in four hours.' The problems were particularly acute when what she calls 'our corporation' decided to combine the portering and housekeeping work. On the night shift she works alone, feels at risk, and suffers the strain. Another housekeeper describes the back pain she suffers as a result of putting up four eight-foot tables by herself. The 'men used to set up the tables and now, in their wise decisions, [they] have decided that maintenance, that isn't under their job description. So they used to set up tables, now they don't. The workload has been put on housekeeping.' She goes on to explain that the housekeepers are women, while the maintenance workers are men. When the men did this work, 'two of them would go together. There's one woman now and it was two guys before' (LTCb 2006).

So you might porter. You might clean. And then they found what was happening was that the portering part was priority, which is to take patients to tests. But the housekeeping was not being done because ... we downsized so much. There just wasn't enough time in the day to do the housekeeping.

It was, from her perspective a 'terrible, terrible disruption' for her, for other staff, and for patients. Another housekeeper reports that she is often 'the only housekeeper in the building. And you get called to OB 'cause someone needs the bed because they're going to deliver a baby. And you're there gowned and gloved in the middle of a double clean. That's stressful!' (LTCb 2006).

Like job strain and employment strain, new forms of work organization can have consequences for the mental health of staff in health care (Woodward et al. 1999). Health care workers suffer from mental stress caused by 'work overload, pressure at work, lack of participation in decision making, poor social support, unsupportive leadership, lack of communication/feedback, staff shortages or unpredictable staffing, scheduling or long work hours and conflict between work and family demands' (Yassi and Hancock 2005, 35). Lack of full-time employment increases the stress, as does casual and temporary work. So does constant switching between work areas when workers have little control over the switching. Such stress helps explain why mental disorders are 'the fastest growing cause of long-term disability' among health care workers. Stress can also have physiological consequences, including increased blood pressure and stress hormone response (Fox, Dwyer, and Ganster 1993; Theorell et al. 1993). Although most of the research identifying these causal factors in mental disorders has been done with nursing staff, there is no reason to believe that such factors do not contribute to ill health among ancillary workers.

Indeed, in our long-term care study (Armstrong, Armstrong, and Daly 2007), employees repeatedly wrote in about the stress they face on a daily basis. Some of the stress results from the nature of their work. 'We become very attached when they hurt. When they die, a piece of us dies. I cry in the night for the loved ones that are dying and are gone. I can't explain the stress that we endure.' Some stress comes from increasing workloads. 'The work we do is so very demanding. I am sometimes so stressed that I don't sleep well worrying about the work. The work we do is so physically demanding that I am so tired that I am grouchy when I go home.' And some of the stress comes from not having the time to do the job they see needs to be done. 'I wish I had quality time to spend with the residents. The only time there is any real conversing is when you feed someone or washing or toileting them. It doesn't give much time for the resident who is upset.' 'Health care is not like it used to be many years ago. Aides had time for residents. We now have too many residents to look after. We now have too much paper work, which takes time away from residents.'

The evidence we do have on ancillary work indicates the same health problems arise in those jobs. Research on those working in private homes, for example, shows that the combination of multiple tasks that must be done in shorter time periods with poor equipment and in isolation from other workers takes a heavy toll (Bleau 2003). Unpaid care providers face similar problems (Morris 2004). The difficulties of completing the work are exacerbated both by demands from those who need the service and by the workers' desire to respond to their needs. This complexity of demands is unique to health care, where the way in which a worker responds can mean the difference between health and illness.

Workers employed in Ontario long-term care facilities who were surveyed about working conditions wrote about residents 'not getting what they deserve' (Armstrong and Daly 2004, 22), a problem that contributed to their stress, low morale, and feelings of lack of support from management. Listen to a dietary worker:

> I work in the kitchen; it's a pretty busy place at most times. We have had a lot of cutbacks. People [are] losing their jobs after working for twenty-two years. I myself may lose mine after working for nineteen years. Because of all these cutbacks we have to work sometimes doing the job of five people, and we're tired and stress[ed] out because there is more work put on us than there should be. All of this makes it hard to enjoy our work. I remember the time when we enjoyed our job. Now you have hardly anytime to even go to say hello to residents. (Armstrong and Daly 2004, 22)

The same workers also wrote about the work–family conflicts created by inflexible and unpredictable schedules, a particular problem for women. One woman, asked if her paid work caused problems in carrying out her other responsibilities, offered a list: younger child at home, sick father, dependent neighbour's spouse recently passed away, working husband (Armstrong and Daly 2004, 16). Work and family commitments were frequently at odds, adding to their stress. While both women and men can face such conflicts, women face more of them because of the heavy load they bear in terms of unpaid work.

Work has too often been reorganized solely on the basis of managerial theories rather than through consultation with those who do the work. Quebec cleaners interviewed by Messing (1998a) complained of not being consulted by hospital administration, even when changes had important consequences for their work and when their knowledge of the cleaning environment could help in the reorganization. Their British Columbia counterparts interviewed by Kahnamoui (2005) similarly complained that the new work schedules and the timing of tasks had not been based on any discussion with them about what was actually involved in the work. In both cases, the result was an underestimation of the work involved and significant stress on the cleaners.

It is not only the paid workers who are suffering as a result of work reorganization. With restructuring has come increasing pressure on women to take up unpaid care work at home and in facilities. The food service worker interviewed for this book volunteers her time to feed patients when she is not at her paid job doing the same work (LTCb 2006). Others participate in compulsory volunteerism, working extra hours without pay or choice. Donna Baines' research with social service workers found that overtime 'was structured by management to remain officially invisible and, of course, unpaid' (2006, 138). The demands, which are particularly heavy on women, 'drain our energy, affect our health and undermine our productivity' (Hunsley 2006, 3). Workplace organization can reflect workers' knowledge of what needs to be done and how it can be done. Such consultation can have the twin benefits of improving work organization and improving work relations (Rasmussen 2004). It can allow workers to develop social relations that create social supports for them in their work.

With the exception of staff shortages and work overload, the numerous factors Annalee Yassi and Tina Hancock (2005, 5??) have identified as significant in causing worker stress are all about managerial strategies that could be fixed without adding new costs. And the shortages would in fact be reduced with better management and more attention paid to women's double workload, with cost savings in the long run. Moreover, even infection exposure, itself a cause of stress, can be linked to 'key organizational and job stress variables' (Yassi and Hancock 2005, 35), suggesting better management could make a difference in this area as well.

Workplace Violence, Bullying, Sexual Harassment, and Racism

Violence is common in health care (Pizzino 1994). Canadian research indicates that in 2004, one-third of all workplace violence involved a victim who was working in health and social services (De Léséleuc 2007). According to the International Labour Organization (2003, 2), 'Health sector personnel are particularly at risk of violence in their workplace. Violence finds its expression in physical assaults, homicide, verbal abuse, bullying/mobbing, sexual and racial harassment and psychological stress.' Similarly, research on nurses working in Alberta and British Columbia found that 'patients were the main source of violence, particularly for physical assaults and threats of assault' (Hesketh et al. 2002, 314). An investigation of a U.S. health care organization found that both mental and physical violence increased with patient contact, regardless of job category (Findorff et al. 2004). A survey of Ontario long-term care workers indicated that all but a few had witnessed violence in their workplace. Almost three-quarters had had violence directed towards them in the most recent three-month period (Armstrong and Daly 2004, 29).

Health care involves particular forms of violence related to the specific nature of health care work. One aspect is neatly summarized by the title Donna Baines (2006) chose for her article on violence in social services: 'Staying with People Who Slap You Around.' Much of the violence comes from patients for whom workers continue to provide care. It often occurs in the course of providing intimate personal care, perhaps reflecting the pain and lack of control as well as the embarrassment of those needing care. Or it may result from frustration with the lack of care or the terms of care in the wake of restructuring (Baines 2006). Personal support workers interviewed for this book talked about patients lashing out when the diapers were changed, and especially when they were changed long after the patient had requested the change but before workers were allowed to do so. In any case, workers often have to return to work with the same person the next day.

A personal support worker in a nursing home reports that there are physical conflicts among residents 'practically every day' and intervening in these conflicts, as they must do, means 'sometimes we get hurt doing that' (LTCb 2006). They even have a code red for such violence. In British Columbia, a survey of those working in emergency reported violence rates of 92 per cent (*Guardian* 2005c, 13). The Occupational Health and Safety Agency for Healthcare in British Columbia reports that 'violence and aggression result in the third highest number of claims in the health care and social service sub-sector in B.C., and are factors which can lead to increased sick time, long term disability and staff turnover, as well as lower morale' (quoted in *Guardian*, 2005c, 13). The violence comes from patients, from families of patients, and from other workers. One worker in long-term care provided a brief glimpse of the daily violence:

> This is very, very hard on your physical body with the resistive and uncooperative residents that come into these homes for care. [Patients with]Alzheimer's and dementias sometimes just don't understand what you are doing to them. They can hit, kick, scream. And this sort of thing goes on when you are changing a diaper or bathing a resident. (LTCa 2006)

> Those who work alone in households face particular risks, often walking into violent relationships or even drug deals. Those who are employed by the homeowner may be particularly vulnerable, especially if they are immigrants without contacts in this country. (LTCa 2006)

That women are often the victims of violence is now widely acknowledged. However, a recent Statistics Canada (2006c) report, *Measuring Violence vs Women*, pays little attention to violence in paid workplaces and little to that related to care in the home. Yet there is research indicating that workplace violence is highly gendered, and that women face significant levels of violence in their paid and unpaid care workplaces (Baines 2006; Santana and Fisher 2002; Wigmore 1995). Women are especially vulnerable to sexual harassment from employers, other workers, patients, and families. Harassment is common, although often unreported because women fear they will not be believed or will lose their jobs. As Lesley Doyal (1995, 168) points out, women who are harassed remain in a constant state of vigilance. The result can be 'long-term physical problems such as high blood pressure, ulcers or heart disease. In addition, mental health problems may well result from the need to deny fear, suppress anger and cope with the irrational guilt that many harassed women feel.' Donna Baines (2006) found significant sex differences in violence experienced by social service workers, with women much more likely to face violence than men. She suggests a number of factors that contribute to this violence. Women work more closely and intimately with clients, exposing them more to acts of violence, while men do more physical activities with clients, perhaps serving to dissipate frustrations that lead to violence. Women are also seen to be more vulnerable and are particularly vulnerable to attacks on body parts related to their sex. 'However, women involved in this study were made even more vulnerable through work organization factors that antagonized and frustrated clients, such as a constantly changing workforce and a lack of resources to meet their needs' (Baines 2006, 145).

Racism creates similar problems. In her article on racism in nursing, Tania Das Gupta (1996) lists targeting, scapegoating, excessive monitoring, marginalization, infantilization, bias in work allocation, underemployment, and denial of promotion among the manifestations of racism within health care. Although her focus is on nurses, there is every reason to believe that ancillary workers face racism as well. Indeed, given the fact that those identified as visible minorities are over-represented in ancillary work and that ancillary workers have less power than nurses, especially in terms of ease of replacement, it seems likely that racism is an even bigger problem for these workers. Neysmith and Aronson (1997, 482) document the particular forms of racism experienced by home care workers. 'Specifically, the parallels between home care and domestic service reveal how racism unfolds in home-based care work in ways it does not in institutionally based care work,' where workers at least have some protection gained from visibility and from organizational structures. Working alone in households, racialized workers have little protection. Because the racism often comes from those needing care, it may be even more difficult to protest against those who are frail.

Violence, harassment, and racism are not new for women. However, education and training, job and employment security, unions, and effective compliance structures can help reduce the incidence. So can workplaces that promote social support and provide appropriate staffing. Indeed, lack of staff may well be the major cause of escalating violence, as patients and families frustrated by lack of care lash out and overburdened workers lose control (Baines 2004c). Supervisors too can make a difference. A U.S. study of a health care organization found that increased supervisor support was associated with decreased violence, suggesting that managers can play a critical, positive role. And it is in the interests of everyone that they should. Research undertaken with food service workers in the United States shows that sexual harassment is not only a problem for the individual, it is also an issue in the way teams function and in overall performance (Raver and Gelfand 2005).

Sexual harassment can thus have an impact on productivity for the workforce and the organization as a whole. Similarly, racism can have an impact on the health of workers and their work.

Lack of Respect

In research on Quebec cleaners (Messing, Chatigny, and Courville 1998, 454), lack of respect was identified by both cleaners and supervisors as a major problem with health consequences. In identifying lack of respect, women are in some ways summarizing the health hazards they face as well as the invisibility of their skills, effort, and responsibilities.

Respect for ancillary workers would mean a recognition of their skills, of their job demands, and of the importance of training. It would also mean responsibility that allowed workers the right to exercise more control over their work (Rasmussen 2004). In our long-term care study, worker after worker wanted policy makers, governments, and families to 'walk a mile in my shoes'; 'do what we do, see what we see'; 'actually see how hard we work and what it's like to be a resident' (Armstrong, Armstrong, and Daly 2007). Research with hospital clerical workers in Manitoba indicates that workers gain the most satisfaction from relationships with other health care providers and with patients, indicating the importance of participating in teams (Dunton 1997). Pride in using their skills and the opportunity for personal growth ranked high with these clerical workers, suggesting that both skill recognition and the chance to further develop them are also critical to respect.

Respect for health care workers would be manifested in decent pay, benefits, schedules, and working conditions, in access to safe equipment and chemicals, in the provision of adequate resources and time. It would be evident in meaningful consultation and effective mechanisms for complaint. It would mean recognizing and addressing the many hazards women face in health care work. And it would mean recognizing women's unpaid care work and the contribution it makes to individuals as well as to the country as a whole.

Conclusions

The specific characteristics of health care work lead to specific conditions and specific health hazards in the work, although some of these hazards are common to women's work throughout the labour force. The overlap with women's work in the home contributes both to notions of safety and to the failure to document and address hazards. So does the fact that many of the injuries and illnesses develop over time, rather than suddenly, and often get attributed to female complaints rather than to the structure and relations of work. Although attention is increasingly paid to safety (primarily as a consequence of medical errors), the spread of infections in health services, and the shortage of registered nurses willing to work under these conditions, most research and action has focused on those defined as direct providers, not on ancillary workers, and has failed to take gender into account. An initiative in British Columbia has, however, concluded that 'ample evidence has already been obtained to indicate that looking after the well-being of health care workers results in safer and better quality patient care' (Yassi and Hancock 2005, 32). Improving conditions for health care workers can also save money for the system in the long run through lower rates of absenteeism, worker turnover, and work compensation claims.

7 Challenging the Construction of Ancillary Work

Reforms that have an impact on ancillary health care workers in care are not simply local. They are found throughout the world and need to be understood within this global context. Several factors have combined to make ancillary workers a target for change over the last couple of decades. In the first section of this chapter, we look at the international pressures and developments that are shaping ancillary work. In order to successfully challenge both the definition of who is a health care worker and the conditions of the work, it is necessary to understand these international forces and question their construction of ancillary work.

International Contexts and Trends

Rising Health Care Expenditures

One pressure on ancillary work is the growth in public sector spending on health care. For more than two decades, there has been a great deal of discussion throughout the world about dramatic increases in health spending. Economist Åke Blomqvist, writing in 1994, argued that health care had been singled out throughout the globe as 'an area in need of productivity improvement and better cost control' (4) because of the rapid rise in the rate of expenditure growth. Among 29 countries in the Organization for Economic Cooperation and Development (OECD), between 1960 and 1998 the average annual rate of growth in health care spending ranged from 2.2 per cent in New Zealand to 7.5 per cent in Spain (Anderson and Sotir 2001, exhibit 5). Between 1975 and 1991, Canadian spending grew by 3.8 per cent, dropping to only 0.8 per cent each year between 1991 and 1996 (CIHI 2006, iii).

Undoubtedly, governments across the industrialized world have been spending more in real terms on health care in almost every year since 1960. However, these growth rates alone cannot explain the concern with productivity and cost. 'In most countries the rate of increase in real health care spending was highest during the 1960s and generally has been declining since then, and the percentage of GDP spent on health care has been relatively stable since the early 1980s' (Anderson and Sotir 2001, 228). From 1992 to 2004, the average annual growth rate in Canada's total real per capita spending on health was 2.3 per cent, compared with an average of 4.0 per cent for 29 industrialized countries in the Organization for Economic Cooperation and Development (calculated from OECD 2006). In 2004, Canada stood fifth out of 30 OECD countries in total spending on health on a per capita basis, and ninth as a share of GDP. But if only public spending on health is considered, the picture changes appreciably. At about 70 per cent, Canada had the ninth *lowest* public share of total health spending. And only six of the 28 countries reporting had reduced their public shares more between 1990 and 2004. Indeed, 14 had increased their public shares (OECD 2006). The proportion of public sector health care spending has declined from 77 per cent to 70 per cent since 1975 (Yates 2006). So scepticism is needed when we are warned that public spending on health care is out of control, or that we spend so much more than other countries do.

As Thomas Bodenheimer (1995, 29) explains, falling profits in the United States in the 1970s coincided with rising health care costs paid by employers. As a result, 'individual health care consumers, business, and government gradually became concerned with the accelerating flow of dollars into the health care industry.' Canadian businesses and individual Canadians were not as concerned about the rising costs, primarily because Canada has a publicly financed health care system for hospital and doctor care, which means individuals and businesses do not bear the costs alone. Moreover, expenditures were much lower in Canada than in the United States, in large measure because our health system is much more administratively efficient, as well as more equitable. However, Canadian governments have for a decade or more faced pressure from growth in health care costs. This growth was combined in some years with declining revenues resulting from falling profits as well as from reductions in corporate tax rates. Indeed, tax reductions may have been a bigger factor. 'Expenditures on social programs did not contribute significantly to the growth of government spending relative to GDP' between 1975 and 1991, according to two Canadian government economists (Mimoto and Cross 1991, 3.1). Now the federal government no longer has a deficit and several provincial ones have significant surpluses, largely as a result of a growing economy based on exports of oil and other natural resources. Nevertheless, Canadians have become very familiar with arguments that health care budgets are no longer sustainable.

The wages, salaries, and benefits of health care workers account for a significant proportion of the costs in care. According to a former Director of Health Services Provision with the World Health Organization, health human resources consume between 60 and 80 per cent of health care budgets (Conference Board of Canada 2005, 15). In cleaning, for example, staff costs account for up to 93 per cent of total costs (Davies 2005, 4). And these costs have risen with unionization in the sector, beginning in the 1970s. Not surprisingly then, staff costs have been targets of reforms in health care.

However, it would be a mistake to see unreasonable demands from labour as a primary cause of cost increases. 'Census data show that, on average, employment incomes for full-time workers in health occupations rose at about the rate of inflation between 1995 and 2000. That compares to almost a 6 per cent after-inflation increase for all earners' (CIHI 2005b, 17). Moreover, there are huge disparities in incomes among health care workers (16) and in their wage gains in recent years. Ancillary workers are the lowest paid of all those employed in this sector. Eliminating jobs or reducing wages for these workers saves much less money than would doing the same for managers or physicians, although this has not prevented ancillary workers from being targets for change.

In Canada, much of the recent growth in health expenditures is attributable to spending on drugs. In 2004, $8.5 billion was paid by the public sector for prescription drugs (CIHI 2005b, 61). Spending on retail drugs rose from 9 per cent of total health spending in 1984 to 16 per cent in 2004 (39). New technologies, especially information technologies, also accounted for a significant share of these new costs, although it is much more difficult to measure their contribution to expenditure growth. Spending on drugs and information technologies continues to grow rapidly, even though many of these technologies have not proven to improve patient care or to increase efficiency. According to an editorial in the *Journal of the American Medical Association* (Wears and Berg 2005, 1261), 'roughly 75% of all large IT projects in health care fail,' and the problems 'are not simply bits of bad programming or poor implementation.' Similar conclusions have been reached about drug effectiveness (Angell 2004, chapters 4–6).

In sum, the evidence does not support either the argument that health care costs are out of control or that health care labour costs are the major driving force. Even if both were the case, it would not make sense to target the ancillary workers who are the lowest paid of all workers. However, a lack of evidence and logic has not prevented a focus on cost cutting that has resulted in major changes in ancillary work.

New Public Management

A second pressure that is changing ancillary work comes from a new philosophy and practice concerning the role and functioning of governments. Over the past two decades or so, there has been a major shift in approaches to government in Canada and throughout the industrialized world. Particularly influential in promoting this shift were the two U.S. authors of a best-selling book entitled *Reinventing Government: How the Entrepreneurial Spirit Is Transforming the Public Sector* (Osborne and Gaebler 1993).The central tenet of the 'reinventing government' movement is that governments should restrict themselves to 'steering' and leave 'rowing' the ship of state to others, on the basis of competitively awarded contracts. In other words, governments should focus on the development of innovative policies, leaving the delivery of programs to efficient agents in the market. And in their remaining operations, governments are to act like businesses. Such an approach removes the principle of governments operating on the basis of a commitment to public service and replaces it with the application of market principles across the public sector (Exworthy and Halford 1999).

A complementary, if more systematic, approach to this shift towards marketization in government has been labelled New Public Management (Hood 1991). New Public Management (NPM) insists on a sharp distinction between the policy-making roles of politicians and the policy implementation and routine management roles of public servants. The former are to set explicit goals, standards, and performance measures, while the latter are to ensure that these objectives are realized in the most economical, efficient, and effective manner possible. This not only means the allocation of program delivery to successful competitors in the market but also the adoption of private-sector practices within what remains of the public sector itself. As a result, politicians rely increasingly on private-sector management consultancy firms for policy development advice instead of on government policy analysts and senior public servants.

NPM assumes that the private sector is more efficient and effective than the public sector in policy development as well as in delivery. NPM also assumes that those with careers inside the public sector cannot be counted upon to concentrate on the state's 'core businesses,' as they will instead try to build up their own 'empires.' Under NPM, the accountability and responsiveness of the state apparatus both to politicians and to citizens – who are increasingly thought of as clients, customers, and consumers – is said to be enhanced.

There are several grounds for challenging the assumptions of NPM, both in general and with specific reference to health care (see for example Savoie 1995; Shields and Evans 1998; Johnson 2002, chapter 11). The most obvious criticism is that the impact of shifting the delivery of services to competing agencies with short-term contracts falls most directly and negatively on the workers. One of the main purposes of changing service delivery is to lower costs, and given that labour absorbs most of the costs, NPM usually means lower pay and poorer working conditions for the mainly female labour force. As Christopher Pollitt puts it with reference to such practices in the United Kingdom: 'Considerable economies can usually be made by compulsory contract tendering of services such as building cleaning, catering, refuse collection and so on. These savings are made principally at the expense of the terms and conditions of the work force, but from the taxpayers' viewpoint they are real nonetheless' (Pollitt 1998, 62, citing Kerr and Radford 1994).

This emphasis on the taxpayers' viewpoint is problematic in health care, however, given that almost all taxpayers can anticipate needing health care for themselves and for their families. And women in particular can anticipate an increase in unpaid care they provide to family and friends at some point in their lives. Overworked and low-paid health care workers who lack stable jobs are less likely to be in a position to provide sensitive, high-quality care to those taxpayers who become health care recipients (Rasmussen 2004). Moreover, eliminating perceived waste can mean eliminating important aspects of care, such as the relationships that develop over time that can benefit both patients and providers (Piercy 2000). 'In schemes tried, for example, in the U.S., the U.K., and Sweden, home care workers are assigned to clients on random or rotating bases so that time-consuming relationships cannot develop and tasks can be accomplished with assembly line efficiency' (Aronson and Neysmith 1997, 56, citing Chicin and Kantor 1992; Qureshi and Walker 1989; and Szebehely 1995, respectively).

The NPM focus on efficiency and the elimination of waste, narrowly defined, often translates into the offloading of paid care work from one agency to another at the expense of integrated services. It frequently means offloading from the health care system in general, primarily at the expense of women who have to pick up the unpaid care work, whatever their other responsibilities, interests, and skills. Paradoxically, the NPM focus on efficiency and the elimination of waste also means that it is often inefficient even in narrow terms, because the elimination of waste reduces services to the minimum required based on average or regular use. As a result, the service usually lacks the surge capacity to deal with the irregular waves of patients who show up at hospital emergency departments, much less to deal with major and virulent outbreaks of infections such as avian flu or SARS, or with major accidents.

The NPM approach emphasizes managerial control at the expense of administration and thus of stability and fairness; at the expense of politics and thus of using values to shape public services. NPM is therefore consistent with the language of 'taxpayers' and indeed of 'customers' and 'consumers,' as against that of 'citizens' and 'residents.' It involves more decisions made by management experts, through market competition, and on the basis of purchasing power. Yet it was as a result of popular political pressure, not management strategy, that Canada established medicare. Medicare is Canada's best-loved social program because it provides quite high-quality care on the basis of need rather than on the basis of market principles. Its maintenance and improvement in the future will require that such pressure continue.

A final critique of NPM relevant here is that the separation of 'steering' from 'rowing' entails contracts between the state and private concerns. To the extent that these contracts contain what are successfully claimed to be trade secrets, they not only reduce transparency and public accountability, but they also blur the public–private distinction, and make it more difficult to mobilize informed public opinion in favour of medicare. This criticism applies with particular force to so-called public–private partnerships, or 'P3s,' by which for-profit enterprises provide some combination of the design, financing, construction, operation, and ownership of facilities such as hospitals that are ultimately paid for from the public purse. The public, however, is bound by rigid contractual provisions for 25 years or more. Under P3 arrangements, ancillary workers are particularly subject to becoming employed, if at all, by the private consortia rather than by the public sector.

They may well lose their union protections and the pay, benefits, and working conditions they have fought for years to achieve. Indeed, this may well be part of the motivation of those who advocate and implement the P3 mechanism.

Meanwhile, P3 facilities are more expensive than traditionally financed public facilities. The private sector must pay more than the public sector does to borrow capital funds, it seeks to secure profits from the arrangement, and there are substantial transaction costs involved in the complex negotiations and ongoing monitoring of P3 projects. If service levels are to be maintained at anything close to the levels in place before the introduction of a P3 project, something or someone has to receive less (Auerbach et al. 2003; Pollock, Shaoul, and Vickers 2002). Ancillary workers are a prime target.

Health Care as an Opportunity for Profit

Another pressure on ancillary workers comes from the opportunities in health care created by its location primarily in the non-profit sector. This is particularly the case when governments following the principles of NPM seek to shed their operations and to promote business. Some aspects of health care, such as pharmaceuticals, have always been in the main produced on a for-profit basis by investor-owned corporations. Until recently, however, investor-owned companies in health care services were virtually unknown. Indeed, there is still a great variety in ownership of health services and in 'no country is the "for-profit" firm dominant' (Cookson, Goddard, and Gravelle 2005, 123). Health services have thus offered, and continue to offer, a new frontier for investment by for-profit firms, especially given that firms had run out of many other places to invest.

Speaking of the emerging for-profit health maintenance organizations in the United States, Ellwood and others suggested that these 'could stimulate a course of change in the health industry that would have some of the classical aspects of the industrial revolution – conversion to larger units of production, substitution of capital for labor, vigorous competition, and profitability as the mandatory condition of survival' (quoted in Bodenheimer 1995, 26). All that is missing from this list is the fragmentation of work into identifiable tasks that would allow the substitution of lower paid labour for higher paid labour, an issue of particular importance to ancillary workers given that their work is assumed to resemble much of that already done in the for-profit sector. As Donna Baines (2004a, 275) notes, 'In the past, these manage-rialist, routinistic forms of work organization would have been seen as antithetical to public and non-profit service delivery.' Now the reverse is the case.

Health education, health information and technologies, insurance coverage, supplies, equipment, laboratories and testing facilities, man-agement, consulting, and service delivery all offer opportunities for investment (WHO 2005b). These opportunities have grown as govern-ments have withdrawn from the field or have failed to cover new developments. In some cases, governments pay the private sector for work or products, based on NPM assumptions that the for-profit sector is more efficient and effective than governments. By the 1990s, many for-profit firms had moved into the health care field, often with the assistance of governments. In *Bitter Medicine*, Jeanne Kassler (1994) doc-uments the huge expansion and the enormous profit growth in health care services in the United States. Colleen Fuller (1998) has done the same for Canada, showing that for-profit companies are growing stron-ger and more profitable here, albeit at a slower pace than in the United States. And the expansion is still going on. 'According to the president of the American Association of Health Plans, 450 million Latin Ameri-cans constitute a health-care market of $120 billion a year' (WHO 2005b, 128).

However, as a number of economists have pointed out, the health care sector is not the same kind of market as other sectors (Mintzberg 1989; Cookson, Goddard, and Gravelle 2005). Disease is unpredictable both in terms of timing and of who gets sick for how long. Some ill-nesses can be very expensive, distorting the equilibrium of markets. Doctors and patients differ significantly in their access to necessary information, much more so than in the case of purchasing consumer goods. Moreover, demand for health services is almost always local, and many areas, even in the United States, have populations too small to support competition between services (Himmelstein and Woolhan-dler 1994, 231). Furthermore, unregulated health care provision can lead to low-quality service, resulting in death or injury, as well as to sig-nificant inequalities in access to care.

As a result of problems arising from unregulated health care ser-vices, their supply, demand, and delivery have been heavily regulated in every country. Those countries shifting to more private investment have often had to introduce new regulations to address problems cre-ated by the conflicts between markets and care. In Ontario, for example, the government had to manage competition for home care services rather than simply let the market operate (Armstrong 2001). But even then, problems arose in terms of continuity of care, costs, and quality. New regulations were introduced to limit the market even more, in an attempt to address the particular characteristics of health care. In Manitoba, the private management firm American Practice Management (or APM as it was called in Canada) failed in its attempt to achieve large savings by applying for-profit techniques to the hospital sector. The firm failed in part because the sector was already quite efficient and in part because it was hard to substitute machines for labour. The solution of reducing staff mainly meant a reduction in service. Manitoba also invited Olsten, the largest U.S. for-profit home care firm, to operate 10 per cent of the province's home care. But Olsten soon left when it became clear that its for-profit methods cost more than the public system (Willson and Howard 2002). These economic realities and these regulations, along with the factors that gave rise to them, help account for the limited penetration of for-profit firms in some areas of care.

Although differences between the health sector and other services are perhaps visible when it comes to life-and-death care provided by doctors and nurses, it is less obvious in the case of ancillary services. Indeed, much of ancillary work seems comparable to work done in the for-profit sector, and as we have noted, it is often described as hotel. work in order to suggest such a comparison (Cohen 2001). Assuming such equivalencies and seeking opportunities for investments, large international organizations have pressed both for the privatization of these services and for international agreements that would allow them to provide the services anywhere in the world. Many companies that provide services to universities and hotels now also cater to hospitals and nursing homes. Some have contracts with these facilities to do the work. Increasingly, public–private partnerships mean that for-profit organizations build and manage the health care facility and provide all the services defined as ancillary, while the public sector manager directs clinical care.

At the same time, technology is being used to replace workers, speed up the work process, and relocate the work. Clerical work provides an obvious example. As Ann Eyerman explains in her book on the globalization of clerical work, the 'computer did not just replace our typewriter as the tool of our trade, it has transformed the structure of our work itself' (2000, 35). It has also eliminated thousands of clerical jobs

(De Wolfe and Associates 2000), while moving others off-shore to countries such as Jamaica and India (Bueckert 1993). Patients talk mainly to an answering machine when they call the hospital and may have their doctor's notes transcribed by someone living in another country. Some patients even check themselves in at the doctor's office, inserting their health card into an automated machine and punching in their own information.

Food production is another sector that has been distanced from the local context. In her book on the global production of food, Deborah Brandt (2004, 14) argues that the 'experiences of women in the food system offer a window on the restructuring of work in the new global economy.' Food services in health care are no exception to this restructuring. Many hospitals and other care facilities no longer have kitchens. Food may even be made in another province and merely reheated in the location where it is consumed. The work that remains at the facility level has become increasingly mechanized, often creating work on an assembly line (Gunnarsdóttir and Björnsdóttir 2003) and removing dietary workers from contact with patients and residents (CUPE 2007a). Similarly, laundry has been centralized into large corporate enterprises, with sheets and other materials often trundled far away for cleaning. In North Bay, Ontario, for example, 26 laundry workers faced the possibility of job loss when only nine of them could be moved to Sudbury to the new laundry facility (CUPE 2007b). In both food and laundry work, the process has been transformed by technologies that speed up production and do some of the heavy labour.

Technology has made less of an impact on cleaning, in part because cleaning has to be done at the local level. Spaces, as well as patients, make machines difficult to use. When machines have been introduced to speed up the work, it is usually men who operate them (Messing 1998a). However, information technology has been used to estimate and control the amount of time each cleaning task takes (Armstrong et al. 1997; Messing 1998a), and those programs may be developed in another region or even another country without regard to the specific characteristics of the work or without knowledge of the workers.

Health care services, then, have offered an opportunity for profit just as other areas for investment have been disappearing. Ancillary services seem particularly appropriate for delivery by for-profit firms, based on their assumed similarity to service work in the private sector of the economy and the assumed efficiencies that come with a competitive private sector. Pressure from global corporations has met with support from those promoting less government and from those seeking to reduce costs. While there is little research evidence to indicate that these organizations provide better or cheaper services, more of this work has moved into the for-profit sector and more is being moved every day. Research does indicate that food and accommodation services in the private sector are among those with the lowest job quality and lowest pay (Maxwell 2002; Hughes, Lowe, and Schellenberg 2003, 22), suggesting a grim future for those who have their jobs moved to the for-profit sector.

Global Markets and Workers

Another means of lowering labour costs in health care is to pit workers from around the world against each other. Workers, like corporations, seek opportunities in other countries, especially in the face of global restructuring. There has long been a global market in workers, but it has grown with the increased emphasis on free trade and global markets. This is particularly the case with those recognized as health care workers. Health care professionals are in high demand in many areas, although their movement from east to west and south to north has been far from free (Bourgeault 2006).

Doctors have particularly strong professional organizations in the West, reflecting the long dominance of white men and reinforced by visible skills obviously acquired through formal training and by their control over admission to the profession (Witz 1992). Nurses, too, have quite strong professional organizations and unions, skills acquired through formal training and protected by credentials, as well as some control over admission. In the West, both doctors and nurses enjoy strong public support as well as high prestige. Both groups have used their power to limit entry from the foreign educated. Nurses' power has been more limited, because doctors are in control and because nurses are women. While the currently perceived and certainly looming shortage of health care professionals not only in Canada but throughout much of the world has strengthened the position of nurses, doctors and nurses in the wealthy countries are being pressured to open the doors to more professionals from abroad.

By 2002, nearly one-quarter of Canadian doctors were foreign trained, while immigrants and non-permanent residents made up just under 20 per cent of the overall labour force. Those trained in the United Kingdom were most common (17 per cent of all foreign trained), with another

11 per cent from South Africa and 9 per cent from India (Mullan 2005, table 14 and figure 5). In spite of the presence of large numbers of foreign-trained doctors in Canada, it should be recognized that medical associations have considerable power over admission to practise. It is difficult to get accurate data on the number of doctors living in Canada who have foreign credentials but are not practising medicine because they have been refused admission to the profession. Some may be working at ancillary jobs in health care.

Compared to doctors, the foreign training of nurses is less consistently recorded, in part because entry is less carefully controlled. Although the criteria that foreign-trained registered nurses must meet are somewhat less restrictive than those for doctors, there is a significantly smaller proportion who are foreign trained. Half of the 8 per cent of registered nurses known to graduate outside Canada are from the Philippines (29 per cent) or the United Kingdom (21 per cent), with another 7 per cent from the United States (CIHI 2005e, table 14 and figure 19). Given the large number of nurses compared to that of doctors, however, there are approximately as many foreign-trained doctors as there are RNs working in Canada.

Licensed practical nurses are even less likely to be foreign trained. Less than 3 per cent received their nursing education outside Canada. Like the RNs, they were mainly trained in the United Kingdom, the Philippines, or the United States. Unlike the RNs, however, nearly 40 per cent of LPNs trained in the United Kingdom while only 17 per cent came from the Philippines (CIHI 2005d, table 7 and figure 12). As is the case with doctors, we do not know how many nurses with foreign credentials are doing ancillary work. Research in British Columbia (Rivers 2000) indicates that there are many nurses with foreign credentials who now work as personal support and home care workers, as cleaners, cooks, and administrative staff. Another study in the same province found that the costs of language training, tests, and upgrading, combined with wage loss during the process and family responsibilities, prevented many foreign nurses from working as nurses. These nurses were from a wide variety of Asian and eastern European countries, as well as from Central and South America.[1]

---

1 This study is reported in a Proposal for the Development of a Pilot Project for Underemployed Foreign Trained Nurses in the Lower Mainland (Hospital Employees Union 2000).

In her study of global nurse migration, Mireille Kingma (2006, 5) reports that many nurses may leave their home countries by choice, but 'when we delve deeply, we see the social and economic conditions in their homelands may oblige them to abandon their homes and families.' She goes on to show how the cost is high for the individuals, their families, and their countries. Such migrations, she argues, 'threaten the sustainable development of health care systems' (4).

While it is possible to develop a general picture of where doctors and nurses are trained, existing sources tell us nothing about where ancillary workers are trained. In contrast to doctors and nurses, ancillary workers are less likely to have collective representation that regulates entry. As we have seen, they are more likely to have skills acquired informally and assumed to be part of what any woman can do. Ancillary workers also have significantly less public visibility. As a result, there is no perceived shortage and no attempt to track where they acquired their skills. Nevertheless, it is clear that many come from other countries, with few of the kinds of controls there are for professionals (see appendix). Many may also have training that goes well beyond what is explicitly required in ancillary work, and they may use this unrecognized training in their work.

In sum, there are global pressures to transform health care into a for-profit service. The pressures have been particularly strong in the case of ancillary work, which has been defined out of care and into the accommodation and food for-profit sector. This transference has been supported by governments committed to a new philosophy and by the international movement of workers, themselves pressured by the increasing emphasis on market techniques.

The Health Policy Context in Canada

Health care reforms in Western countries share many similarities that go beyond the drive to make profit from the delivery of services and beyond concerns over costs as well as over shortages of providers. These common themes have to do with ideas about the principles for change. Privatization, teamwork, evidence-based decision making, accountability, regionalization, and an emphasis on public health have all been promoted in health care reforms in and outside Canada. This section reviews these common themes from within the Canadian context, seeking to show how many of their principles are contradicted by the practices affecting ancillary workers.

Public Health Care in Canada

All health care reforms in Canada take place within the context of the complex public system and are limited by its structure and, some would contend, its popularity. In order to understand current reforms and their impact on ancillary work, it is thus appropriate to rehearse the development and structure of public health care.

Under the Canada Health Act (CHA), health care is primarily a provincial or territorial responsibility. The federal government still screens immigrants, provides some care to First Nations and Inuit peoples as well as to the armed forces, and regulates drug and food safety. But most of the rest is left to the provinces and territories. Nevertheless, the federal government has used its ability to raise money through taxes as a way to influence public health care in Canada. This influence is most obviously evident in the Canada Health Act and related financial arrangements.

The federal government began the process of building a public system by offering, in 1948, to pay for half the cost of hospital construction. In the late 1950s, under the Hospital Insurance and Diagnostic Services Act, the federal government offered to pay for half the cost of specified services offered in hospitals if the provinces met certain criteria. A decade later, the federal government followed this successful strategy a third time with the Medical Care Act. This Act covered the services of allopathic doctors and some dentists working in hospitals. These two pieces of legislation were brought together in the 1984 Canada Health Act (CHA). This short document set out clearly and simply the five principles that provinces must follow if they are to receive their money for what is called medicare.

The CHA requires that all medically necessary services provided in hospitals and by doctors or nurses paid under the provincial or territorial plans must be universal, accessible, comprehensive, and portable. Some aspects of extended care services are also covered. In addition, the government insurance plans must be administered by a non-profit, public agency. These principles are not defined in much detail. However, it is made clear that services must be provided under uniform terms and conditions and that a wide range of services are covered under the definition of hospitals, including all drugs and tests as well as all cleaning, food, and laundry provided in them. The federal government, then, contributes funds for services provided under provincial jurisdiction but does not deliver them. The provinces in turn mostly pay for services delivered by agencies that are not directly government-owned. Until recently, almost all of them were non-profit.

This approach to public care has a number of consequences that are relevant for the analysis of ancillary work. First, and most obviously, public health care services expanded enormously as they became more accessible to those who previously could not afford them. This expansion meant paid jobs in health care grew as well, especially for women. Second, services became more equally distributed not only among individuals but also across jurisdictions. Greater equity was, and is, particularly important to women and minority groups who need the system more but have fewer resources to use for payment. Third, although there was a more uniform approach to providing health care, provinces and territories continued to have a great deal of leeway in determining what services are provided and how they are provided. As a result, there are considerable variations among jurisdictions in terms of such things as length of stay in hospital, and the numbers of doctors, nurses, and ancillary workers per capita. The regulation of these workers is also left to the provinces. Fourth, doctors' power grew along with the health care system, in large measure because they determined what doctor or hospital care was medically necessary and thus covered by the public system. Clinical care and prevention based on medical perspectives dominated, rather than perspectives based on a determinants of health approach. Fifth, the emphasis was on doctor and hospital care because these were the services most clearly funded by the federal plan. This encouraged the development of large facilities, facilities which in turn had a high demand for ancillary workers. Other services, such as home care and drugs provided outside hospitals, remained largely private responsibilities and ones that were often privately delivered, even though the Canada Health Act does mention extended health care services. Conditions for both patients and workers in these privately delivered services varied enormously. The extent to which these services were regulated also varied enormously. Sixth, many facilities remained non-profit, non-government institutions, albeit ones considered to be part of the public sector and heavily regulated as well as funded by the various governments.

Under this approach, federal health care costs were determined in large measure by what provinces and territories decided to spend. Costs continued to rise and so did federal concern about expenditures. These cost increases reflected in part the enormous expansion in the number of beds and thus in the number of health care workers. By the mid-1970s, the federal government began moving away from its commitment to pay for half of the medically necessary care provided by doctors or hospitals. Limits were put on the total amounts to be contributed, and the cash portion reduced. Part of this reduction was replaced by the federal government transferring some of its tax 'room' to the provinces and territories. In the mid-1990s, the federal government collapsed all their contributions to health, social services, and higher education into one package called the Canada Health and Social Transfer (CHST) and significantly reduced the overall amount it contributed. The CHST reduction was not simply about rising government debts, however. It was also about the increasingly dominant neoliberal understanding of governments that considered smaller states, for-profit management techniques, and more personal responsibility as important in health as in other sectors.

The federal government thus reduced the amount of money available to provinces and territories for health care at the same time as it made the federal contribution significantly more difficult to calculate. The changes in funding had an important impact on public care, although the impact was not immediately obvious. Perhaps most importantly, the lack of clarity about how much the federal government contributed to health care, combined with reductions in funding, made it more difficult for the federal government to use its financial clout to enforce the five principles of the Canada Health Act. Provinces and territories increasingly challenged the federal government's right to have a say in public care. Facing rising costs and falling federal contributions at the same time as they began embracing neoliberal strategies, provincial and territorial governments turned to privatization as a means of reforming public care, as we shall see in the next section.

In recent years, the federal government has started to make up for some of the money lost to health care under the CHST, partly at least in response to public pressure. But it has not used this increase to enforce the principles of the Canada Health Act, and most provinces and territories continue to resist any such move. The federal government has now moved to a Canada Health Transfer that identifies money going to health and has increased the funding, but there is still no evidence of enforcement. Meanwhile, the move towards privatization continues, especially in terms of for-profit delivery and methods of work organization (Armstrong and Armstrong 2003; Gilmour 2002).

It is important to remember, however, that some kinds of care have never been part of the public health system. The Canada Health Act explicitly covers only doctors and hospitals and some extended health care services. Provinces and territories have made some drugs and some home care, along with some dentistry, part of the public system. Some jurisdictions have also added midwifery. However, coverage for services other than doctors and hospitals has been much more uneven and tends to be the first to be shed by public systems seeking to reduce costs. This is particularly the case with rehabilitation services at the moment.

So why is this history relevant for studying ancillary work? It shows how the expansion of public sector health services meant many more paid jobs for women doing ancillary work and greater access to health services. This expansion also brought women together in ways that encouraged unionization and the application of human rights principles that are part of government commitments, as we shall see in a later section. The organizations delivering publicly funded services have been highly regulated by the state in ways that helped, at least for a period, to improve conditions of work. But this history is also meant to show that the complex system of what Canadians think of as public health care makes categorization difficult and analysis confusing. In particular, the system's complexity makes it difficult to understand the impact of reforms that came in the wake of New Public Management and cutbacks in health care budgets. These reforms are changing the location, ownership, and structure of care services in ways that have profound consequences for work and employment relations, as we shall see in the next section on privatization.

Privatization

Privatization is not a single process. Nor is it a simple one. It is about much more than determining ownership and making a distinction between public and private sectors. Indeed, the move to a new government philosophy and practices has blurred the lines between what is public and what is private in terms of both ownership and responsibility. This section explores various forms of privatization in order to make their impact on ancillary work more visible.

Canada's public health care system has, from the beginning, been characterized by a separation between purchaser and provider. The federal, provincial, and territorial governments usually pay other individuals and organizations to deliver care. Before medicare, almost all institutional care was provided by local governments or more commonly, by independent, non-profit organizations. The five principles of the Canada Health Act apply explicitly to doctors and hospitals, but it is not clearly stated that other services must conform to them and that delivery must be non-profit. This lack of clarity has important implications for privatization in its various forms.

Pressures to reform health care were also present from the beginning of medicare. As Malcolm Taylor (1987) put it, hospitals and doctors were handed a blank cheque when they were promised payment for care determined by them to be medically necessary. Governments quickly became concerned about controlling costs, a concern that escalated in the 1990s. Those worried about the medicalization of daily life, about the quality of care, and about the authoritarian nature of health services also called for reforms. Women's groups were particularly vocal in pushing for changes that would result in fewer people in institutions, less power for doctors, and more external evaluation of care procedures. By the 1990s, governments in Canada became increasingly disenchanted with public health care services and more enamoured with private ones.

These pressures were central in the reforms of recent years, reforms characterized by privatization. Privatization can take multiple forms (Armstrong, Armstrong, and Connelly 1997; Armstrong 2001), and one form is a change in where care is provided. Less and less care is offered in the hospital, where the Canada Health Act principles clearly apply and where most workers are unionized. More services are offered in facilities and homes, where fees are usually charged or where individuals are required to pay for care, or provide it without pay. This shift of locations not only means a privatization of both costs and care work, it also means more of the paid work is done by those termed ancillary workers who often work alone and are less likely to have union protection. The farther care moves away from hospitals, the more care work is unpaid as well. Because most of these ancillary workers are women, more of them take on this additional unpaid care work.

In addition to privatizing costs and care work, governments have been contracting out services to for-profit concerns and entering into public–private partnerships that alter the nature and conditions of ancillary work, as the earlier discussion of New Public Management indicated (CUPE 2007c). In order to initiate this process, governments had to first define this work out of care. The discourse of 'hotel services' both laid the groundwork for and reflected the privatization of these services. In the process, the employment of these workers becomes a private concern, with their employment contract usually hidden from public view so profit-making companies can maintain confidentiality as they compete with each other (McGillis Hall 1999). It is worth noting, however, that the Canada Health Act explicitly includes all such work in the detailed description of what is covered in hospitals, suggesting it is understood as central to health care rather than constituting a 'hotel service.'

Even when these services have remained part of non-profit organizations, there has been significant pressure to follow the lead of for-profit management. In another form of privatization, governments moved to adopt for-profit business practices within their own organizations and to require such practices from others receiving their funding. Especially in the case of ancillary workers, considerable effort has been directed towards making work in health care similar to work outside health care (Stinson, Pollack, and Cohen 2005). Those who work in kitchen, laundry, housekeeping, caregiving, and clerical jobs in the for-profit sector are among the lowest paid and most precariously positioned in terms of benefits, pensions, hours of work, union coverage, and job security (Armstrong and Laxer 2006). Privatization through the adoption of private sector practices means moving to such conditions within public institutions as well.

Research has begun to show the impact of the privatization of ancillary services through contracting out, public–private partnerships, and the application of for-profit methods to this work. Carol Kushner (2005) looked at the contracting out of three services in Toronto hospitals: housekeeping, supplies and logistics, and food services. All three contracts were ended for several reasons. First, savings were short-term and quite small, both because these services were already quite efficient and because the wages were already quite low. Since these services involve the lowest-paid workers, three or four of them would have to be laid off to make up for the wages of one nurse, seven or eight of them to equal the loss of one manager. Second, systems developed in the private sector were not easily adapted to the public one. Third, contracting out added costs to administer the contracts, for severance and retraining, in capital developments such as renovating kitchen spaces, and in staff morale. Kushner (2005, slide 11) concluded that there is 'no scope for savings without serious compromises to quality.' When housekeeping services in Kushner's study were returned to the public sector, there was agreement that staff levels increased, the hospital was cleaner, and the cleaning materials were less toxic, creating a healthier workplace. A joint hospital plan was developed through a non-profit organization to buy and store supplies, and kitchens were re-established in-house.

According to the Hospital Employees Union, a seniors' home in British Columbia cancelled a cleaning and food services contract with a private company because of 'the declining state of cleanliness and food' (*Guardian* 2005b, 6). A 2005 audit of health facilities in British Columbia by a private firm (Westech Systems) had found that half of the facilities were not being cleaned well enough. And this was after the large move to privatize these services in the province.

In the United Kingdom, a 2001 investigation by the National Health Service found that the overwhelming majority of the filthiest hospitals were those cleaned by private contractors (Butler and Batty 2001). Three years later, inspections found that the worst hospitals – 'the three hospitals whose cleaning was rated as unacceptable – had already contracted out their cleaning to private providers' (McGauran 2004, 1361). That year, 2004, the health secretary announced that cleaning would be brought back into the public sector (Mulholland 2004).

And there may be other, less visible problems related to the contracting out of cleaning and other ancillary services. A Quebec man, hired by a private company to manage hospital cleaning, took the unusual step of going public about his lack of training in health care. He reported being exposed to biohazardous waste without any knowledge of how to deal with it, and being sent to clean an isolation room without receiving any education for the task (Toth 2004). The Canadian Union of Public Employees also points to the hidden costs to taxpayers, who have lost their public investment in existing kitchens and laundries and must also pay for the new ones, as well as pay for the replacement of old ones if the new ones do not prove to be effective. Ensuring that the contracts are fulfilled costs taxpayers money in terms of supervisors and lawyers (CUPE 2007a). Moreover, the centralization of services means job loss at the local level not only for ancillary workers but also for those who produce goods locally.

Research also indicates that working conditions deteriorate with privatization. In Hamilton, Ontario, the contracting out of home care services meant that two-thirds of the home support workers who kept their jobs saw their pay and benefits deteriorate. Many lost their jobs, and 3,500 clients lost their services. The four for-profit organizations that received contracts paid almost a dollar an hour less than was the case before privatization, while the not-for-profit one paid slightly more. All of the workers lost their sense of security and most experienced 'heightened anxiety about providing for themselves and their families' (Aronson, Denton, and Zeytinoglu 2003, 2). Equally important, privatized workers may no longer interact with patients and residents in ways that provide social support and other care. At the same time, work injuries may escalate. After the cook-chill method of centralized food production was introduced in a Vancouver hospital, 'the injury rate in the dietary department increased on average 28 per cent per month' (CUPE 2007a, 3).

Privatization in its many forms thus has a significant impact on ancillary workers. Even when the work remains part of the public sector, managerial techniques taken from the for-profit sector are applied to their work in ways that fail to recognize ancillary workers' contribution to health care while undermining their working conditions.

Integration and Teamwork

Another common theme in health care reform is the emphasis on integration and teamwork. According to a report published by the Health Council of Canada (El-Jardali and Fooks 2005, 4), virtually all the organizations and governments they surveyed 'recognize the importance of multidisciplinary teams' and call for 'training on team-based care' (2005, 5). The Canadian Institute for Health Information report on providers has chapters on 'Teamwork in Health Care' and 'Working in Health Care.' Its focus is primarily on doctors and nurses, although other regulated professions are also mentioned.

The Canadian Health Services Research Foundation in its report 'Teamwork in Healthcare' defines teams as 'a collection of individuals who are interdependent in their tasks, who share responsibility for outcomes, *who see themselves and are seen by others* as an intact social entity embedded in one or more large social systems and who manage their relationships across organizational borders' (CHSRF 2006, 3; emphasis in original). Clinical providers are the only ones considered in the team, however, even though the work of the ancillary staff is critical both to care and to the work of that team. Nurses and doctors cannot put someone in a bed that is not clean, for example, and they cannot leave a patient unfed. As a housekeeper interviewed for this book explained, 'We're part of the team. And when they need help, when they need a bed moved or when they need a patient's stuff moved, you're part of the team' (LTCb 2006).

Ancillary workers are not only left out of the teams described in the policy papers. In Karen Messing's educational session with cleaners, they 'mentioned their invisibility in answer to the questions on their relations with coworkers' and the lack of consultation on their work (1998a, 172). The contracting out of services such as cleaning and laundry further separates these workers from each other, making teamwork difficult if not impossible. Research indicates it also separates the various services, making integration within the system equally difficult.

In England, a report describes the apartheid created by the contracting out of services. In his investigation of infection control and the contracting out of public services, Steve Davies (2005, 4) concluded that 'the contract culture atomises functions within a hospital and contributes to the breakdown of a team-based approach that unifies clinical and non-clinical staff, thereby damaging flexibility and overall effectiveness.' The result was a two-tier and even three-tier workforce among ancillary workers. The first two tiers were created by the division of the workforce between those working under public sector conditions and those working under for-profit ones that are significantly worse. The third tier was made up of immigrant workers, hired under even more inferior conditions. Celia Davies (1995, 26), also on the basis of British research, argues that 'the new arrangements, by stressing market competition, lay bare the notion of hostility and warring, encourage it, celebrate it and aim to work with it rather than seeking to contain, hide or transcend it in some way.'

In her study of cleaning work that was contracted out in a British Columbia hospital, Kahnamoui (2005) found disruption of both services and teams, resulting in inefficient organizations and poor care. The log book, where cleaning requests were written by clinical staff and then read by the cleaning staff on the floor, had been replaced by a call centre at the corporation. Clinical staff reported waiting on the line for requests that had to go through the private employer rather than directly to the cleaners. The private centre would then page the cleaner, who disrupted her work to respond to the call. Indeed, clinical staff could no longer directly ask cleaners to do work that needed to be done, as a result of changes caused by the regular irregularity of health care. Calling the private employer took clinical staff away from their caring work. New ancillary staff was hired by the new employer and those with years of experience and relationships on the floor dismissed. Tensions, rather than teamwork, were the result. And Christmas decorations disappeared, because the ancillary workers who had undertaken the responsibility for putting them up in the past were no longer allowed to take the time.

Separating ancillary from clinical work, in policy and in practice, conflicts with the emphasis on integration and teamwork. At the same time, it creates logistical problems and adds more work for the rest of the staff while making the support networks among workers more difficult to maintain.

Evidence-Based Decision Making

Evidence-based decision making is yet another central theme in health care reforms. The National Forum on Health, a group appointed by the Canadian prime minister to advise on how to improve health and care, devoted an entire section of their report to evidence-based decision making. The section begins by explaining that 'the National Forum on Health believes that one of the key goals of the health sector in the 21st century should be the establishment of a culture of evidence-based decision-making. Decision-makers at all levels – health care providers, administrators, policy-makers, patients and the public – will use high-quality evidence to make informed choices about health and health care' (National Forum on Health 1997, 3). Research has become increasingly important with the call for evidence-based decision making, and there is a renewed emphasis on research that is interdisciplinary.

The term 'evidence-based medicine' was coined by Dr Gordon Guyatt and others at McMaster University in 1991, and the approach was recently listed by the *British Medical Journal* as one of the 15 most important milestones in medicine since 1840 (Godlee 2007; see also Dickersin, Straus, and Bero 2007). Yet there is very little evidence produced on ancillary workers in Canada or elsewhere. It is difficult to find research on the workers or their work. The multitude of documents on health care providers largely ignores them. There is little that either documents or analyses their work in relation to patient care or to the health of the ancillary workers themselves. Statistics Canada makes it harder to track them, now that the industrial classification system no longer counts them as part of the health care sector if their employer is a for-profit firm.

The Romanow Report argues that ancillary work 'could be the domain of private providers' (Commission on the Future of Health

Care in Canada 2002, xxi), without offering any evidence to support this claim or even a clear definition of who the ancillary workers are. Indeed, the Report did not even provide any evidence on how the division between ancillary and clinical work could be determined. Who is counted as a health care worker varies significantly from setting to setting, leaving considerable ambiguity and little means of assessing this recommendation and other policy on the basis of evidence.

Governments across Canada have been reorganizing the work without much evidence that this is a safe and effective practice for patients and providers, and without doing sufficient follow-up research to examine the impact on services, providers, and patients. They have also been contracting out the work, based on a belief in the superior efficiency and effectiveness of the for-profit sector rather than on evidence.

Even when the research has been done, there is little evidence that the evidence drives the practices. There is a great deal of social science literature demonstrating the importance, for example, of social networks and control over the labour process for both worker health and worker productivity. But the literature from these disciplines is seldom integrated into health care reform policies. The scan of views on health human resources prepared for the Health Council of Canada points out that 'despite robust evidence which suggests that improving working conditions in the short and long term is key to maximizing productivity and meeting growing service demands, stakeholders recognize that there has not been a lot of action in this regard' (El-Jardali and Fooks 2005, 7). This report goes on to say that 'much of the focus' has been on retaining nurses and physicians but that little attention has been paid to other providers. While there is little indication that this report intends to extend the definition of health care providers beyond professionals, it is clear that issues linked to the quality of workplaces for ancillary workers is not on the agenda.

Emerging evidence suggests that separating out ancillary work for privatization is a mistake on all grounds. Most of this research has been done on cleaning services, perhaps because cleaning is obviously connected to infection rates. A study conducted in the United Kingdom concluded that 'in the long term, cost-cutting on cleaning services is neither cost effective nor common sense' (Rampling et al. 2001, 115). In the U.K. survey of contract cleaning cited earlier (Davies 2005, 18), the researcher concluded that there is poor performance in contract cleaning because most, and perhaps all, of the savings came from poorer conditions of employment (21). But little research has been done by policy makers on how these changing conditions impact on the health of the ancillary workers.

Research in British Columbia (Cohen and Cohen 2004, 4) shows that in the wake of contracting services out, the wages of ancillary workers 'have been cut almost in half, and all these workers have no pension, long-term disability plan, parental leave or guaranteed hours of work.' Wages for this mainly female labour force are now equivalent to those paid in 1968. Male-dominated jobs have fared better, but that has created a larger wage gap among ancillary workers. The government has not, however, produced evidence on the impact this has on the women, their families, or the services they provide. Nor has it produced evidence to show that the immediate cost savings for the government will offset any additional costs incurred from dealing with the lack of pensions, disability insurance, and loss in income for these workers.

The British Columbia government did hire a consulting firm to conduct a 'quality audit' for facility cleanliness, including the contracted cleaning services. The B.C. Nurses' Union argued that the evidence from the audit was not reliable, given that both the health authority and the facility knew when the audit was to be conducted and that the auditing tool itself was inadequate (British Columbia Nurses Union and the Health Services Association 2004, 49). Nevertheless, the audit reported that a quarter of the facilities did not meet their standards (Westech Systems 2005). What this means in terms of the health of workers was not considered in the audit and it is not clear what action, if any, will result from this evidence.

In sum, evidence-based decision making in everything is a much-touted but little-practised approach when it comes to ancillary workers. The evidence that does exist suggests that ancillary work is critical to care and that cost-cutting strategies can have long-term negative consequences for both patients and providers. So does contracting out services. At the same time, research has focused on those who provide clinical care while reforms have proceeded without much evidence to support the strategies in relation to ancillary work or to assess the financial or health consequences for patients and workers.

Accountability

Calls for accountability are also at the heart of health care reforms and of government reforms in general (Gendron et al. 2007; Morris and

Zelmer 2005; Townley et al. 2003). The Canadian Policy Research Networks, for example, launched a seven-part series as a response to what they see as a demand from citizens for accountability (Fooks and Maslove 2004). Citizens' forums and national reports have repeatedly identified accountability as a critical and priority issue. .

Accountability seems to have a variety of meanings. According to the 2005 Ontario Budget, accountability 'involves setting out expectations about the outcomes to be achieved; monitoring and reporting publicly on progress; using the information to improve performance; and working to achieve results and taking responsibility for them' (Ontario 2005, 87).

'Accountability, like most character-building processes, is more bracing when applied to other people' (Stewart 2004, 127). It is usually about the exercise of power and the assignment of blame (Harber and Ball 2003). Moreover, it tends to be understood as being about financial counting, managerial control, and marketization within the public sector. Mark Exworthy and Susan Halford explain, in their book on the new managerialism in the public sector, that financial decentralization divides public sector organizations internally into purchasers and providers who are expected to operate like businesses, with transparency and accountability strictly defined in market terms. 'The development of cost-centres allows abstract space inside organizations to become "calculable" and therefore comparable: "calculative technologies make it possible to render visible [the] activities of individuals, to calculate the extent to which they depart from the norm of performance and to accumulate such calculations in computers and files and to compare them"' (Exworthy and Halford 1999, 5, quoting Peter Miller). This is what the province of Ontario (2005, 87) seems to mean as well, defining progress in terms of bottom-line financial results from hospitals, value-for-money audits, and the like. Such notions of accountability can come at the cost of care. The U.K. Healthcare Commission, investigating the death of 41 seniors in a hospital, concluded that members of the trust board 'mistakenly prioritized other objectives such as the achievement of government targets, the control of finances and their configuration of services' over infection control in areas such as cleaning (quoted in Carvel 2006, 1).

Accountability has been a theme in recent federal/provincial/territorial agreements on health care funding. Most recently, the way this notion of accountability was translated into practice was through a number of indicators that provinces and territories agreed to report on for their federal funding. The focus is on primary health care, cata-strophic drug coverage, and home care. According to the federal/provincial/territorial ministers' joint statement (Canada 2003, 3), their reporting 'will inform Canadians on progress achieved and key out-comes. It will also inform Canadians on current programs and expen-ditures, providing a baseline against which new investments can be tracked, as well as service levels and outcomes.' The indicators do move beyond money to focus on access, satisfaction, and perceived overall quality. Leaving aside the fact that not all indicators were fully reported, the indicators fail to define quality and satisfaction in ways that allow either improvement in care or an assessment of ancillary work. Indeed, we have little idea from these indicators what contrib-utes to either satisfaction or assessments of quality, and no idea of what role ancillary work plays. Moreover, the hospitals that employ a major-ity of these workers are not covered by the indicators.

Inadequate indicators are not the only problem. Accountability is made difficult when services are contracted out and when public–pri-vate partnerships of the sort that are increasingly common for ancillary services are formed. Lines of responsibility are blurred, making it diffi-cult to determine who is responsible for what (Toynbee 2003). Transpar-ency is an issue, because many aspects are held to be confidential in order to maintain necessary commercial secrets. There is no reporting we could find on the impact of reforms on the health of Canadian ancil-lary workers or on their work in health care delivery. There is little reporting on comparable costs or on quality assessments of privatized ancillary work.

Ownership is integrally related to decision making and accountabil-ity. Public facilities are responsible to governments and ultimately to citizens, creating at least the possibility for transparency and demo-cratic control. Private organizations are responsible mainly to their members or their shareholders, making it possible to claim that much of their decision making should be kept confidential and exclusive to those members or shareholders. When organizations need to make a profit over and above what they receive in funding, there is greater pressure to reduce costs. Given that by far the greatest expenditures in ancillary work are labour costs, the pressure to reduce both the number of workers and their wages and benefits is greater for private organiza-tions than it is for public institutions. Accountability to those who do the work is not part of the plan.

Often patient satisfaction surveys are used as a means of assessing

citizens' assessments of care services and are considered to be participation linked to accountability. Completing surveys, however, is a form
of participation that fits better with the notion of citizen as consumer
than citizen as democratic participant, and even in these terms is a limited means of participation. The content of surveys is primarily determined by experts, and so are the options for response. Such surveys can
provide an indication of whether services look good or feel good to
patients and families – and these are not irrelevant considerations. But
the patients and families who fill in surveys are often not in a position
to assess whether a bed is full of germs or know if records are accurate,
for example. And the assessments of dissatisfaction may lead to blame
being placed on the workers rather than on the management or structure of the work.

Even if we understand accountability in narrow accounting terms,
the cost-benefit analysis of reforms in terms of ancillary workers is simply not done. Nor are there reports on the impact on their families, or
the overall costs of this impact on the health system or on the larger
society.

Public Health

In the wake of the 2003 SARS outbreak and in the face other epidemics,
public health has been identified as a priority area in health care. The
World Health Organization defines public health as 'the science and art
of preventing disease, prolonging life, and promoting health through
the organized efforts of society' (WHO 2005a, 45). A public health perspective means 'the health care workforce must be engaged in the full
range of advocacy, disease prevention and health promotion activities
relevant to the population served' (45).

The public health movement of the nineteenth century focused on
food, clothing, shelter, and water. This was the period when regulations
about the handling, preservation, preparation, and inspection of food
were introduced. Clothes made in infested tenements were recognized
as contributors to diseases such as tuberculosis, and union labels
became a symbol of garments made in factories rather than in households (Johnson and Johnson 1982). Poor housing conditions were identified as a problem, not only for those whose clothes were made in
tenements but also for those living in them. As a result, new regulations
for tenements were introduced. Water and sewage systems were built
and monitored. Records and recording also gained prominence as a

health tool that allowed disease to be tracked and individuals to be treated (Jorland, Opinel, and Weisz 2005). A Royal Commission on Capital and Labour investigated working conditions and wages in Canada, revealing both discrimination against women and the role poor wages played in health. The knowledge gained about public health was applied in hospitals as well.

Nevertheless, although the implications of poor housing and working conditions were clearly identified in the nineteenth century, very little of the current discussion about public health focuses on the ancillary workers in facilities and households, or on the role their work plays in preventing injury and illness. Recall that health care workers are in general 50 per cent more likely than other workers to miss work because of injury or illness (CIHI 2002, 87) and ancillary workers even more likely, but neither the Canadian Institute for Health Information nor other sources discuss the specific occupational health and safety of ancillary workers. This oversight is in contrast to the increasing, and welcome, attention being paid to the serious dangers nurses face at work (see especially Shields 2006a). There is even less discussion about how the injuries and illnesses experienced by ancillary workers can be prevented. In spite of the fact that the main strategies to prevent further outbreaks of SARS, such as ensuring clean environments and accurate records, involve ancillary work, the focus of public health discussions remains on clinical aspects of care. And there is virtually no discussion of the health hazards faced in the household, even at a time when more care is being provided there.

Regionalization and Decentralization

All provinces except Ontario decentralized some of their decision making in the 1990s. Regionalization of health authorities became the norm, and recently Ontario has been moving cautiously in this direction as well with the establishment of 14 Local Health Integration Networks or LHINs. Provincial governments have retained the authority in setting standards, overall policies, and budgets while regional organizations were held responsible for the management of services within their geographical areas (CIHI 2005b, 43).

On the one hand, regionalization brings some decision making closer to those who need the services and allows programs to be designed for local needs. It also creates the possibility of sharing services such as laundry across local facilities. On the other hand, regionalization means local authorities are left with the tough decisions about what to cut in response to provincial limitations on resources. Moreover, it is also up to these regional authorities to decide whether 'to directly provide or contract out some services – such as meal services, laundry and cleaning for health care facilities – to for-profit companies' (Willson and Howard 2002, 221). Forced to find cost savings, many regions have looked to competitive bidding and the for-profit sector as a means of saving on labour. The result is uneven conditions for those who do ancillary work, often with different conditions of employment in each jurisdiction.

While regionalization suggests not only local responses but also local impact, this is not necessarily the case under the free trade agreements Canada has signed (Hankivsky and Morrow 2004). When a local authority opens the market to for-profit provision, it may be doing so for Canada according to international agreements such as the North American Free Trade Agreement (NAFTA). This could mean that foreign corporations can bid on the contract, and that it would then be very difficult to return the service to the public sector if the for-profit provision turns out to be a poor option. Decisions made at a local level about services such as home care, cleaning, food, and laundry, in response to immediate financial pressures, could mean that the decisions about these services are no longer in local hands for any region.

Regionalization and decentralization thus have consequences for ancillary work. They may allow for the more effective organization of local services and the integration of these services within the overall health care plan. But they may also promote the separation of ancillary workers from other health care providers and encourage strategies that lead to deteriorating working conditions.

Conclusions

In sum, reforms in health care often ignore ancillary work, leaving it out of discussions about teams and integration, about evidence-based decision making and accountability, as well as discussions about public health. At the same time, ancillary work has been the focus of privatization strategies and defined out of care, even though a determinants of health approach would make these services central to safe and effective care. This contradiction can be linked to the failure to understand health care as different from other services and the failure to understand that ancillary work is critical to care.

8 Developing Options

Feminist political economy, the theory that guides this book, teaches us to understand women's work from the standpoint of political, ideological, and economic forces that operate across a range of interrelated contexts, from global and national to local and household levels. At the international level, investors are searching for new sources of profit and seek to make that profit both by selling more and by paying less, especially for labour. Health care has offered and continues to offer an unmined source for profit, given that services are primarily provided on a non-profit basis. Canadian governments, operating at home and abroad, have supported and even promoted this mining for profit through their commitment to the market principles central to New Public Management. At the heart of these developments in the political economy is the explicit but unsubstantiated assumption that market competition necessarily improves efficiency and choice. Less explicit, but nonetheless central, is the assumption that women bring innate skills to their work and will necessarily take on the extra, unpaid caring tasks that are unprofitable yet required for profit and for a decent society. This assumption about women's work is perpetuated through managerial practices and the failure of governments to provide services, or through the way these services are provided.

Along with NPM, the research supporting a determinants of health approach has been promoted by governments and used as a justification for cutbacks in health services. Yet applying this same literature within health services would suggest that ancillary work plays a central role in health protection and that costly infections or errors can result from new managerial practices and the privatization of the work (CUPE 2007c; Lister 2005). Indeed, work injuries and work absences among ancillary workers have increased significantly under these new practices, as has the number of people hired to enforce contracts and coordinate for-profit services with the rest. Thus, in direct contradiction to the claims, costs rise not only in financial terms but also in terms of individual workers' health. Although the new management practices have also been justified as a means of saving money for taxpayers, taxpayers lose both as payers and as those with care needs.

Feminist political economy also reminds us that investors, governments, and ideas about women and race are not the only factors determining current reforms. In Canada, unions, professional associations, and various other organizations have played critical roles in the development of health care and work organization. Individuals have worked actively to protect health within health services and to protect their own health. As is the case with actions by investors and governments, the consequences of these collective and individual initiatives have often been contradictory for the women who do ancillary work. Indeed, current practices can be understood in some ways as a response to the success of collective action in defending worker rights and as strategies intended to undermine them. Similarly, the success of nurses has meant both a wider and perhaps more interesting range of tasks for ancillary workers, and greater pressure to define their work out of care. And while the actions taken by individual women to make up for the care deficit improve care, they can hide system failure and undermine the health of the individual woman.

Finally, feminist political economy helps us see the skills involved in women's work and the relationship between the work they do in the household and the work they do in the labour force (Armstrong and Armstrong 2004b). This is particularly the case with the ancillary work, where the skills are often not made visible through formal credentials and formal education, even when the work is done for pay. Employers – and governments – count on women combining their informally learned caring skills with their other paid and unpaid tasks. They get two for one in the paid labour force and two for no pay in the home.

Implications for Policy, Research, and Action

The analysis in this book based on theory, data, and experience is intended to be more than an intellectual exercise, however. It is also designed to provide a platform for the development of strategies to recognize the critical contribution ancillary workers make to health care and to alter conditions in ways that make it possible for them to provide quality care for appropriate rewards. In this final chapter, we suggest some of the strategies prompted by our analysis. But of course it is up to workers and patients, and to citizens more generally, to create and implement actual plans for change.

First, We Need an Active State

On the basis of their research in long-term care, Jane Aronson and Sheila Neysmith (1997, 61) argue that an active state is required to address the rights and responsibilities of both those who need care and those who do care work. We would add that an active state is necessary to control costs throughout the health care system and in private homes as well. An active state is one that not only steers but also rows in order to ensure safe, appropriate, and supportive care environments for workers and for those with care needs. This call for a state active in supporting the right to care flies in the face of many global and national pressures but confirms the research on both health care and public health.

Active states investing in public health systems provide the most effective and efficient health care (Armstrong et al. 2003). Single, non-profit employers in health care services are in the best position to integrate ancillary and other care work in ways that promote health both for workers and for those with care needs (Rachlis 2004). The research overwhelmingly confirms the superiority of non-profit health services supported collectively through taxes, and of public sector employers (see for example Devereaux et al. 2004; Relman 2002). Public health care services can also lead to a more equitable distribution of work and care across the country, rather than to an allocation based on local demand and ability to pay.

In terms of public investment, states can support workers through other services not so obviously linked to health care. Childcare is an obvious example, given that it is primarily women's responsibility. Public transit is another, perhaps less obvious example, given women's reliance on transit to get to work and to care. Unpaid caregivers want respite care, information, and financial compensation to support their work, all of which are most effectively provided by the state (Pyper 2006, 43). Workers want more access to public education and on-the-job training leading to credentials and recognition of skills so they are in a better position to improve their care and the conditions of their work.

Other programs, such as workers' compensation, maternity leave, and disability payments also play a critical role and need to be reformed in ways that support ancillary workers returning to their jobs.

States are also in the position to legislate, monitor, and regulate conditions for work and conditions for care. Without state support in this form, other strategies may be less effective (Bourgeault and Khokher 2006). We need not only recognition of the skills, effort, and responsibilities involved in ancillary work but also the establishment and enforcement of standards for training, entry, and conditions in this work. Health and safety regulations that recognize the particular nature and conditions of the work are also required.

Women who are unpaid caregivers would like more flexible work arrangements and job protection, both of which could be promoted by the state through regulation (Pyper 2006, 43). This unpaid work has direct consequences for the ways women participate in paid work, just as the conditions of their paid work have direct consequences for their life and care work at home. Ancillary workers in particular often go home to face the same job they just did all day or all night in the labour force. Recognizing their double or even triple workload is only a necessary first step in developing state-supported strategies to address this load in collective and equitable ways.

Pay and employment equity legislation can help address inequalities linked to gender and racialization, if they are appropriately developed and effectively enforced. Minimum wages and minimum standards for vacations and for health and safety have been particularly important to women in these kinds of jobs, sometimes providing the only protection they have. Both kinds of legislation need to be reformed and enforced in ways that ensure decent conditions of work under the reforms that follow the principles of New Public Management (Fudge and Owens 2006). The state also significantly influences who enters Canada under what conditions, with what education, and to which jobs (Bourgeault 2006). Together, these interventions could simultaneously promote equity and better care by ancillary workers, both of which would encourage a more productive society.

However, it cannot simply be assumed that states always act in the best interest of us all or that states are always good employers. Indeed, although ancillary workers fare better in the public sector than they do in the for-profit one, they still too often face low pay, precarious employment, and hazardous conditions. Indeed, public sector employers are increasingly acting like private sector ones. Neysmith and Aronson caution that 'an active state would always be formulating policy among unequal participants with conflicting interests' and that such policy making is always a 'huge challenge' (1997, 61). In that challenge, the weakest – most often women and too frequently women identified as visible minority or immigrants – often lose. New Public Management strategies mean that work is either contracted out to employers who lower pay and security or that the work stays in the public sector but is subjected to for-profit methods that lead to deteriorating conditions for workers and care recipients. Keeping jobs in the broader public sector, in non-profit firms, is a necessary but not sufficient condition for decent work and care. We need to develop working conditions that not only recognize the determinants of health for those with care needs but also for workers. We also need conditions that build on and enhance skills associated with women's work. And we have to monitor how policy is put into practice, given the current political economy context. As Marilyn Waring cautions, 'when social policy suggests "family-friendly" alternatives, from childcare to flex-time to family leave, the implementation of these policies is often skewed by patriarchy and the market-place' (2004, 112).

Equally important, states have been active in moving towards less regulation, monitoring, and democratic control over other employers not only at home but around the globe. This deregulation can undermine efforts in and outside the public sector to ensure decent work, and thus decent care. Meanwhile, states have become more active in protecting employers' rights and enforcing regulations that protect them, with patent rights for drug manufacturers and the imposition of competitive bidding providing two examples among many. In the process, worker is often pitted against worker, within Canada and among countries. Indeed, the intent is to increase competition among individual workers and reduce the power that comes from collective efforts. Partly as a result of the growing free trade in people, 'countries with the lowest relative need have the highest numbers of health workers,' because so many workers are leaving the countries that educated them and because their countries cannot offer employment (WHO 2006, 8). Global government efforts are required to address this imbalance in jobs and protections, and to support appropriate conditions for work in health care everywhere.

We need better mechanisms to ensure that states and managers are accountable both to the public and to workers. This means greater transparency, which can only be attained if health services remain in the public realm and the secrecy inherent in competitive contracts is avoided. It means more opportunity to influence directly and continually health care decision making and not just to receive more information on indicators chosen by governments or to be the subject of satisfaction surveys designed by those governments. Accountability has to mean much more than counting. Accountability requires the means – including the time, the education, and the energy – to participate fully. Tired workers pushed to their limits, as many ancillary workers are, cannot take advantage of even the very limited possibilities they are given for consultation. Workers have considerable experiential knowledge to contribute, and the failure to involve them in decision making is inefficient as well as undemocratic.

Second, We Need Better Management

Facing a shortage of nurses willing to take work as nurses, states and managers have started to look at the factors that keep people at jobs in health care (Baumann et al. 2001). Although little attention has been paid to ancillary work or workers or to a gender analysis of these factors, many of the lessons from this nursing research can be applied to ancillary work. Other health care research is focused on sources for infections and errors in health care (United Kingdom, Parliamentary Office of Science and Technology 2005). A third area of research, in this case in the social sciences field, examines the factors that contribute to healthy workplaces (Koehoorn et al. 2002). It is time to bring all three areas together with a gender analysis of the management of ancillary work.

Managers should be trained not only in health care but also in the determinants of health as they relate to both care work and worker health. The two are centrally linked. According to the World Health Organization (WHO 2002), for example, infectious and blood-borne diseases are largely preventable with good management and staff training. Managing on the basis of such evidence means paying attention to the organization of work. 'The design of jobs and how they are integrated into organizational systems provides the foundation for a high-quality workplace' (Koehoorn et al. 2002, 8). Teams have been identified as essential to care work. In designing these workplaces, however, the focus has been on the medical and nursing staff. Good design, based on the evidence, would integrate ancillary work in these teams.

The evidence suggests as well that one of the best sources of information about workplaces is the people who do the work. The 'health care field,' as more than one long-term care worker (LTCa 2006) wrote, 'is steadily getting worse because no one asks the people who would know what would work; i.e., the people who work daily with these residents.' We have heard very similar complaints over the years from ancillary workers in all health care workplaces. Listening to workers and acting on their advice can improve both work relations and conditions for care. Ancillary workers account for as much as half of the health care labour force, and they are often in a position to see what is happening on a daily basis in care, to see what may not be visible to others working in care. Their voices need to be heard. As Phil Hassen (2005, 9), President and CEO of the Canadian Patient Safety Institute explains, 'Being able to report adverse events without blame or retribution, to participate in addressing causes and to disseminate the lessons learned is part of the solution' to adverse events that cause injury and illness in health care. It is equally important for workers to be able to shape the workplace in ways that promote their health. A recent edition of Health Canada's *Health Human Resource Connection* reports that health care workers 'want to feel valued, have performance appraisals, have communication on a regular basis, and they want their managers to be visible' (Health Canada 2006, 6). There is no indication, however, that the definition of health care worker goes beyond the registered nurses, licenced practical nurses, doctors, and managers named in the publication.

Better management also means recognizing skills, teaching them in more formal ways, and protecting these skills when work is reorganized. This requires resources, resources that can be understood as promoting health and preventing diseases for workers and care recipients. Particular attention should be paid to the skills and needs of those with disabilities and of older workers. Davezies (2003, 273) argues that task shifting, which allows managers to adjust tasks to the particular skills and age of the worker, can make it possible for older workers to fully contribute without injury. Such work shifting requires trust earned over longer term relationships and counters 'managerial mobility policy which inevitably puts a greater focus on abstractly defined work organization' (274). And providing ancillary workers with more interesting tasks and allowing them more decision making could improve care as well as the conditions of work (Rasmussen 2004).

Equally important, states and managers need to promote employment security and decent conditions of work. High turnover creates high costs in terms of administration, continuity of care, training, and workers' health. Piercy's research (2000) shows the benefits for clients and workers of continuity over time that comes from stable employment and work. Based on their research with those who left work in home care, Denton and others argue that the key to keeping workers is 'good working conditions where employees have some predictability in their lives in terms of pay, hours of work and work scheduling' (Denton et al. 2005, 16). For these workers, such conditions not only provide the basics for survival but also indicate the value we place on their work.

Decent conditions mean, among other things, appropriate staffing levels based on a recognition of care needs and workers' contributions. A long-term care worker summed up her solution to stress and bad care by saying that the staffing problem could be solved by providing full-time rather than part-time employment. 'Many employees in health care juggle two or three part-time jobs just to get by' (LTCa 2006). As another put it, 'Staff are too time-pressured in a day to be able to provide the support that our elderly and challenged people need' (LTCa 2006). We need regulation of staffing and other conditions to promote health.

Good conditions are in turn related to good health. The high illness and injury rates in health care work come at a high price for the workers as well as for the system. They are the result of poor management, poor job design and poor working conditions, precarious employment and lack of training, no recognition, exclusion from teams, and little control over work (Yassi and Hancock 2005). The high rates of injury and illness can be addressed and reduced, with good management and state action playing a central role.

None of this will be possible if managers are not also educated about gender and about racism. As we have argued, the workforce is profoundly gendered and racialized. Without an understanding of the pervasive impacts of gender and racism, managerial strategies are bound to fail, especially for women and visible minorities and especially in the long term. This means education in what is often called cultural competency; it also means education about the structural conditions and relations that create inequities and discrimination.

Third, We Need to Promote Unions and Other Forms of Collective Organization

Research clearly shows that all workers fare better with unions, and this is especially the case for women (Jackson 2005; White 1980; White 1993). Unions not only help protect employment and conditions, they also give women the right to say no to unfair demands and to sexual harassment. Unions can give women a voice and the capacity to enforce existing legislation, regulations, and standards in areas such as pay equity and anti-discrimination principles. Unions also allow management to deal with workers in a collective and consistent manner, promoting more stable work relations.

In recent years, government policy and managerial practices have been directed at reducing the role of unions and altering the conditions of collective agreements. Workplace reorganization has meant that many of the existing laws and regulations no longer apply. As a result, women are losing the protection that unions and labour standards provided in the past. New legislation and regulations are required to address the gaps and to allow women to organize collectively to defend their rights (Fudge and Owens 2006). In the process of doing so, they will also help protect those who need care by creating better conditions for care.

In promoting unions, it is equally important to develop strategies that take gender and racism into account. Unions have become increasingly conscious of the roles gender and racism play and are making an effort to include analysis of these factors in their practices. Indeed, unions have played a central role in the adoption of anti-discrimination legislation and in ensuring its application. Yet there is still a need to require gender and racialization analysis and action within workplaces in order to make change on these issues a priority. Unions also need to recognize the skills involved in ancillary jobs and ensure they are visible and valued. And as is the case with states, unions must be subjected to measures that would ensure accountability to their membership and to the public. Unions often and increasingly face employers and governments seeking to reduce their power, making them ineffective. This in turn can undermine faith in unions (Aronson and Neysmith 2006). The Supreme Court decision makes it clear that workers have the right to organize and to have employers and governments negotiate with them in good faith, respecting collective agreements (*Health Services and Support – Facilities Subsector Bargaining Association v. British Columbia*, 2007). That the unions had to go to the Supreme Court to make this clear emphasizes the extent to which their power is being undermined.

Unions can divide workers from each other, given that membership is based on workplace and often, occupation. As economist Nancy Folbre (2006, 20) points out, we need to encourage links among health care sector workers. Given that many women work in the health care sector because they want to support others, it is possible to build on these shared values to promote conditions that in turn promote good care. Doing this will require women to confront the dismissal of jobs associated with domestic work as unskilled and with little value. It is not only managers and health planners who have done so. Many nurses and other professionals have as well, so it is important to identify the shared interests as well as shared values in exposing the skills, effort, responsibilities, and working conditions involved in ancillary work. Breaking down the walls among unions and other organizations to allow this kind of recognition and teamwork will take considerable effort and new strategies to protect skills and jobs while promoting effective care.

The links among health care workers need to be made with unpaid caregivers as well. It is in the home that many of these skills are developed. It is in the home that the work is combined, with ancillary and direct care delivery inextricably mixed. It is in the home where the skill, effort, responsibilities, and conditions are hidden and undervalued. Addressing the nature and conditions of the work means addressing the gender baggage that makes care in the home so difficult to see and to value as work.

Other forms of collective organizing are also required. The women's movement, often benefiting from working with unions, has been important for women's right to take and keep jobs, to say no to sexual and racial harassment, and to demand equal pay. Unfortunately, the Canadian government has cancelled or cut support for several programs that grew out of the women's movement, such as Status of Women Canada, leaving a number of women's groups much weaker as a result. Other civil society groups, such as the Canadian Health Coalition, have been contributing to the defence of the public system in ways that support ancillary work. The Council of Canadians has played a crucial role in limiting some of the most harmful aspects of free trade that had the potential to further undermine public care. And the Canadian Centre for Policy Alternatives has produced essential research on related areas of health care and work. Such organizations are necessary to address global and national issues that influence ancillary work.

While collective organizing is often the most effective, we also need to protect individual workers who speak out against poor conditions in care. Whistle-blower protection is one means for an individual to be heard, one long overdue in a public system that talks about accountability. Other forms of protection are legal aid and financial supports programs, all of which need to be considered in terms of this health care work.

Fourth, We Need More and Better Research

Governments and researchers are promoting evidence-based decision making. However, little research has been done in Canada on ancillary work. The research we have in Canada and from abroad often contradicts the direction of policy and practices. The problem is not simply one of absence. It is also one of perspective and assumptions. What we need, then, is more research that begins with a determinants of health approach *within* health care, recognizing the integral relationship among these determinants and their location within a specific political economy. This would mean making both gender and racialization critical components in research and in recommendations for action, and understanding the ways they are influenced by global and local forces. It would mean making the invisible visible. As Ana Maria Seifert and Karen Messing explain, 'If the work activity has aspects that are not visible to the people in charge of planning, these aspects will not be considered in the allocation of resources, particularly in the service sector, which has many aspects of caring necessary for quality of care, patient well-being and even, in some cases, patient safety' (2004, 13).

In particular, we need more research focused on organizational practices related to ancillary work, including contracting out, and their consequences for the health of workers and the quality of care. As a recent review of research on mental health indicates, we need to 'acquire a further understanding of, and monitor the effects on, the mental health of prominent trends in organizational practices' as well as find the means 'to address stigma and discrimination' (Lesage et al. 2004, 8). This process includes developing an understanding of the undervaluing of women's work, and it holds true for all areas of health, not just mental health.

Such research should begin by listening to workers. UNISON (2005, 7–9), the union voice for ancillary workers in the United Kingdom, did. They interviewed cleaners and on that basis proposed ten steps to cleaner hospitals. Cleaning, as the Infection Control Nurses Association in Britain and UNISON define it, includes 'hand hygiene, decontamination of patient equipment, linen and waste handling, clinical practice, the environment and ward kitchens' (Infection Control Nurses Association 2004, 10). In other words, 'cleaning' refers to most of the jobs considered in this book. In addition to making cleaning a priority, the British study recommends more staff and more hours, more and better resources, staff involvement to ensure contracts match needs, effective teams that include the full range of workers in care, respect for all health care workers and improved communications, training for all, scope to respond to criticism, bringing cleaning services back in-house, and finally, better pay and conditions. We need similar research here on the full range of ancillary work.

Health hazards cost employers and workers, and those taxpayers we hear so much about. We also need further research on health hazards, research that recognizes gender as central to the investigation of these hazards. And we need research that points to action. There are some necessary risks to working in health care. But we know from the existing research that a focus on hazard prevention strategies related to violence and equipment, along with return to work initiatives, can significantly reduce time lost from work (Yassi, Gilbert, and Cvitkovich 2005, 325). Much more work is necessary to make health care safe for patients and providers.

Conclusions

This book makes a simple argument. Those jobs labelled as ancillary play a critical role in health care and those who do this work are health care workers. Moreover, the health of these workers is integrally related to the effectiveness of the care they provide. Our argument means applying a determinants of health framework within health care and recognizing that these determinants are interpenetrating rather than independent factors. A feminist political economy analysis helps us see how and why this work remains invisible and undervalued. Understanding ancillary work within the context of global developments reveals the forces contributing to the privatization of the work. Applying recent health policy priorities to ancillary work exposes the gaps in research and in practice.

As the World Health Organization (2006, 4) puts it, excluding the full range of workers 'from official counts results in a substantial underestimation of the size of the health workforce and its potential to improve health. Such undercounting also prevents consideration of the complex labour market links between different sectors that could inform planning, recruitment, retention and career paths.' In short, we need to include ancillary workers as health care workers, because they are critical to care.

Appendix: A Guide to Canadian Data on Ancillary Workers in the Health Care Sector

Introduction: Interpret Data with Care!

The general aim in assembling the data used in this book is to produce an empirical portrait of ancillary workers in the health care field in Canada, using available public and custom data sources from Statistics Canada. Although some strong trends emerge from the data, the portrait produced thus far is a partial one. Data are scanty in some areas and inappropriately aggregated or presented in others. Therefore, the data in this book have the following specific objectives:

- to augment the analytical component of research into ancillary workers;
- to identify what characteristics of ancillary workers can be measured with current data sources;
- to identify what *cannot* be measured, or not fully measured, with current data sources; and
- to suggest areas for further research.

Despite the importance of knowing more about ancillary health care workers in Canada, obtaining accurate, detailed data about them is an ongoing challenge (see for example Armstrong and Laxer 2006). This is due to many factors, including

- the way in which ancillary work is (inaccurately) conceptualized as external to health care and thus rarely mentioned in studies of health care workers or health care work;
- the way in which occupational and industrial data is collected and represented by Statistics Canada;

- the difficulty in settling on definitions and criteria for ancillary workers;
- the invisibility of many forms of work that are endemic to ancillary occupations, such as privatized, contracted, or subcontracted work;
- the demographics of the ancillary labour force, which is largely female, and for many occupations often racialized, often immigrant, and typically involved in lower-status service work ; and
- the frequent ambiguity of ancillary work's status as paid or unpaid work. For example, does a family member's caregiving in the hospital count? does work that falls outside of a worker's job description count (for example, a cleaner assisting a patient)?

Data quality notes available from Statistics Canada usually focus on issues of statistical methodology (such as how to calculate the coefficient of variation) and neglect the theoretical issues of how the data itself is conceptualized, collected, and organized – precisely the issues we take up in this work.

In this book, we have assembled a collection of data from which we can infer particular things about the character and organization of ancillary work. We have used multiple surveys and multiple paths into the data. Such a project is rather like putting together a puzzle in which holes remain: although there are significant gaps, we can discern the general form of the puzzle's gradually emerging image. Because of these issues of data precision, any figures cited *should be regarded as rough estimates at best*, and further considered as indicators of where more (and more useful) data are needed.

While it presents a temporary research limitation, the absence of adequate data should nevertheless be regarded as a research challenge and a guide to further work in this area. For example, where data suppression renders quantitative data from Statistics Canada unavailable, researchers might consider augmenting these absences with critical qualitative work. Throughout the book, we have occasionally provided some suggestions for additional investigation.

Methodology and General Overview

We used multiple data sources from Statistics Canada to produce a composite portrait of ancillary workers in the health care field. The two main surveys we used were the *Labour Force Survey* and the 2001 *Census of Population* (Statistics Canada 2001a; 2005b; 2005c; 2006b). We obtained survey data in both aggregate form from published sources as well as from custom microdata runs. Because of the difficulty in obtaining accurate data on ancillary workers, data in this report should be regarded as *approximate estimates only*.

Notes on the Labour Force Survey

The *Labour Force Survey* (LFS) is widely available in public use microdata files (PUMF) and CANSIM tables. It is useful to obtain time series data, along with richer work- and income-based data on dimensions such as earnings and absence from work. However, industry is rarely cross-tabulated with occupation in any published aggregate data from LFS. Additionally, the LFS PUMF provide no data on important dimensions of social location such as immigrant status and period of immigration, place of birth, or ethnicity (see below for more on obtaining data concerning migration and race-ethnicity).

OCCUPATIONAL AND INDUSTRIAL CLASSIFICATION
The LFS now uses the 2001 National Occupational Classification (NOC-S 2001) system to code occupations. This makes comparison with 2001 Census-based data easier, as until relatively recently only the 1991 Standard Occupational Classification (SOC91) was available from the LFS.

Both the LFS and the Census share the use of the North American Industry Classification System (NAICS). However, publicly available LFS microdata use a highly aggregated occupational and industrial breakdown, which inhibits precision and obscures occupational and industrial heterogeneity. For the importance of occupational and industrial detail, see below.

Notes on Census Data

Like the LFS, Census aggregate data is broadly disseminated in both data table and PUMF format. The Census is particularly useful for obtaining data on race-ethnicity, immigrant status and period of immigration. However, also like the LFS, the Census PUMF provides highly aggregated occupational and industrial categories, and the few detailed data tables that cross-tabulate industry and occupation are of limited utility, as they cover only full-time, full-year workers (more on this below).

ROUNDING

To preserve confidentiality, aggregate data that are publicly available from the Census are randomly rounded to '0' or '5' in its final digit. For example, the figure 3,784 may be rounded down to 3,780 or up to 3,785. Thus, when 'drilling down' into data categories (for instance, cross-tabulating occupation by sex), category totals may not always add up precisely to totals provided by Statistics Canada. This may also result in figures with a relatively larger margin of error (+/− a few per cent), especially when calculating percentages in cross-tabulated data.

In cases where there are fewer than ten observations, Statistics Canada represents the number as '0.' This is a particularly critical point to remember when using very small numbers. Very small numbers should not be broadly generalized or interpreted. While nevertheless useful in that they may indicate significant absences (for example, the lack of men in a highly female-dominated occupation, or the lack of health care workers in certain geographic regions), such small numbers should be understood as approximate estimates only.

Defining Ancillary Occupations in Health Care

The first task in generating a portrait of ancillary occupations in health care is to establish what exactly those occupations are. Establishing criteria for inclusion of ancillary workers means that defining ancillary work involves understanding both the division of labour in health care provision, as well as the *status* (both the ascribed social value as well the practical characteristics of job status, such as compensation and presumed skill) frequently associated with such a division of labour. This requires exclusion of occupational tasks typically associated with health care professionals such as doctors and nurses – namely, that of diagnosis and direct treatment (for example, performing surgery or giving injections).

Based on this conceptual framework, we devised the following occupational categorization for the ancillary group:

- workers who directly or indirectly support the diagnosing and treating work of health care professionals and paraprofessionals (for example, dental assistants or medical laboratory technicians);
- workers who develop and administer health care policy, research, and regulation (for example, inspectors in public health or health policy researchers)

- workers who maintain the physical infrastructure of health care delivery (for example, cleaners or laundry workers);
- workers who maintain the information infrastructure of health care delivery (for example, clerical workers);
- workers who maintain the interpersonal and organizational infrastructure of health care delivery (for example, orderlies or managers); and
- workers who provide additional services critical to the smooth maintenance of a health care enterprise (such as food service workers and security personnel).

Although there was some ambiguity about a few specific occupations, we attempted to exclude all occupations defined as providing direct diagnosing, treatment, and care.

We reviewed the occupations listed in the National Occupational Classification for Statistics (NOC-S) 2001 and developed the following list grouped by occupational categories (table A.1). For more detailed descriptions of what each occupation involves, please refer to Statistics Canada, *National Occupational Classification for Statistics, 2001*, Catalogue 12-583-XPE.

Where the available data permitted, we used as detailed an occupational category as possible, because larger groups often contained occupations that should be excluded. For instance, in the case of the D21 group, most occupations met the criteria. However, a few did not, such as veterinary assistants (D213). Wherever possible, we used a three-digit level of detail (e.g., D211). Unfortunately, publicly available data rarely permits such detail in the desired configuration. This is a key methodological issue for researchers studying ancillary occupations.

Additionally, although occupational groups are handy for conceptual organization, it is essential to note the heterogeneity within these groups. For example, compare the gender composition of two types of cleaners (all industries):

	Men	Women	Total
G931 Light duty cleaners	28.6%	71.4%	100.0%
G933 Janitors, caretakers, and building superintendents	70.5%	29.5%	100.0%

(Statistics Canada 2001a).

Table A.1 List of ancillary occupations

NOC-S 2001 Code	Job title
Managers	
A014	Senior Managers – Health, Education, Social and Community Services, and Membership Organizations
A321	Managers in Health Care
A331	Government Managers – Health and Social Policy Development and Program Administration
Policy, research, and administration	
C163	Inspectors in Public and Environmental Health and Occupational Health and Safety
E039	Health Policy Researchers, Consultants, and Program Officers
Clerical	
B41	Clerical Supervisors
B213	Medical Secretaries
B214	Court Recorders and Medical Transcriptionists
B513	Records Management and Filing Clerks
B514	Receptionists and Switchboard Operators
Technical Occupations in Health Care	
D211	Medical Laboratory Technologists and Pathologists' Assistants
D212	Medical Laboratory Technicians
D215	Medical Radiation Technologists
D216	Medical Sonographers
D217	Cardiology Technologists
D218	Electroencephalographic and other Diagnostic Technologists, n.e.c.
D219	Other Medical Technologists and Technicians (except Dental Health)
D223	Dental Technologists, Technicians, and Laboratory Bench Workers
Supporting Occupations in Health Care	
D31	Assisting Occupations in Support of Health Services Subtotal
D311	Dental Assistants
D312	Nurse Aides, Orderlies, and Patient Service Associates
D313	Other Assisting Occupations in Support of Health Services
Personal Care and Home Support	
G811	Visiting Homemakers, Housekeepers, and Related Occupations
Cleaning	
G015	Cleaning Supervisors
G931	Light Duty Cleaners

Table A.1 (*Concluded*)

NOC-S 2001 Code	Job title
G932	Specialized Cleaners
G933	Janitors, Caretakers, and Building Superintendents
Food services and retail	
G012	Food Service Supervisors
G3	Cashiers
G412	Cooks
G961	Food Counter Attendants, Kitchen Helpers, and Related Occupations
Laundry	
G014	Dry Cleaning and Laundry Supervisors
G981	Dry Cleaning and Laundry Occupations
G982	Ironing, Pressing, and Finishing Occupations
Protective Services	
G63	Security Guards and Related Occupations

These two types of cleaners differ not only by gender but also by dimensions such as status, perceived skill, earnings, and the organization of work. To aggregate them would result in overlooking crucial differences. Thus wherever possible, occupational detail should be retained in order to fully represent the differences within occupational groups. This is not always practical, of course, given sample sizes when combining other dimensions, but nevertheless one should not make the error of assuming that all supporting occupations are exactly alike.

The Importance of Industry

'Industry' refers to the main economic activity of a business or enterprise, while 'occupation' refers to the particular jobs done within that enterprise. We used four main industry categories under the broad sectoral heading of the North American Industry Classification System (NAICS) code 62, 'Health Care and Social Assistance Industries' (see table A.2).

For more detailed descriptions of what each industry category involves, please refer to Statistics Canada, *North American Industry Classification System – NAICS Canada*, Catalogue 12-501-XPE.

Table A.2 List of health care and social assistance industry categories (NAICS 1997 and 2002)

NAICS Code	Industry category
621	*Ambulatory Health Care Services*
6211	Offices of Physicians
6212	Offices of Dentists
6213	Offices of Other Health Practitioners
6214	Out-Patient Care Centres
6215	Medical and Diagnostic Laboratories
6216	Home Health Care Services
6219	Other Ambulatory Health Care Services
622	*Hospitals*
6221	General Medical and Surgical Hospitals
6222	Psychiatric and Substance Abuse Hospitals
6223	Specialty (except Psychiatric and Substance Abuse) Hospitals
623	*Nursing and Residential Care Facilities*
6231	Nursing Care Facilities
6232	Residential Developmental Handicap, Mental Health and Substance Abuse Facilities
6233	Community Care Facilities for the Elderly
6239	Other Residential Care Facilities
624	*Social Assistance*
6241	Individual and Family Services
6242	Community Food and Housing, and Emergency and Other Relief Services
6243	Vocational Rehabilitation Services
6244	Child Day-Care Services

In her research, Kate Laxer indicates the difficulty of using the NAICS to obtain a precise picture of ancillary workers, noting that 'the NAICS has not been designed to take account of the range of integrated production processes in complex enterprises' such as hospitals (Laxer 2004). She argues that because of shifts in classification and representation, as well as the process of privatization and contracting out, workers whose actual jobs involve support tasks within health care industries will be invisible because of the ways in which their occupations become classified. For instance, a privatized food service worker who works in a hospital cafeteria may be classified as part of that hospital or may be classified as belonging to the food service company, which would be listed under a different industry group. This divergence between how and where work is actually done and the way in which it is recorded for data collection purposes illustrates the methodological problems in relying on empirical data alone.

Nevertheless, industry remains an important, if problematic, element of representing ancillary work, if only because it is one of the only tools we have for interpreting Statistics Canada data. Because many ancillary occupations are not explicitly health related and are found in other industries (such as cleaners or food service workers), it is essential to cross-tabulate occupation with industry in order to obtain a more accurate estimate. With a few exceptions (noted below), occupation alone should *not* be used to produce a portrait of ancillary workers in health care. However, occupation can be useful for comparison and inference. Based on our knowledge of the composition of an occupation, we can begin to develop educated hypotheses about the composition of that occupation in the health care field.

Form of Employment

Form of employment for the purposes of these data may be understood as operating along three axes:[1]

- class of worker: employee (wage and salary earner), self employed (with or without employees), and unpaid family worker;
- job tenure: permanent (or full year) and temporary (or part year);
- job status: full time or part time.

However, because of data availability and accuracy, not all of these can be fully explored. For instance, unpaid family workers are understood by Statistics Canada to include only workers in a family business/ enterprise or farm. This does not count work such as domestic or caregiving work, which would be understood as ancillary work if the same tasks were done for pay but which does not count as 'unpaid family work' if done for the members of one's own household or on a volunteer basis (e.g., for a neighbour or an organization).

---

1 For more on the role of form of employment in shaping paid work, refer to Vosko (2006).

Publicly available aggregate data from the 2001 Census on paid work often counts only a subset of workers; namely, full-time, full-year workers. While in some industries and occupations, this subset would cover most workers, using this form of employment as the normative form effectively hides much of the work in ancillary occupations. First, many types of ancillary work tend to be part-time or temporary. Second, many types of women's work also tend not to follow the full-time, full-year model. Given that many ancillary occupations in the health care field tend to be precarious as well as female-dominated, the choice to represent only full-time, full-year workers has a significant impact on collecting and representing data on ancillary occupations.

Compare, for example, the following aggregate Census data showing the number of workers in two occupations, one technical and one clerical. What is evident is that not only are these occupations highly female-dominated (81 per cent and 99 per cent women, respectively), but also that including only full-time, full-year work fails to capture a large segment of them.

D211 Medical laboratory technologists and pathologists' assistants	Male	Female
Total all industries, number of all workers in the labour force	3,590	14,885
62 Health and social assistance industries		
All workers	2,670	13,335
Full-year, full-time workers	2,030	8,625
Per cent of workers in health care captured in full-year, full-time work category alone	76%	65%

B213 Medical secretaries	Male	Female
Total all industries, number of all workers in the labour force	545	44,105
62 Health and social assistance industries		
All workers	510	41,705
Full-year, full-time workers	190	23,115
Per cent of workers in health care captured in full-year, full-time work category alone	34.9%	52.4%

Source: Statistics Canada, *Census of Population*, custom tabulation using data from two published aggregate tables: 97F0012XCB2001049 and 97F0012XCB2001050 (Statistics Canada 2001b).

Published Census data that cross this full-time, full-year worker group with other outcomes such as average annual earnings thus results in misleading figures. For instance, using occupational category B213 in the example above, full-time, full-year workers in all industries earn an average annual salary of $28,380, whereas when all workers are considered, the average annual salary drops to $23,321.

However, since Census data are often highly detailed, with a sample size unmatched by other surveys and with useful cross-tabulations (such as detailed industry combined with class of worker combined with annual earnings), we have nevertheless included some published aggregate data on full-time, full-year workers. These data should simply be understood as provisionally useful, rather than as a definitive depiction of the full scope of ancillary work in health care.

CLASS OF WORKER

The majority of ancillary workers are employees. In most occupations, self-employed workers are a small proportion of the total. This is because of the intersection between work type and work location: many of these ancillary workers are traditionally employees and not self-employed, and aside from professionals in health care, most health care workers are also employees. Notable exceptions include medical transcriptionists (approximately 20 per cent are self-employed) and dental technicians (about 18 per cent are self-employed), but even these figures are small, and the proportion of self-employment tends to be much smaller in health care work than in other occupations. Because of this low proportion of self-employed workers in the selected occupations, we have not included an examination of the self employed in this book.

Immigrant and Visible Minority Status

Obtaining detailed data on racialization, immigrant status, and the selected ancillary occupations in the health care industry is an exceedingly difficult task with currently available public data. The Census PUMF provide rich data on elements such as place of birth, citizenship, immigrant status, and period of immigration, but the level of detail available in the PUMF for occupations and industry is poor. Running cross-tabulations here yields many missing values and small numbers, which are then unreliable (although they can be loosely correlated with other data sources). Additionally, the Census does not collect data on many aspects of work and earnings.

Conversely, while the LFS and its companion survey the SLID (Survey of Labour and Income Dynamics is an excellent source of data on work and earnings, the LFS PUMF provide no data on important dimensions of social location such as immigrant status and period of immigration, place of birth, or ethnicity. The smaller sample sizes of non-Census surveys are also likely to result in data suppression when cross-tabulations are applied. In 2001, immigrants made up approximately 19 per cent of the Canadian population, while visible minorities made up about 13 per cent (Statistics Canada 2001a). Given that cutoffs for data suppression in SLID and LFS are 13,000 and 1,500 respectively,[2] it is evident that combining immigrant and visible minority dimensions with industry and occupation presents possible problems with suppression.

Without the benefit of custom data runs, the best one can do is make informed assumptions regarding these dimensions and ancillary occupations, drawing on aggregate cross-tabulations as well as relevant literature. Researchers interested in pursuing this area of inquiry should recommend custom runs that achieve the required level of detail.

The category of 'immigrant' or 'visible minority' is often used as a blunt instrument. When it comes to publicly available data that present immigrant status merely as a bivariate dimension (e.g., immigrant versus non-immigrant), a wealth of diversity is lost. The experiences of a white British-born worker differ greatly from the experiences of a dark-skinned, non-anglophone, South Asian-born worker, due to a variety of factors. The same might be said of the category that Statistics Canada calls visible minority, which is a self-declared status that interestingly excludes Aboriginal people. Thus it is also important to examine dimensions such as place of birth, period of immigration, and the region of destination for immigrants, as well as ethnicity and language for visible minorities. Crossing visible minority and ethnicity with immigrant status is also useful. Reflection on the conceptualization and methodological relevance of these dimensions is largely outside the scope of this appendix, but such things should nevertheless be noted.

---

2 Suppression refers to 'hiding' certain elements of published data, generally either because to show a small number of specific cases would compromise anonymity, or because the group is too small for the researcher to draw accurate conclusions from the sample.

References

Abraham, Carolyn. 2007. Ontario lapses linger four year after SARS. *Globe and Mail*, 10 January, A1, A6.

Anderson, Gerard, and Peter Sotir. 2001. Comparing health system performance in OECD countries. *Health Affairs* 20 (3): 219–32.

Anderson, Joan M., Connie Blue, and Annie Lau. 1998. Women's perspectives on chronic illness: Ethnicity, ideology and restructuring of life. In *Health and Canadian society*, 3rd ed., ed. David Coburn, Carl D'Arcy, and George Torrance, 163–86. Toronto: University of Toronto Press.

Andrew, Caroline, et al., eds. 2003. *Studies in political economy: Developments in feminism*. Toronto: Women's Press.

Angell, Marcia. 2004. *The truth about drug companies*. New York: Random.

Arat-Koc, Sedef. 1995. The politics of family and immigration in the subordination of domestic workers in Canada. In *Gendering the 1990s: Images, realities and issues*, ed. E.D. Nelson and B.W. Robinson, 413–42. Toronto: Nelson.

Armstrong, Hugh. 1977. The labour force and state workers in Canada. In *The Canadian state: Political economy and political power*, ed. Leo Panitch, 289–310. Toronto: University of Toronto Press.

– 2001. Social cohesion and privatization in Canadian health care. *Canadian Journal of Law and Society* 16 (2): 65–81.

Armstrong, Hugh, Pat Armstrong, and M. Patricia Connelly. 1997. The many forms of privatization. *Studies in Political Economy* 53 (Summer): 3–9.

Armstrong, Pat. 1987. Women's work: Women's wages. In *Women and men: Interdisciplinary readings on gender*, ed. Greta Hofmann Nemiroff, 354–76. Toronto: Fitzhenry and Whiteside.

– 1993. Professions, unions or what? Learning from nurses. In *Women challenging unions*, ed. Linda Briskin and Patricia McDermott, 304–24. Toronto: University of Toronto Press.

Armstrong, Pat, et al. 2002. *Exposing privatization: Women and health care reform in Canada*. Aurora, ON: Garamond Press.

Armstrong, Pat, and Hugh Armstrong. 1983. *A working majority: What women must do for pay*. Ottawa: Supply and Services Canada for the Canadian Advisory Council on the Status of Women.

– 1994. *The double ghetto: Canadian women and their segregated work*. 3rd ed. Toronto: McClelland and Stewart.

– 2003. *Wasting away: The undermining of Canadian health care*. 2nd ed. Toronto: Oxford University Press.

– 2004a. Planning for care: Approaches to health human resource policy and planning in health care. In *Changing health care in Canada*, ed. Pierre-Gerlier Forest, Gregory P. Marchildon, and Tom McIntosh, 117–49. Toronto: University of Toronto Press.

– 2004b. Thinking it through: Women and caring in the new millennium. In Grant et al. 2004, 5–43.

– 2005. Public and private: Implications for care work. *Sociological Review* 53 (2): 167–87.

Armstrong, Pat, Hugh Armstrong, Ivy Lynn Bourgeault, Jacqueline Choiniere, Joel Lexchin, Eric Mykhalovskiy, Suzanne Peters, and Jerry P. White. 2003. Market principles, business practices and health care: Comparing the U.S. and Canadian experiences. *International Journal of Canadian Studies* 28 (Fall): 13–38.

Armstrong, Pat, Hugh Armstrong, Jacqueline Choiniere, Gina Feldberg, and Jerry White. 1994. *Take care: Warning signals for Canada's health system*. Toronto: Garamond.

Armstrong, Pat, Hugh Armstrong, Jacqueline Choiniere, Eric Mykhalovskiy, and Jerry P. White. 1997. The promise and the price: New work organization in Ontario hospitals. In *Medical alert: New work organizations in health care*, ed. Pat Armstrong et al., 31–68. Toronto: Garamond.

Armstrong, Pat, Hugh Armstrong, and Tamara Daly. 2007. The thin blue line: Long-term facility care as an indicator of equity in a welfare state. Paper presented at Stockholm University, Stockholm, May.

Armstrong, Pat, Hugh Armstrong, and Krista Scott-Dixon. 2006. Critical to care: Ancillary workers in health care. Canadian Women's Health Network. http://www.cwhn.ca/.

Armstrong, Pat, Madeline Boscoe, Karen R. Grant, et al. 2006. It's about time: Women-defined quality care. Paper presented at the American Sociological Association Meetings, Montreal, August.

Armstrong, Pat, and M. Patricia Connelly, eds. 1999. *Feminism, political economy and the state: Contested terrain*. Toronto: Canadian Scholars' Press.

Armstrong, Pat, and Tamara Daly. 2004. *'There are not enough hands': Conditions in Ontario's long-term care facilities.* Toronto: CUPE.

Armstrong, Pat, and Irene Jansen. 2003. Assessing the impact of restructuring and work reorganization in long term care. In *Head, heart and hands: Partnerships for women's health in Canadian environments,* ed. Penny Van Esterik, 1:175–217. Toronto: National Network on Environments and Women's Health.

Armstrong, Pat, and Kate Laxer. 2006. Precarious work, privatization, and the health-care industry: The case of ancillary workers. In *Precarious employment: Understanding labour market insecurity in Canada,* ed. Leah Vosko, 115–38. Montreal: McGill-Queen's University Press.

Aronson, Jane. 2004. 'Just fed and watered': Women's experiences of the gutting of home care in Ontario. In Grant et al. 2004, 167–84.

Aronson, Jane, Margaret Denton, and Isik Zeytinoglu. 2003. 'I really can't afford to stay in home care': A follow-up study of Hamilton home support workers laid off in 2002. Hamilton: McMaster University.

Aronson, Jane, and Sheila M. Neysmith. 1996a. Home care workers discuss their work: The skills required to 'use your common sense.' *Journal of Aging Studies* 10 (1): 1–14.

– 1996b. 'You're not just in there to do the work': Depersonalizing policies and the exploitation of home care workers' labour. *Gender and Society* 10 (1): 59–77.

– 1997. The retreat of the state and long-term care provision: Implications for frail elderly people, unpaid family caregivers and paid home care workers. *Studies in Political Economy* 53 (Summer): 37–66.

– 2006. Obscuring the costs of homecare: Restructuring at work. *Work, Employment and Society* 20 (1): 27–45.

Attewell, Paul. 1990. What is skill? *Work and Occupations* 17 (4): 422–48.

Attree, Moira. 2001. Patients' and relatives' experiences and perspectives of 'good' and 'not so good' quality care. *Journal of Advanced Nursing* 33: 456–66.

Auerbach, Lewis, et al. 2003. Funding hospital infrastructure: Why P3s don't work, and what will. Ottawa: Canadian Centre for Policy Alternatives.

Avison, William R. 1998. The health consequences of unemployment. In *Determinants of health: Adults and seniors,* 3–42. Papers Commissioned by the National Forum on Health, vol. 2. Sainte-Foy: Éditions MultiMondes.

Badgley, Robin. 1975. Health workers' strikes. *International Journal of Health Services* 5 (1): 1–19.

Baines, Donna. 2004a. Caring for nothing: Work organization and unwaged labour in social services. *Work, Employment and Society* 18 (2): 267–95.

- 2004b. Losing the eyes in the back of your head: Social service skills, lean caring and violence. *Journal of Sociology and Social Welfare* 31 (3): 31–50.
- 2004c. Seven kinds of work – only one paid: Raced, gendered and restructured care work in the social services sector. *Atlantis: A Women's Studies Journal* 28 (2): 19–28.
- 2004d. Women's occupational health in social services. *Canadian Woman Studies* 23 (3/4): 157–64.
- 2006. Staying with people who slap you around: Gender, juggling responsibilities and violence in paid (and unpaid) care work. *Gender, Work and Organization* 13 (2): 129–51.

Bakker, Isabella. 1998. *Unpaid work and macroeconomics: New discussion, new tools for action*. Ottawa: Status of Women Canada.

Basen, Gwynne, Margrit Eichler, and Abby Lippman, eds. 1993. *Misconceptions: The social construction of choice and the new reproductive and genetic technologies*. Quebec: Voyageur.

Bates, Christina, Dianne Dodd, and Nicole Rousseau, eds. 2005. *On all frontiers: Four centuries of Canadian nursing*. Ottawa: University of Ottawa Press.

Baumann, Andrea, et al. 2001. *Commitment to care: The benefits of a healthy workplace for nurses, their patients and the system*. Ottawa: Canadian Health Services Research Foundation and the Change Foundation.

BC Nurses' Union Update. 2007. Brutal attack on Chilliwack RN highlights urgent need to protect health care workers from violence. April/May, 19–22.

Beaupré, Marie-Andrée. 1991. Petites misères des services alimentaires. Adapted from *Guide de prévention pour le service alimentaire*. ASSTSAS, 313.

Belkin, N.L. 1998. Aseptics and aesthetics of chlorine bleach: Can its use in laundering be safely abandoned? *American Journal of Infection Control* 26 (2): 149–51.

Benner, Patricia. 1984. *From novice to expert: Excellence and power in clinical nursing practice*. Menlo Park, CA: Addison-Wesley.

Benoit, Cecelia, and Dena Carroll. 2005. Canadian midwifery: Blending traditional and modern practices. In Bates, Dodd, and Rousseau 2005, 27–42.

Bleau, Julie. 2003. L'Entretien ménager à domicile: Un nétier à risque? *Objectif prévention* 26 (3): 10–11.

Blomqvist, Åke. 1994. Introduction: Economic issues in Canadian health care. In *Limits to care: Reforming Canada's health system in an age of restraint*, ed. Åke Blomqvist and David M. Brown, 3–50. Ottawa: C.D. Howe Institute.

Bodenheimer, Thomas. 1995. The industrial revolution in health care. *Social Justice* 22 (4): 26–42.

Borg, M.A., and A. Portelli. 1999. Hospital laundry workers – An at-risk group for hepatitis A? *Occupational Medicine* 49 (7): 448–50.

Bourgeault, Ivy Lynn. 2006. *On the move: The migration of health care providers in Canada.* http://strateggis.ic.gc.ca.

Bourgeault, Ivy, and Patricia Khokher. 2006. Making a better living from caregiving: Comparing strategies to improve wages for care workers. *Canadian Review of Sociology and Anthropology* 43 (4): 407–26.

Bradbury, Bettina. 1997. Women's workplaces: The impact of technological change on working-class women in the home and in the workplace in nineteenth-century Montreal. In Strong-Boag and Fellman 1997, 154–69.

Brandt, Deborah, ed. 2004. *Women working in the NAFTA food chain: Women, food and globalization.* 2nd ed. Toronto: Sumach Press.

Breen, Mary J. 1998. Promoting literacy, improving health. In *Determinants of health: Adults and seniors,* 47–87. Papers Commissioned by the National Forum on Health, vol. 2. Sainte-Foy: Éditions MultiMondes.

British Columbia Nurses' Union and the Health Services Association. 2004. *Falling standards, rising risks: Issues in hospital cleanliness with contracting out.* Vancouver: BCNU & HSA.

Bueckert, Lynn. 1993. The impact of off-shore office work on women workers globally and locally. In *Women and social location,* ed. Marilyn Asheton-Smith and Barbara Spronk, 157–66. Ottawa: Canadian Research Institute for the Advancement of Women.

Butler, Patrick, and David Batty. 2001. 'Filthiest' NHS hospitals cleaned by private contractors. *Guardian,* 10 April. http://society.guardian.co.uk/nhsperfomance/story/0,,471423.00.html.

Canada. 2003. 2003 First Ministers' accord on health renewal. Press release, September.

Canada, Health and Welfare Canada. 1986. *Achieving health for all: A framework for health promotion* [Ottawa Charter]. Ottawa.

Canada, Minister of National Health and Welfare. 1974. *A new perspective on the health of Canadians* [Lalonde Report]. Ottawa.

Canadian Nurses Association. 2004. Nursing staff mix: A literature review. Ottawa: CNA.

Carvel, John. 2006. Hospital's focus on waiting times targets led to 41 superbug deaths. *Guardian,* 25 July. http://society.guardian.co.uk.

Carver, Virginia, and Charles Ponée, eds. 1995. *Women, work and wellness.* Toronto: Addiction Research Foundation.

CBC. 2006. Jobs axed after pay doubles at Ottawa nursing home. 5 December. http://www.cbc.ca/canada/story/2006/12/montfort.html.

Cesana, G., et al. 1998. Risk evaluation and health surveillance in hospitals: A critical review and contributions regarding experience obtained at S. Gerardo dei Tintori Hospital in Monza. *Medical Law* 89 (1): 23–46.

Chicin, E., and M.H. Kantor. 1992. The home care industry: Strategies for survival in an era of dwindling resources. *Journal of Aging and Social Policy* 4 (1/2): 89–105.

[CHSRF] Canadian Health Services Research Foundation. 2006. *Teamwork in healthcare: Promoting effective teamwork in healthcare in Canada.* Ottawa: CHSRF.

Chung, Jinjoo, Donald Cole, and Judy Clarke. 2000. Women, work, and injury. In *Injury and the new world of work,* ed. Terrence Sullivan, 69-90. Vancouver: UBC Press.

[CIHI] Canadian Institute for Health Information. 2002. *Canada's health care providers.* Ottawa: CIHI.

– 2004. *Health personnel trends in Canada.* Ottawa: CIHI.

– 2005a. *Canada's health care providers: Charts.* Ottawa: CIHI.

– 2005b. *Exploring the 70/30 split: How Canada's health care system is financed.* Ottawa: CIHI.

– 2005c. *Improving the health of young Canadians.* Ottawa: CIHI.

– 2005d. *Workforce trends of licensed practical nurses in Canada 2004.* Ottawa: CIHI.

– 2005e. *Workforce trends of registered nurses in Canada 2004.* Ottawa: CIHI.

– 2006. *National health expenditure trends.* Ottawa: CIHI.

– 2007. *Canada's health care providers 2007.* Ottawa: CIHI.

Cloutier, Esther, Elise Ledoux, Madeleine Bourdouxhe, Hélène David, Isabelle Gagnon, and François Ouellet. 2007. Restructuring of the Québec Health Network and its effects on the profession of home health aides and their occupational health and safety. *New Solution: A Journal of Environmental and Occupational Health Policy* 17 (1/2): 83–95.

Coburn, Judi. 1987. 'I see and am silent': A short history of nursing in Ontario, 1850–1930. In *Health and Canadian society,* 2nd ed., ed. David Coburn et al., 441–62. Toronto: Fitzhenry and Whiteside.

Cochrane, Jeanette. 1995. Stress and the working woman. In *Women, work and wellness,* ed. Virginia Carver and Charles Ponée, 127–40. Toronto: Addiction Research Foundation.

Cohen, Marcy. 2006. The privatization of health care cleaning services in south-western British Columbia, Canada: Union responses to unprecedented government actions. In *The dirty work of neoliberalism: Cleaners in the global economy,* ed. Luis Aguiar and Andrew Herod, 195–213. Oxford: Blackwell.

Cohen, Marcy, et al. 2004. Workload as a determinant of staff injury in intermediate care. *International Journal of Occupational Environmental Health* 10:375–83.

Cohen, Marjorie Griffin. 2001. Do comparisons between hospital support workers and hospitality workers make sense? Report prepared for the Hospital Employees Union (CUPE), Burnaby, BC.

Cohen, Marjorie Griffin, and Marcy Cohen. 2004. *A return to wage discrimination: Pay equity losses through privatization in health care*. Vancouver: Canadian Centre for Policy Alternatives.

Coleman, Ronald. 2003. The economic value of civic and voluntary work in Atlantic Canada. Halifax: GPI Atlantic.

Commission on the Future of Health Care in Canada. 2002. *Building on values: The future of health care in Canada* [Romanow Report]. Ottawa: Commission on the Future of Health Care in Canada.

Compass Group Canada. 2006. Milton Cook Chill Facility wins CCPPP silver award. http://www.compass-canada.com/home/default.asp?action. 12 December.

Conference Board of Canada. 2005. *Unleashing innovation in health systems: Alberta's symposium on health*. Ottawa: Conference Board of Canada.

Connelly, M. Patricia, and Pat Armstrong, eds. 1992. *Feminism in action: Studies in political economy*. Toronto: Canadian Scholars' Press.

Copp, Terry. 1981. Public health in Montreal, 1870–1930. In *Medicine in Canadian society: Historical perspectives*, ed. S.E.D. Shortt, 395–416. Montreal: McGill-Queen's University Press.

Cook, Ramsey, and Wendy Mitchinson. 1976. *The proper sphere: Women's place in Canadian society*. Toronto: Oxford University Press.

Cookson, Richard, Maria Goddard, and Hugh Gravelle. 2005. Regulating health care markets. In *Health policy and economics: Opportunities and challenges*, ed. Peter C. Smith, Laura Ginnelly, and Mark Sculpher, 121–47. New York: Open University Press.

Corley, Mary C., and Hans O. Mauksch. 1988. Registered nurses, gender, and commitment. In *The worth of women's work*, ed. Anne Stratham, Eleanor M. Miller, and Hans O. Mauksch, 135–51. Albany: State University of New York Press.

Cranford, Cynthia. 2005. From precarious workers to unionized employees and back again? The challenges of organizing personal care workers in Ontario. In Cranford, Fudge, Tucker, and Vosko 2005, 96–135.

Cranford, Cynthia, Judy Fudge, Eric Tucker, and Leah F. Vosko, eds. 2005. *Self-employed workers organize*. Montreal: McGill-Queen's University Press.

[CUPE] Canadian Union of Public Employees. 2007a. Fact sheet – Shared food services. http://cupe.ca/udir/shared%20service%20-%20food%20sheet.doc.

– 2007b. Hundreds tell Liberal MPP to defend her community in health services restructuring showdown. http://cupe.ca/laundry/hundreds_ tell_libera.

– 2007c. Innovation exposed. An ongoing inventory of major privatization. July. http://cupe.ca/privatization.

Danylewycz, Marta. 1991. Domestic science education in Ontario, 1900–1940. In *Gender and education in Ontario*, ed. Ruby Heap and Alison Prentice, 127–46. Toronto: Canadian Scholars' Press.

Das Gupta, Tania. 1996. Anti-black racism in nursing in Ontario. *Studies in Political Economy* 51 (Fall): 97–116.

Davezies, Philippe. 2003. France: Prevention of work-related wear and tear in aging hospital staff. In Vogel 2003, 264–76.

Davies, Celia. 1995. Competence versus care? Gender and caring work revisted. *Acta Sociologica* 38:17–31.

Davies, Steven. 2005. Hospital contract cleaning and infection control. January. www.cf.ac.uk/soci/CREST.

Decima Research. 2002. *National profile of family caregivers in Canada 2002*. Ottawa: Health Canada.

De Léséleuc, Sylvain. 2007. *Criminal victimization in the workplace*. Ottawa: Minister of Industry.

Denton, Margaret, Isik Uria Zeytinoglu, Sharon Davies, and Danielle Hunter. 2005. Where have all the home care workers gone? Paper presented at the Canadian Sociology and Anthropology Annual Meetings, University of Western Ontario, June.

Des Meules, Marie, et al. 2003. *Women's health surveillance report*. Ottawa: Health Canada and Canadian Institute for Health Information.

Devereaux, P.J., et al. 2004. Payments for care at private for-profit and private not-for-profit hospitals: A systematic review and meta-analysis. *Canadian Medical Association Journal* 170 (12): 1817–24.

De Wolfe, Alice, and Associates. 2000. *The impact of e-business on office work*. Toronto: Office Workers' Career Centre and Human Resources Development Canada.

Diamond, Timothy. 1988. Social policy and everyday life in nursing homes: A critical ethnography. In *The worth of women's work*, ed. Anne Stratham, Eleanor M. Miller, and Hans O. Mauksch, 39–56. Albany: State University of New York Press.

Dickersin, Kay, Sharon E. Straus, and Lisa A. Bero. 2007. Evidence based medicine: Increasing, not dictating, choice. *British Medical Journal* 334, Suppl. 1: 510.

Doyal, Lesley. 1995. *What makes women sick: Gender and the political economy of health*. New Brunswick: Rutgers University Press.

Doyal, Lesley, S. Payne, and A. Cameron. 2003. Promoting gender equality in health. Manchester: Equal Opportunities Commission.

Doyal, Lesley, and I. Pennell. 1979. *The political economy of health*. London: Pluto.

Ducki, Antje. 2003. Germany: Women, health and work – Main finding of the First Federal Report on Women's Health. In Vogel 2003, 213–22.

Dunton, D.E. 1997. Sources of job satisfaction and dissatisfaction for unit clerks employed in acute care settings. PhD thesis, University of Manitoba, Winnipeg.

El-Jardali, Fadi, and Cathy Fooks. 2005. *An environmental scan of current views on health human resources in Canada*. Toronto: Health Council of Canada.

European Agency for Safety and Health at Work. 2003. *Gender issues in safety and health at work*. Luxembourg: Office for Official Publications of the European Communities.

Evans, Robert G., Morris L. Barer, and Theodore R. Marmor. 1994. *Why are some people healthy and others not? The determinants of health of populations*. New York: Aldine De Gruyter.

Executive Housekeeping Today. 1991. Housekeepers suffer highest sharp-object injury rate. Vol. 2 (February 12): 10.

Exworthy, Mark, and Susan Halford. 1999. *Professionals and the new managerialism in the public sector*. Philadelphia: Open University Press.

Eyerman, Ann. 2000. *Women in the office: Transitions in a global economy*. Toronto: Sumach Press.

Faragher, E.B., M. Cass, and C.L. Cooper. 2005. The relationship between job satisfaction and health: A meta-analysis. *Occupational Health and Medicine* 62 (2): 105–12.

Farmer, Paul. 2005. *Pathologies of power: Health, human rights, and the new war on the poor*. Berkeley: University of California Press.

Feldberg, G., et al. 1996. *Ontario women's work-related health survey: Descriptive summary*. Toronto: Centre for Health Studies and Institute for Social Research, York University.

Findorff, M.J., et al. 2004. Risk factors for work related violence in a health care organization. *Injury Prevention* 5 (October 10): 296–302.

Folbre, Nancy. 2006. Demanding quality: Worker/consumer coalitions and 'high road' strategies in the care sector. *Politics and Society* 34 (1): 1–32.

Fooks, Cathy, and Lisa Maslove. 2004. Rhetoric, fallacy or dream? Examining the accountability of Canadian health care to citizens. Ottawa: Canadian Policy Research Networks.

Fox, M., D.J. Dwyer, and D.C. Ganster. 1993. Effects of stressful job demands and control on physiological and attitudinal outcomes in a hospital setting. *Academy of Management Journal* 36:289–318.

Freidson, Eliot. 1970. Dominant professions, bureaucracy and client services. In

Organizations and clients, ed. W.R. Rosengren and M. Lefton, 71–92. Columbus, OH: Merril.

Fudge, Judy, and Rosemary Owens, eds. 2006. Precarious work, women and the new economy: The challenge to legal norms. Oxford: Hart Publishing.

Fuller, Colleen. 1998. *Caring for profit: How corporations are taking over Canada's health care system.* Ottawa: Canadian Centre for Policy Alternatives.

Fuller, T., and S. Bloom. 2005. Occupational exposure to dimethyl sulphide in the health care setting. http:www.aiha.org/abs05/po 103.htm.

Galarneau, Diane. 2003. Health care professionals. *Perspectives on Labour and Income* 4 (12): 14–27.

Gaskell, Jane. 1991. What counts as skill? Reflections on pay equity. In *Just wages: A feminist assessment of pay equity,* ed. Judy Fudge and Patricia McDermott, 141–59. Toronto: University of Toronto Press.

Gelber, Steven. 2005. The healing potential of food. Medscape *General Medicine* 7 (3): 1–3. http://www.medscape.com/. 16 August.

Gendron, Yves, David Cooper, and Barbara Townley. 2007. The construction of auditing expertise in measuring government performance. *Accounting, Organizations and Society* 32:101–29.

Gilmour, Joan. 2002. Creeping privatization in health care: Implications for women as the state redraws its role. In *Privatization, law and the challenge to feminism,* ed. Judy Fudge and Brenda Cossman, 267–310. Toronto: University of Toronto Press.

Godlee, Fiona. 2007. Milestones on the long road to knowledge. *British Medical Journal* 334, Suppl. 1: s2.

Grant, Karen, et al., eds. 2004. *Caring for/Caring about: Women, home care, and unpaid caregiving.* Aurora, ON: Garamond Press.

Guardian. 2005a. The critical roles we play on the health care team. 23 (4): 11.
– 2005b. Newsbites. 23 (2): 6.
– 2005c. Violence, harassment and bullying in the workplace. 23 (4): 13.

Guberman, Nancy. 1999. *Caregivers and caregiving: New trends and their implications for policy.* Ottawa: Health Canada.

Gunnarsdóttir, S., and K. Björnsdóttir. 2003. Health promotion in the workplace: The perspective of unskilled workers in a hospital setting. *Scandinavian Journal of Caring Sciences* 17 (1): 66–78.

Guruge, S., G.L. Donner, and L. Morrison. 2000. The impact of Canadian health care reform on recent woman immigrants and refugees. In *Care and consequences: The impact of health care reform,* ed. D.L. Gustafson, 222–42. Halifax: Fernwood.

Haiven, Larry. 1995. Industrial relations in health care: Regulation, conflict and transition to a wellness model. In *Public sector collective bargaining in Canada,* ed. G. Swimmer and M. Thompson, 236–71. Kingston, ON: Industrial Relations Centre, Queen's University.

Haj-Younes, L.S., S. Sanchez-Politta, et al. 2006. Occupational contact dermatitis to mikrobac extra in 8 hospital cleaners. *Contact Dermatitis* 54 (1): 69–70.

Hall, E.M. 1989. Gender, work, control and stress: A theoretical discussion and an empirical test. *International Journal of Health Sciences* 19:725–45.

Hamilton, Roberta. 1978. *The liberation of women*. London: George, Allen and Unwin.

Hammerstrom, A. 1994. Health consequences of youth unemployment: Review from a gender perspective. *Social Science and Medicine* 38 (5): 699–709.

Hankivsky, Olena, and Marina Morrow. 2004. *Trade agreements, home care and women's health*. Ottawa: Status of Women Canada.

Harber, Bruce, and Ted Ball. 2003. From the blame game to accountability in health care. *Policy Options* 24 (10): 49–54.

Harder, Lois. 2003. *State of struggle: Feminism and politics in Alberta*. Edmonton: University of Alberta Press.

Hassen, Phil. 2005. Canadian patient safety institute. *Healthcare Quarterly* 8 (Special Issue): 9–10.

Hawley, Gordon. 2004. Canada's health care workers: A snapshot. *Health Policy Research* 8 (May): 8–11.

HCHSA. 2004. Fast facts. Ergonomic tips for dietary staff. www.hchsa.on.ca/ products/ffacts_e/lap_172pdf. 4 October 2005.

Health Canada. 2005. *External 2005 environmental scan* (July). Ottawa: Health Canada.

– 2006. *Health human resource connection* (December). Ottawa: Health Canada.

Healthcare Quarterly. 2005. Special issue on patient safety. Vol. 9 (October).

Health Policy Research Bulletin. 2006. Building social capital: A role for public policy? Vol. 12 (September): 3–5.

Health Services and Support – Facilities Subsector Bargaining Association v. British Columbia, 2007 SCC 27.

Hennessy, Trish. 2006. CCPA launches major project to promote equality in Canada. *CCPA Monitor* 13 (7): 1, 6, 7.

Herod, Andrew, and Luis Aguiar. 2006. Introduction: Cleaners and the dirty work of neoliberalism. In *The dirty work of neoliberalism: Cleaners in the global economy,* ed. Luis Aguiar and Andrew Herod, 11–15. Oxford: Blackwell.

Hesketh, Kathryn, Susan M. Duncan, Carole A. Eatabrooks, Marlene A. Reamer, Phyllis Giovanetti, Kathryn Hyndman, and Sonia Acorn. 2002. Workplace violence in Alberta and British Columbia hospitals. *Health Policy* 63:311–21.

Heyes, Anthony. 2004. The economics of vocation, or 'Why is a badly paid nurse a good nurse?' *Journal of Health Economics* 24:561–69.

Himmelstein, David, and Steffie Woolhandler. 1994. *The national health program book*. Munroe, ME: Common Courage Press.

Hochschild, Arlie. 1985. *The managed heart: Commercialization of human feeling*. Berkeley: University of California Press.

Hollander, M.J., and A. Tessaro. 2001. *Evaluation of the maintenance and preventive function of home care*. Ottawa: Home Care/Pharmaceuticals Division, Policy and Communication Branch, Health Canada.

Home Care Sector Study Corporation. 2003. Canadian home care human resources study: Synthesis report. Ottawa: Home Care Sector Study Corporation.

Hood, Christopher. 1991. A public management for all seasons? *Public Administration* 69 (Spring): 3–19.

Hospital Employees' Union. 2000. Proposal for the development of a pilot project for underemployed foreign trained nurses in the lower mainland. Vancouver, BC, May.

Hughes, K., G.S. Lowe, and G. Schellenberg. 2003. *Men's and women's quality of work in the new Canadian economy*. Ottawa: Canadian Policy Research Networks.

Hunsley, Terrance. 2006. Work-life balance in an aging population. *Horizons* 8 (3): 3–13.

Hunter, David. 2003. *Public health policy*. Oxford: Polity.

Illich, Ivan. 1976. *Limits of medicine*. London: Penguin.

Infection Control Nurses Association. 2004. *Audit tools for monitoring infection control standards*. London: Infection Control Nurses Association.

International Labour Organization. 2003. *Workplace violence in the health sector: Country case study research instruments*. Geneva: ILO.

Jackson, Andrew. 2005. *Work and labour in Canada: Critical issues*. Toronto: Canadian Scholars' Press.

Jensen, Phyllis. 1988. The changing role of nurses' unions. In *Canadian nursing faces the future*, ed. A. Baumgart and J. Larsen, 557–72. Toronto: Mosby.

Johnson, David. 2002. *Thinking government: Public sector management in Canada*. Toronto: Broadview.

Johnson, Laura, and Bob Johnson. 1982. *The seam allowance: Industrial home sewing in Canada*. Toronto: Women's Press.

Johnson, Terrance. 1972. *Professions and power*. London: Macmillan.

Jorland, G., A. Opinel, and G. Weisz, eds. 2005. *Body counts: Medical quantification in historical and sociological perspectives*. Montreal: McGill-Queen's University Press.

Kapsalis, Constantine. 1998. An international comparison of employee training. *Perspectives on Labour and Income* 10 (1): 23–8.

Karasek, R.A. 1979. Job demands, job decision latitude and mental strain: Implications for job design. *Administrative Science Quarterly* 24:285–308.

Karasek, R.A. and T. Theorell. 1990. *Healthy work: Stress, productivity, and the reconstruction of working life*. New York: Basic Books.

Kassler, Jeanne. 1994. *Bitter medicine*. New York: Birch Lane Press.

Keddy, Barbara, and Dianne Dodd. 2005. The trained nurse: Private duty and VON home nursing (late 1800s to 1940s). In Bates, Dodd, and Rousseau 2005, 43–56.

Kahnamoui, Niknaz. 2005. *After outsourcing: Working collaboratively to deliver patient care*. MA thesis, Faculty of Arts and Sciences, Simon Fraser University, Burnaby, British Columbia.

Kelleher, David, Jonathan Gabe, and Gareth Williams, eds. 2006. *Challenging medicine*. London: Routledge.

Kerr, A., and M. Radford. 1994. TUPE or not TUPE: Competitive tendering and the transfer laws. *Public Money and Management* 14 (4): 37–45.

Kingma, Mireille. 2006. *Nurses on the move: Migration and the global health care economy*. Ithaca, NY: Cornell University Press.

Kirkwood, L. 2005. Enough but not too much: Nursing education in English language Canada (1874–2000). In Bates, Dodd, and Rousseau 2005, 183–95.

Koehoorn, Mieke, Graham S. Lowe, Kent V. Rondeau, Grant Schellenberg, and Terry H. Wager. 2002. *Creating high-quality health care workplaces*. Ottawa: Canadian Policy Research Network.

Kushner, Carol. 2005. Inside-outside-in. Slide presentation to Conference on Progressive Health Reform, Ontario. Based on Inside-outside-in: Three tales of outsourcing at a Toronto hospital, 21 March 2002.

La Duca, P.N. 1987. Medical facilities, environmental concerns and the role of the hospital sanitarian. *Journal of Environmental Health* 50 (3): 146–9.

Lakeman, Lee. 2006. Linking violence and poverty in CASAC Report. In *Canadian woman studies: An introductory reader*, ed. Andrea Medovarski and Brenda Cranney, 380–89. Toronto: Inanna Publications.

Langton, H.H., ed. 1950. *A gentlewoman in Upper Canada*. Toronto: Clarke-Irwin.

Laperrière, E., K. Messing, V. Couture, and S. Stock. 2005. Validation of questions on working posture among those who stand during most of the day. *International Journal of Industrial Ergonomics* 35:371–8.

Laxer, Kate. 2004. Where are all the healthcare workers? The North American industrial classification system and ancillary workers. Paper presented at Gender and Work: Knowledge Production in Practice conference, 1–2 October, York University, Toronto.

Lee-Treweek, Geraldine. 1997. Women, resistance and care: An ethnographic study of nursing auxiliary workers. *Work, Employment and Society* 11(1): 47–63.

Lesage, Alain, et al. 2004. Guest editorial. Mental health and the workplace: Towards a research agenda in Canada. *Healthcare Papers* 5 (2): 1–8.

Lippel, K. 1995. Watching the watchers: How expert witnesses and decision-makers perceive men's and women's workplace stressors. In *Invisible: Occupational health problems of women at work/Invisible. La santé des travailleuses*, ed. K. Messing, B. Neis, and L. Dumais. Charlottetown, PEI: Gynergy Books.

– 2003. Compensation for musculo-skeletal disorders in Quebec: Systemic discrimination against women workers? *International Journal of Health Services* 33 (2): 253–81.

Lile, J. 1994. Occupational health services. In *Mental health at work*, ed. M. Floyd, M. Povall, and G. Watson, 77–9. London: Jessica Kingsley.

Lister, John. 2005. Cleaners' voices: Interviews with hospital cleaners. London: UNISON.

Louther, J., et al. 1997. Risk of tuberculin conversion according to occupation among health care workers at a New York City hospital. *American Journal of Respiratory Critical Care Medicine* 156 (1): 201–5.

LTCa. 2006. Long-term care study: Write-in comments added to survey of long-term care workers conducted by Pat Armstrong, Hugh Armstrong, and Tamara Daly.

LTCb. 2006. Long-term care study: Interviews with long-term care workers, conducted for this book by Lynn Spink.

Luffman, Jacqueline. 2006. The core-age labour force. *Perspectives on Labour and Income* 18 (4): 5–11.

Mahon, Ann, and Ruth Young. 2006. Health care managers as a critical component of the health care workforce. In *Human resources in health in Europe*, ed. Carl-Ardy Dubois, Martin McKee, and Ellen Nolte, 116–39. New York: Open University Press.

Manitoba Law Reform Commission. 1994. *Regulating professions and occupations*. Manitoba: Law Reform Commission.

Marmot, M.G. 1986. Social inequalities in mortality: The social environment. In *Class and health: Research and longitudinal data*, ed. R.G. Wilkinson, 21–33. London: Tavistock.

Marmot, M., et al. 1999. Health and the psychological environment at work. In *Social determinants of health*, ed. Michael Marmot and Richard G. Wilkinson, 105–31. Oxford: Oxford University Press.

Marshall, Katherine. 2006. Converging gender roles. *Perspectives on labour and income* 7 (7): 5–23.

Maxwell, Judith. 2002. Working for low pay. Canadian Policy Research Networks, presentation to Alberta Human Resources and Employment, 4 December.

McCulla, Karen. 2004. A comparative review of community health representatives scope of practice in international indigenous communities. Paper prepared for the National Indian and Inuit Community Health Representatives Organization.

McGauran, Ann. 2004. Government tells hospitals to tighten up cleaning contracts. *British Medical Journal* 329 (11 December): 1361.

McGillis Hall, Linda. 1999. The use of unregulated workers in Toronto hospitals. *Canadian Journal of Nursing Administration* 11 (1): 8–30.

McMullen, K., and R. Brisbois. 2003. *Coping with change: Human resource management in Canada's non-profit sector.* Ottawa: Canadian Policy Research Networks.

McKinlay, John B. 1984. *Issues in the political economy of health care.* London: Tavistock.

McPherson, Kathryn. 2003. *Bedside matters: The transformation of Canadian nursing, 1900–1990.* Toronto: University of Toronto Press.

– 2005. The Nightingale influence and the rise of the modern hospital. In Bates, Dodd, and Rousseau 2005, 73–88.

McWilliam, C.L., C. Ward-Griffin, D.B. Sweetland, C. Sutherland, and L.O. O'Halloran. 2001. The experience of empowerment in home service delivery. *Home Health Care Services Quarterly* 20 (4): 49–71.

Merck Frosst Canada. 2007. SARS Commission final report tabled. *Health Edition* 11 (12 January): 1–2.

Messing, Karen. 1998a. Hospital trash: Cleaners speak of their role in disease prevention. *Medical Anthropology Quarterly* 12 (2): 168–87.

– 1998b. *One-eyed science: Occupational health and women workers.* Philadelphia: Temple University Press.

– 2004. Physical exposure in work commonly done by women. *Canadian Journal of Applied Physiology* 29 (5): 639–56.

Messing, K., C. Chatigny, and J. Courville. 1998. 'Light' and 'heavy' work in the housekeeping services of a hospital. *Applied Ergonomics* 29:451–9.

Messing, K., and D. Elabidi. 2003. Desegregation and occupational health: How male and female hospital attendants collaborate on work tasks requiring physical effort. *Policy and Practice in Health and Safety* 1 (1): 83–103.

Messing, Karen, Katherine Lippel, Diane Demers, and Donna Mergler. 2000. Equality and differences in the workplace: Physical jobs demands, occupational illnesses and sex differences. *National Women's Studies Association Journal* January 12 (3): 21–49.

Messing, K., and P. Östlin. 2006. *Gender equality, work and health: A review of the evidence.* Geneva: World Health Organization.

Mills, C. Wright. 1961. *The sociological imagination.* New York: Grove.

Mimoto, H., and P. Cross. 1991. The growth of the federal debt. *Canadian Economic Observer* 4 (June): 1–17.

Mintzberg, Henry. 1989. *Mintzberg on management.* New York: Free Press.

Mitchell, Elizabeth B. 1981. *In Western Canada before the war.* Saskatoon, SK: Western Producer Prairie Books. First published 1915.

Mitchinson, Wendy. 1991. *The nature of their bodies: Women and their doctors in Victorian Canada.* Toronto: University of Toronto Press.

Morris, Kathleen, and Jennifer Zelmer. 2005. *Public reporting of performance measures in health care.* Ottawa: Canadian Policy Research Networks.

Morris, Marika. 2004. What research reveals about gender, home care and caregiving: Overview and policy implications. In Grant et al. 2004, 91–114.

Mulholland, Hélène. 2004. NHS cleaning brought in-house amid MRSA fears. *Guardian,* 29 September. http://society/guardian.co.uk/. 13 October.

Mullan, Fitzhugh. 2005. The metrics of physician brain drain. *New England Journal of Medicine* 353 (17): 1810–18.

Mussallem, Helen. 1988. The changing role of the Canadian Nurses' Association in the development of nursing in Canada. In *Canadian nursing: Issues and perspective,* ed. Janet Kerr and Janetta MacPhail, 400–31. Toronto: McGraw-Hill Ryerson.

National Forum on Health. 1997. Creating a culture of evidence-based decision making. In *Canada health action: Building on the legacy.* Vol. 2, *Synthesis reports and issues papers.* Ottawa: Minister of Public Works and Government Services.

– 1998. *Determinants of health: Children and youth.* Papers Commissioned by the National Forum on Health, vol. 1. Sainte-Foy: Éditions MultiMondes.

Naylor, David. 1986. *Private practice, public payment.* Montreal: McGill-Queen's University Press.

Neysmith, Sheila, and Jane Aronson. 1997. Working conditions in home care: Negotiating race and class boundaries in gendered work. *International Journal of Health Services* 27 (3): 479–99.

NHSEstates. 2003. http://patientexperience.nhsestates.gov.uk/bhf/bhf_content/home/home.asp. 28 February.

[OECD] Organization for Economic Cooperation and Development. 2002. Expenditures on health and their financing. In *OECD health data.* Paris: OECD.

– 2004. *Health data 2004: Frequently requested data.* Paris: OECD.

– 2005. *Health at a glance: OECD indicators 2005.* Paris: OECD.

– 2006. *OECD health data: Frequently requested data.* http://www.oecd.org.

Ontario. 2005. *Ontario budget* (11 May), appendix 2.

Ontario Pay Equity Commission. 1988. *Questions and answers: Pay equity in the workplace.* Toronto: Pay Equity Commission.

Ontario Pay Equity Hearings Tribunal. 1991. *Ontario Nurses Association v. Regional Municipality of Haldimand Norfolk* 0001-89 (29 May).

O'Reilly, Patricia. 2000. *Health care practitioners.* Toronto: University of Toronto Press.

Orr, K.E., M.G. Holliday, A.L. Jones, I. Robson, and J.D. Perry. 2002. Survival of enterococci during hospital laundry processing. *Journal of Hospital Infection* 50 (2): 133–9.

Osborne, David, and Ted Gaebler. 1993. *Reinventing government: How the entrepreneurial spirit is transforming the public sector.* New York: Penguin.

Otero, R.B. 1997a. Healthcare environmental services infection control: The basics of microbiology. *Professional Development Services* (May): 1–17.

– 1997b. Healthcare textile services: Infection control. *Professional Development Services* (January): 1–13.

Paris-Seeley, Nancy, Helen Heacock, and James Watzke. 2004. Development and evaluation of an affordable lift device to reduce musculoskeletal injuries among home support workers. *Applied Ergonomics* 35 (4): 1–3.

Parr Traill, Catherine. 1969. *The Canadian settler's guide.* Toronto: McClelland and Stewart. First published 1855.

Patterson, E.A., C. Del Mar, et al. 2000. Medical receptionists in general practice: Who needs a nurse? *International Journal of Nursing Practice* 6 (5): 229–36.

Perry, Ann. 2003. $414 million ends Ontario pay equity case. *Toronto Star,* 14 January, A1.

Perspectives on Labour and Income. 2004. Work absences. *Perspectives on Labour and Income* 16 (2): 59–68.

– 2005a. The labour market in 2004. *Perspectives on Labour and Income* 17 (1): 54–68.

– 2005b. Unionization. *Perspectives on Labour and Income* 17 (3): 61–8.

– 2006a. Unionization. *Perspectives on Labour and Income* 18 (3): 64–71.

– 2006b. Work absences. *Perspectives on Labour and Income* 19 (2): 58–67.

Piercy, Kathleen W. 2000. When it is more than a job: Close relationships between home health aides and older clients. *Journal of Aging and Health* 12 (3): 362–87.

Pizzino, A. 1994. *Report on CUPE's national health and safety survey of aggression against staff.* Ottawa: Canadian Union of Public Employees Health and Safety Branch.

Poland, B., et al. 1998. Wealth, equity and health care: A critique of a 'population health' perspective on the determinants of health. *Social Science and Medicine* 47 (7): 785–98.

Polanyi, Michael F.D., Joan Eakin, John W. Frank, et al. 1997. Creating healthier work environments: A critical review of the health impacts of workplace change. In *Determinants of health: Setting the issues*, 87–137. National Forum on Health, vol. 3. Sainte-Foy: Éditions MultiMondes.

Pollitt, Christopher. 1998. Managerialism revisited. In *Taking stock: Assessing public sector reforms*, ed. B. Guy Peters and Donald J. Savoie, 45–77. Montreal and Kingston: McGill-Queen's University Press.

Pollock, Allyson, Jean Shaoul, and Neil Vickers. 2002. Private finance and 'value for money' in NHS hospitals: A policy in search of a rationale? *British Medical Journal* 324 (19 May): 1205–09.

Pyper, Wendy. 2006. Balancing career and care. *Perspectives on Labour and Income* 18 (4): 37-47.

Quinlan, M.C., C. Mayhew, and P. Bohle. 2001. The global expansion of precarious employment, work disorganization and consequences for occupational health: A review. *International Journal of Health Services* 31 (2): 335–414.

Qureshi, H., and A. Walker. 1989. *The caring relationship: Elderly people and their families*. London: MacMillan.

Rachlis, Michael. 2004. *Prescription for excellence: How innovation is saving Canada's health care system*. Toronto: HarperCollins.

Ramkhalawansingh, Ceta. 1974. Women in the great war. In *Women at work: Ontario 1850–1930*, ed. Janice Acton, Penny Goldsmith, and Bonnie Shepard, 261–307. Toronto: Canadian Women's Educational Press.

Rampling, A., S. Wiseman, L. Davis, P. Hyatt, A.N. Walbridge, G.C. Payne, and A.J. Cornaby. 2001. Evidence that hospital hygiene is important in the control of methicillin resistant staphylococcus aureus. *Journal of Hospital Infection* 49:109–16.

Rasmussen, B. 2004. Between endless needs and limited resources: The gendered construction of greedy organizations. *Gender, Work and Organizations* 11 (5): 506–25.

Raver, Jana L., and Michele J. Gelfand. 2005. Beyond the individual victim: Linking sexual harassment, team processes and team performance. *Academy of Management Journal* 48 (3): 387–400.

Reddy, Madhuri, Sudeep Gill, and Paula Rochon. 2006. Preventing pressure ulcers: A systematic review. *Journal of the American Medical Association* 296 (8): 974–1020.

Relman, Arnold. 2002. For profit health care: Expensive, inefficient and inequitable. Presentation to the Standing Senate Committee on Social Affairs, Science and Technology. http://www.healthcoaltion.ca/relman.html.

Rivers, Elaine. 2000. *Foreign trained nurses in British Columbia: Employment issues and opportunities.* Victoria: BC Ministry of Multiculturalism and Immigration.

Rosenberg, Harriet. 1990. The home is the workplace. In *Through the kitchen window,* ed. Meg Luxton, Harriet Rosenberg, and Sedef Ara-Kroc, 57–80. Toronto: Garamond.

Sachdev, S. 2001. Contracting culture: From CCT to PPPs. London: UNISON.

Saha, A., et al. 2005. Occupational injuries: Is job security a factor? *Indian Journal of Medical Science* 59 (9): 375–81.

Santana, Shannon A., and Bonnie S. Fisher. 2002. Workplace violence prevention programs in West Texas. *S.A.M. Advanced Management Journal* 70 (4): 35–43.

Savoie, Donald J. 1995. What is wrong with the new public management? *Canadian Public Administration* 38 (1): 112–21.

Scott, Kimberly. 1998. Balance as a method to promote healthy indigenous communities. *Determinants of health: Setting the issues,* 147–92. National Forum on Health, vol. 3. Sainte-Foy: Éditions MultiMondes.

Seifert, Ana Maria, and Karen Messing. 2004. Looking and listening in a technical world: Effects of discontinuity in work schedules on nurses' work activity. *PISTES* 6 (1): 1–15.

Sexton, Patricia Cayo. 1982. *The new nightingales: Hospital workers, unions, new women's issues.* New York: Enquiry Press.

Shannon, H.S., C.A. Woodward, C.E. Cunningham, et al. 2001. Changes in general health and musculoskeletal outcomes in the workforce of a hospital undergoing rapid change: A longitudinal study. *Journal of Occupational Health Psychology* 6:3–14.

Sherwin, Susan, et al. 1998. *The politics of women's health.* Philadelphia: Temple University Press.

Shields, John, and B. Mitchell Evans. 1998. *Shrinking the state: Globalization and public sector 'reform.'* Halifax: Fernwood.

Shields, Margot. 2006a. *Findings from the 2005 National Survey of the Work and Health of Nurses.* Ottawa: Health Canada and the Canadian Institute for Health Information.

– 2006b. Stress, health and the benefit of social support. *Health Reports* 15 (1): 9–38.

Sinclair, Sonja. 1969. *I presume you can type.* Toronto: CBC.

Smith, Dorothy. 1990. *The conceptual practices of power: A feminist sociology of knowledge.* Toronto: University of Toronto Press.

– 1992. Feminist reflections on political economy. In Connelly and Armstrong 1992, 1–21.

Smith, Ellen. 2004. *Home support services – cost and effect*. Fredericton: New Brunswick Advisory Council.

Soucie, Riva. 2005. Newschool: The precariousness of workplace learning for new nurses. MA thesis, York University, Toronto.

Spiers, Rosemary. 2000. The growing gap between the rich and the poor. *Toronto Star*, 4 March, H3.

Stasiulus, Daiva, and Abigail Bakan. 2005. *Negotiating citizenship: Migrant women in Canada and the global system*. Toronto: University of Toronto Press.

Statistics Canada. 1992. *Family incomes, census families 1990*. Ottawa: Supply and Services Canada.

– 1998. *Characteristics of dual-earner families*. Ottawa: Ministry of Industry, Science and Technology, table 16.

– 2001a. *Census of population*. Ottawa: Supply and Services Canada.

– 2001b. *The changing profile of Canada's labour force*. Ottawa: Supply and Services Canada.

– 2004. *Women in Canada: Work chapter updates 2003*. Ottawa: Minister of Industry.

– 2005a. *General social survey*. Cycle 19 (Time Use), Public Use Microdata File, Catalogue #12M0019XCB.

– 2005b. *Labour force historical review*. Catalogue #71F0004XCB.

– 2005c. *Labour force survey*. Public Use Microdata File, Catalogue #71M0001XCB.

– 2006a. General social survey: Paid and unpaid work. *The Daily*, 19 July, 1–5.

– 2006b. Labour force survey estimates (LFS), by sex and detailed age group, annual. Canada; Employment rate; Females; 15 years and over. CANSIM table series 2820002, vector 2461686 (1976-01-01–2006-01-01).

– 2006c. *Measuring violence vs women. Statistical trends*. Ottawa: Minister of Industry.

– 2006d. *Women in Canada. A gender-based, statistical report*. Ottawa: Minister of Industry.

Status of Women Canada. 1995. *Setting the stage for the next century: The federal plan for gender equality 1995*. Ottawa: Status of Women Canada.

Steinberg, Ronnie, and Lois Haignere. 1987. Equitable compensation: Methodological criteria for comparable worth. In *Ingredients for women's employment policy*, ed. Christine Bose and Glenna Spitze, 157–82. Albany: State University of New York Press.

Stellman, Jeanne Mager. 1977. *Women's work, women's health*. New York: Pantheon.

– 1998. Foreword to Karen Messing, *One-eyed science*. Philadephia: Temple University Press.

Stellman, Jeanne Mager, and Susan M. Daum. 1973. *Work is dangerous to your health*. New York: Vintage.

Stewart, Jenny. 2004. *The decline of the tea lady*. Kent Town, South Australia: Wakefield Press.

Stinson, Jane, Nancy Pollak, and Marcy Cohen. 2005. *The pains of privatization: How contracting out hurts health support workers, their families, and health care*. Vancouver: Canadian Centre for Policy Alternatives.

Stobert, Susan, and Kelly Cranswick. 2004. Looking after seniors: Who does what for whom? *Canadian Social Trends* 74 (Autumn): 2–6.

Stock, Laura. 2005. LOHP studies home care workers. http://ist-socrates. berkley.edu/~lohp/In_The_Spotlight?Home_Care.

Stone, Deborah. 1988. *Policy paradox and political reason*. New York: HarperCollins.

– 2000. *Reforming Home Health Care Policy*. Cambridge, MA: Radcliffe Public Policy Centre.

Strong-Boag, Veronica. 1985. Discovering the home: The last 150 years of domestic work in Canada. In *Women's paid and unpaid work: Historical and contemporary perspectives*, ed. Paula Bourne, 35–60. Toronto: New Hogtown Press.

Strong-Boag, Veronica, and Anita Clair Fellman. 1997. *Rethinking Canada: The promise of women's history*. Toronto: Oxford University Press.

Szebehely, Marta. 1995. *Vardagens organisering: Om vardbitraden och gamla i hemtjansten* [*The organization of everyday life: On home helpers and elderly people in Sweden*]. Lund: Arkiv Forlag.

Taylor, Malcolm G. 1987. *Health insurance and Canadian public policy: The seven decisions that created the Canadian health insurance system and their outcomes*. 2nd ed. Toronto: Institute of Public Administration of Canada.

Theorell, T., et al. 1993. Influence of job strain and emotion on blood pressure in female hospital personnel during work hours. *Scandinavian Journal of Work, Environment and Health* 19:313–18.

Thompson, Edward Palmer. 1978. *The poverty of theory and other essays*. New York: Monthly Review Press.

Toth, Christina. 2004. More concerns raised about Abby hospital. *Abbotsford Times*, 16 April. http://www.P3watch.ca, accessed 18 June 2004.

Toronto Star. 2004. Hospital wages too high, minister warns: Latest salvo in debate over costs. 21 October, A1.

Torrance, George. 1987. Hospitals as factories. In *Health and Canadian society*, 2nd ed., ed. David Coburn et al., 479–500. Toronto: Fitzhenry and Whiteside.

Townley, B., D. Cooper, and L. Oakes. 2003. Performance measures and the rationalization of organizations. *Organization Studies* 24 (7): 1045–71.

Toynbee, Polly. 2003. *Hard work: Life in low-pay Britain*. London: Bloomsbury.

UNISON. 2005. *Cleaner's voices: Interviews with hospital cleaning staff*. London: UNISON.

United Kingdom, Comptroller and Auditor General. 2004. *Improving patient care by reducing the risk of hospital acquired infections*. London: House of Commons.

United Kingdom, Department of Health. 2004. *Towards cleaner hospitals and lower rates of infection. A summary of action*. London: Department of Health.

United Kingdom, Parliamentary Office of Science and Technology. 2005. Infection control in healthcare settings. *Postnote* 247 (July): 1–4.

United Nations. 1995. *1995 Beijing platform for action*. New York: United Nations.

Valiquette, L. et al. 2004. Clostridium difficile infection in hospitals: A brewing storm. *Canadian Medical Association Journal* 171 (1): 27–9.

Visser, Laura. 2006. Toronto hospital reduces sharp injuries by 80%, eliminates blood collection injuries. *Healthcare Quarterly* 9 (1): 1–7.

Vogel, Laurent, ed. 2003. *The gender gap: Workplace health gap in Europe*. Brussels: European Trade Union.

Vosko, Leah. 2003. The pasts (and futures) of feminist political economy in Canada: Reviving the debate. In Andrew et al. 2003, 305–32.

– ed. 2006. *Precarious employment: Understanding labour market insecurity in Canada*. Montreal: McGill-Queens University Press.

Wa, M. 1995. The role of organized labor in combating the hepatitis-B and AIDS epidemics: The fight for an OSHA bloodborne pathogens standard. *International Journal of Health Services* 25 (1): 129–52.

Waehrer, Geetha, J. Paul Leigh, and Ted R. Miller. 2005. Costs of occupational injury and illness within the health services sector. *International Journal of Health Services* 35 (2): 343–59.

Waring, Marilyn. 2004. Unpaid workers: The absence of rights. *Canadian Woman Studies* 23 (3/4): 109–15.

Wears, Robert I., and Marc Berg. 2005. Computer technology and clinical work. *Journal of the American Medical Association* 293 (10): 1261–3.

Westech Systems. 2005. Report and results for third party independent unannounced housekeeping audit of B.C.'s health care facilities. Vancouver: Westech.

White, Jerry. 1990. *Hospital strike*. Toronto: Thompson.

White, Julie. 1980. *Women and unions*. Ottawa: Minister of Supply and Services Canada.

– 1993. *Sisters and solidarity: Women and unions in Canada*. Toronto: Thompson.

Wigmore, Dorothy. 1995. 'Taking back' the workplace. In *Invisible: Issues in women's occupational health*, ed. K. Messing, B. Neis, and L. Dumais, 321–52. Charlottetown, PEI: Gynergy Books.

Wilcox, Denton M., et al. 2005. Role of environmental cleaning in controlling an outbreak of acinetobacter baumannii on a neurosurgical intensive care unit. *Intensive Critical Care Nursing* 2 (April 21): 94–8.

Wilkinson, Richard. 2005. *The impact of inequality*. London: New Press.

Wilkinson, Richard G. 1992. Income distribution and life expectancy. *British Medical Journal* 304:165–8.

Williams, Cara. 2004. The sandwich generation. *Perspectives on Labour and Income* 16 (4): 7–14.

Willson, Kay, and Jennifer Howard. 2002. Missing links: The effects of health care privatization on women in Manitoba and Saskatchewan. In Armstrong et al. 2002, 217–52.

Wilson, D.M., C. Truman, J. Huang, S. Sheps, S. Birch, R. Thomas, and T. Noseworthy. 2007. Home care evolution in Alberta: How have palliative clients fared? *Healthcare Policy* 2 (4): 58–69.

Witz, Anne. 1992. *Professions and patriarchy*. New York: Routledge.

Women's Health Bureau. 2003. *Exploring concepts of gender and health*. Ottawa: Health Canada.

Woodward, C.A., H.S. Shannon, C. Cunningham, et al. 1999. The impact of reengineering and other cost reduction strategies on the staff of a large teaching hospital. *Medical Care* 37:556–69.

[WHO] World Health Organization. 1991. Sundsvall Conference. http://www.who.ch/.

– 2002. *World health report*. Geneva: WHO.

– 2005a. *Preparing a healthcare workforce for the 21st Century*. Geneva: WHO.

– 2005b. Trade in health services in the region of the Americas. www.who.int/entity/trade/en/Thpart3chap10.pdf.

– 2006. *Health workers*. Geneva: WHO.

Wotherspoon, Terence. 2002. Nursing education: Professionalism and control. In *Health, illness and health care in Canada*, ed. B.S. Bolaria and H.D. Dickinson, 82–101. Scarborough, ON: Nelson Thompson.

Wright, Eric Olin. 2006. Compass points: Towards a socialist alternative. *New Left Review* 41 (September/October): 93–124.

Yassi, A., M. Gilbert, and Y. Cvitkovich. 2005. Trends in injuries, illnesses, and policies in Canadian healthcare workplaces. *Canadian Journal of Public Health* 96 (5): 325–7.

Yassi, Annalee, and Tina Hancock. 2005. Patient safety – worker safety: Building a culture of safety to improve healthcare worker and patient well-being. *Healthcare Quarterly* 8 (Special Issue): 32–8.

Yates, Glenda. 2006. *What Canada spends on health care*. Ottawa: Canadian Institute for Health Information.

Zayed, Joseph, and Luc Lefebvre. 1998. Environmental health: From concept to reality. In *Determinants of health: Setting the issues*, 237–70. National Forum on Health, vol. 3. Sainte-Foy: Éditions MultiMondes.

Zock, J.P. 2005. World at work: Cleaners. *Occupational and Environmental Medicine* 62 (8): 581–4.

Zukewich Ghalam, Nancy. 1997. Attitudes toward women, work and family. *Canadian Social Trends* 46 (Autumn): 13–17.

Index

Aboriginal, 19, 83, 153, 194
absenteeism, 121, 122, 125, 139, 185
abuse, 15, 38, 135
accountability, 12, 144, 145, 152, 164, 165, 167, 169
admission: to hospital, 15, 29
age, 15, 22, 33, 34, 36, 38, 41, 43, 45, 47, 49, 50, 52, 54, 58, 59, 61, 65, 68, 88, 93, 98, 106, 107, 117, 122, 124, 125
agencies, employment. See employment agencies
AIDS, 123
Alberta, 37, 59, 115, 135
Alberta Union of Public Employees (AUPE), 115
allergies, 21, 25
allopathic, 62
Alzheimer's disease, 40
amalgamation: of hospitals, 14, 80
ambulatory care, 36, 40, 42, 43, 53, 56, 104, 190
ancillary: definitions/categorizations of, 3–6, 9, 16, 37, 42, 62, 82, 86, 88, 91, 140, 157, 183, 186, 190, 191
ancillary workers, portrait of 4, 5, 6, 7, 11, 12, 51, 61, 183–94
antibiotics, 84, 97

assignment of work, 14
assisting occupations in health, 36, 37, 40, 41, 42, 45, 60, 112, 188
authority, medical, 62

bacteria, 44, 71, 73; resistant, 45, 78, 97, 98, 99
bathing, of clients/patients, 16, 38–40, 42, 43, 76, 97, 113, 133, 136
bed, 20, 22, 27, 38, 46, 79, 96, 102, 124, 154
bedsores, 80
bias: in research, 123, 137
biology/biological, 67, 68, 69
blood pressure, 30, 38
bookkeeping, 43
British Columbia, 78, 95, 114, 125, 126, 128, 134, 135, 139, 151, 159, 161, 164
bullying. See abuse
burnout, 129, 130. See also mental health; stress

C. difficile, 45. See also bacteria, resistant
Calgary, 115
Canada Health Act, 153–5, 157, 158

Canada Health and Social Transfer, 155

Canadian Institute for Health Information (CIHI), 18, 19, 57, 67, 81, 103, 104, 121, 125, 140, 142, 151, 160, 168

Canadian Nurses' Association (CNA), 111

Canadian Union of Public Employees (CUPE), 114, 115, 149, 157, 159, 160

cancer, 32, 80, 97

capitalism, 64

cardex, 24, 25. *See also* record keeping

cardiac arrest, 23

care/caregivers: informal/unpaid, 67, 82, 90, 191. *See also* unpaid work

care deficit, 118, 120

Caribbean, 15

cashier, 49, 52, 61, 112

Census, 36, 54, 84, 183–94

Central America, 151

certification, 14, 41, 43, 47, 49, 72, 92, 103, 104. *See also* education; skills; training

Charter of Rights and Freedoms, 70, 108, 114

charts. *See* record keeping; cardex

child (children), 15, 19, 21–6, 31, 32, 56–8, 68, 72, 73, 90, 97, 133

childbirth, 84, 97, 111

childcare, 73, 107, 112, 129, 130

chiropractic, 3

class, 4, 7, 8, 65, 66, 73, 83, 88, 89, 105, 193

cleaner, 3, 4, 17, 18, 44–6, 48, 60, 80, 84, 86, 94–9, 111, 112, 114, 123, 125–7, 131, 132, 134, 138, 151, 158, 160, 161, 184

cleaning tasks or services, 3, 14–17,
20, 27, 31, 38, 39, 40, 42–8, 50, 51, 57, 58, 60, 70, 71, 75, 78–80, 82–4, 86, 89–92, 94–102, 104, 114, 115, 122, 123, 126, 127, 131, 132, 134, 142, 144, 149, 153, 158–61, 163–5, 168, 169, 188

clerk/clerical worker, 3, 4, 15, 19, 20, 23, 25–8, 30, 32–7, 41, 44, 60, 61, 80, 86, 93–6, 98, 100, 104, 108, 112, 122, 124, 126, 138, 148, 158, 187, 188, 192; ward clerks, 3, 19, 22, 23, 25, 26, 28, 32, 83, 97, 100, 125, 126

clinics, 16

collective agreement, 27, 112, 114, 116

collective bargaining, 114

community health representatives, 19

community, 65–7, 71, 72, 79, 82, 113, 119, 129

computer, 23, 24, 29, 30, 31, 34, 93, 99, 148. *See also* technology

contracting out, 10–11, 15, 17, 18, 81, 108, 114, 115, 120, 127, 144, 157–9, 161, 163, 164, 166, 184, 190

control over work, 127–30, 138

cook, 18, 48–50, 84, 112, 151

cooking. *See* food preparation

counselling, 32

credentials. *See* skills

culture, 66, 68, 70, 73, 81

data, 6, 13, 16, 17, 18, 19, 36, 42, 47, 50, 52, 54, 56, 57, 58, 59, 69, 99, 107, 108, 122, 142, 151, 183–94; interviews/ qualitative, 6, 13, 19, 194; limitations of, 6, 183–94; numeric/quantitative, 6, 13, 16, 19, 29, 62, 66, 183–94

death/dying, 25, 59; of clients/ patients, 14, 38, 40, 97, 132

demands, 15, 22, 32
dementia, 38
dental assistant, 41, 186
dentist, 40
denturist, 18
depression, 129. *See also* mental
    health
diagnosing and treating, 17, 25, 62,
    186, 187
dialectics, 64
dietary worker, 3, 4, 79, 80, 86, 94, 96,
    97, 100, 111, 118, 123, 124, 125, 127,
    133, 149
diets. *See* nutrition
disability, 4, 8, 70, 79, 80, 96, 100
discharge: from hospital, 20, 29, 46
discourse, 7, 63, 64
discrimination, 70, 108, 168
division of labour, 3, 9, 66, 81, 84–6,
    88, 161, 186
doctor, 3, 18, 20, 23, 24, 25, 26, 29, 30,
    31, 32, 37, 39, 54, 56, 62, 80, 83, 96,
    97, 103, 109, 110, 111, 141, 142, 147–
    9, 150–7, 160, 163, 186
domestic labour, 15, 43, 58, 82–5, 89,
    90, 94, 107, 110, 120, 137, 191
drug. *See* medication

education, 17, 33, 34, 36, 41, 43, 49, 50,
    51, 53, 55, 60, 61, 64, 67, 68, 72, 83,
    85, 91, 92, 94, 95, 104, 110, 111, 112,
    129, 137, 147, 151, 159, 161; college
    diploma or certificate, 14, 33, 38, 41,
    43, 49, 54, 92; high school, 33, 49,
    104; postgraduate, 41; post-second-
    ary general, 33, 36, 42, 47, 49, 50, 51,
    95, 104, 111; university degree, 33,
    41, 49, 54, 92, 95, 110, 111
effort, of work, 9, 88, 96, 100, 103, 119,
    121, 138

elder care, 129,
emergency, 25, 32
emotional labour, 21, 26, 32, 43, 45,
    76
employment: casual, 14, 81, 132; con-
    tract (*see under* employment, tem-
    porary); full-time, 14, 15, 34, 36, 41,
    42, 43, 47, 50, 52, 55, 56, 60, 107, 108,
    113, 114, 130, 132, 142, 185, 191, 192,
    193; irregular, 15, 38, 42; part-time,
    15, 34, 36, 41, 42, 43, 44, 45, 47, 50,
    51, 52, 55, 60, 61, 81, 107, 113, 127,
    128, 191, 192; permanent, 34, 55, 60,
    128, 129, 185, 191, 192, 193; tempo-
    rary, 52, 81, 108, 128, 132, 184, 191,
    192 (*see also* contracting out)
employment agencies, 14
employment benefits, 60, 81, 109, 113,
    114, 127, 128, 134, 138, 142, 146, 158,
    159, 166
employment equity, 70
environment, 8, 67, 68, 71–3, 78, 79,
    99, 115, 127, 134
epidemic, 83
equity, 12, 65, 113, 154
ethnicity. *See* racialization; visible
    minority; whiteness
evidence, 7, 10, 11, 63, 66, 71, 83, 96,
    122, 124, 131, 133, 139, 143, 150,
    152, 155, 162–4, 169
expertise, 62. *See also* skills

family, 14, 15, 20, 21, 22, 25, 26, 31, 39,
    40, 43, 50, 57, 72, 78, 80, 82, 90, 97,
    98, 102, 107, 108, 119, 129, 132, 133,
    136, 137, 138, 144, 151, 152, 160,
    164, 167, 184, 191
feeding: of patients/clients, 16, 38,
    46, 47, 57, 96, 97, 101
female-dominated sectors or jobs, 10,

36, 60, 95, 104, 110, 119, 129, 186, 192

feminism, 4, 8, 62, 63, 66, 68, 75, 87, 88, 89, 91, 108

First Nations. *See* Aboriginal

flu, 22, 79, 145

food and accommodation industry, 15, 17. *See also* hotel services

food preparation, 3, 7, 10, 15–17, 31, 38, 40, 43–52, 57, 60, 61, 64, 68, 71, 72, 78, 79, 83, 86, 89, 90, 92, 94–8, 100–2, 115–17, 125, 134, 137, 144, 149, 150, 152, 153, 158–60, 167, 169, 187, 189, 190, 191

foreign-born. *See* immigrant

formal economy, 7, 65, 66

for-profit (care/models/services), 10, 11, 17, 65, 115, 127, 145–50, 152, 155, 157–63, 169

frailty, 78, 79, 96, 100, 137

gender, 4–10, 12, 47, 48, 65–9, 73, 81, 82, 93, 95, 96, 105, 109, 115, 117, 119, 121–3, 136, 139, 187, 189. *See also* sex

genes (genetic makeup and endow-ment), 8, 67, 68, 73

geography (geographical location), 64, 65, 186

global, 5, 7–8, 10, 66, 69, 71, 74, 75, 140, 148, 149, 150, 152

gloves, 40, 98, 99, 127

government, 10, 16, 17, 22, 29, 56, 96, 103, 115, 119, 120, 138, 141, 143, 146, 147, 148, 150, 152–8, 160, 163–6; federal, 69, 70, 73, 90, 99, 141, 153, 155, 166; provincial/territorial, 114, 116, 142, 153, 155, 156, 164, 165, 166, 168

gown, 98, 99

grievance, 15

hand washing, 15

health, indicator of, 70

health and social service sector. *See* health care and social assistance industry

Health Canada, 67, 68, 70, 72, 73

health care and social assistance industry, 16–18, 33, 37, 43–5, 49, 50, 56, 75, 87, 90, 112, 183, 189, 190

health care costs/expenditures. *See* health spending

health care reforms, 105, 116, 118, 142, 152, 153, 156, 157, 160, 162–4, 166, 167, 169

health care system, 68, 69, 80, 81; public, 11, 12, 65, 84, 141, 147, 153–6

health hazard, 9, 10, 69, 71, 72, 98, 103, 120, 121, 122, 123, 124, 125, 126, 138, 159, 168

health human resources (HHR), 16, 18, 131, 142, 163

health promotion, 67, 70–2

health spending, 8, 10, 140–3, 150, 154–7, 166, 169

hepatitis, 123, 124

history, 7, 9, 11, 63–5, 82, 86, 89, 91, 103, 109, 156

home care, 14, 18, 37, 38, 43, 59, 102, 107, 112, 113, 116, 117, 122, 126, 129–31, 137, 144, 148, 151, 154, 156, 159, 166, 169

homemaker/housekeeper. *See* cleaner

homemaking/housekeeping ser-vices. *See* cleaning

homeopathy, 3

hospital, 12, 14, 15, 16, 17, 18, 19, 21,

26, 27, 29, 30, 32, 36, 37, 40, 42, 43,
45, 47, 48, 49, 52, 53, 54, 76, 78–80,
83–6, 90, 95, 96, 99, 104, 111, 114–
16, 125–8, 131, 134, 138, 141, 145,
148, 149, 153–61, 165, 166, 168, 184,
190
hotel services, 5, 9, 10, 96, 98, 99, 148,
150, 157, 158
household work/housework. *See*
domestic labour
household, 7, 9, 65, 66, 71, 81, 85–9,
90, 91, 94, 107, 108, 124, 125, 127,
129, 136, 137, 168, 191
human rights, 67, 75, 108, 156

iatrogenesis, 78
immigrant, 5, 34, 41–4, 47, 50, 52, 55,
60, 79, 83, 89, 91, 95, 115, 136, 150–3,
161, 184, 185, 193, 194
immigration, 6, 47, 65, 88, 185, 193,
194
income, 67, 68, 70, 72, 85, 107, 108,
110, 129, 142, 164, 185. *See also*
wages and earnings
incontinence, 38
India, 15, 128, 149, 151
indigenous peoples, 73. *See also*
Aboriginal
industrial groups/categories, 16–19,
39, 185, 187, 189–94
inequality/inequity, 5, 7, 63, 65–7, 69,
70, 108, 147
infection, 78, 79, 99, 123, 124, 134, 139,
145, 161, 163, 165
injury, 10, 65, 77, 121, 122, 124–8, 130,
139, 147, 160, 168
institution, 5–8, 53, 63, 66, 68, 79, 85,
91, 95, 104, 111, 116, 154, 158, 166
interruption of work, 30
Inuit. *See* Aboriginal

Jamaica, 149
job loss, 14, 114–16, 122, 149, 159
job search, 14
job security, 11–12, 113, 127, 129, 130,
131, 158
job strain, 128–30, 132

kitchen, 15, 48, 49, 61, 84, 86, 126, 133,
149, 158, 159

lab work/lab tests, 20, 23–5
labour force, 9, 16–18, 33, 34, 36, 41,
43, 47, 49, 50–2, 55–7, 60, 85, 90, 94,
95, 105–8, 112, 120, 122, 138, 144,
150, 164
labour force participation, women's,
9, 106, 107, 108, 109, 120, 132,
167
labour market, 92, 95, 117
Lalonde Report, 67
laundry (tasks/services), 15, 16, 18,
40, 44, 45, 47, 48, 50, 51, 58, 60, 61,
70, 79, 82, 86, 87, 89, 90, 92, 94–6,
100, 101, 113, 115, 122–7, 149, 153,
158, 159, 168, 169
laundry workers, 3, 4, 18, 48, 100,
111, 115, 125, 126, 149, 187, 189
layoff. *See* job loss
legionnaires' disease, 45, 71
legislation, 88, 95, 104, 108, 111, 114
lifting, 102, 125, 126, 127
linen, cleaning or changing of, 15, 31,
46, 125, 127. *See also* bed; laundry
literacy, 72, 93
location of work, 6, 16, 193
long-term care, 13, 16, 37–9, 41–3, 45–
8, 50, 52, 53, 56, 72, 76, 79, 84, 86,
91, 94, 96, 97, 104, 105, 115, 118,
121, 128–30, 132, 133, 135, 136, 138,
190

low-income cut-offs (LICOs), 107. *See also* income; poverty

maintenance staff, 3–5, 16, 46, 48, 57, 59, 68, 115, 131, 145, 146
male-dominated sectors or jobs, 34, 46, 59, 95, 104, 121, 164
malnutrition, 79. *See also* nutrition
manager, 3–5, 14–17, 32, 34, 36, 52–6, 60, 92, 96, 99, 111, 112, 117, 120, 127, 128, 134, 137, 142, 145, 148, 158, 160, 165, 187, 188
Manitoba, 103, 113, 138, 148
market, 7, 63, 64, 143, 145, 147, 148, 150, 152, 161, 165, 169
mask, 40, 98
maternity benefits, 108
mechanical lift, 38, 39, 102, 125
media, 64
medical error, 15, 23, 24, 139
medical information, 21. *See also* record keeping
medical model, 18, 62
medical secretary, 32–7, 192
medical transcriptionist, 32, 33, 60, 192
medicare, 145, 153, 156, 157
medication, 3, 23–5, 30, 38, 40, 65, 96, 102, 103, 131, 142, 153, 154, 156, 166
men, 5, 16, 33–6, 39–44, 47–61, 68, 69, 70, 83, 88, 90, 95, 105, 107–10, 113, 117, 120, 122, 123, 125, 128, 129, 131, 134, 136, 137, 149, 150. *See also* male-dominated sectors or jobs
menstruation, 68
mental health, 38, 127, 130, 131, 132, 136
minimum wage, 14. *See also* wages and earnings
mortality, 71

mother/mothering, 67, 72, 90

National Occupational Classification for Statistics (NOC-S), 185, 187
New Public Management, 10, 143, 144, 145, 146, 147, 156, 157
non-profit (care/models/services), 12, 65, 146, 147, 153, 154, 157, 158, 159
North American Free Trade Agreement (NAFTA), 169
North American Industrial Classification System (NAICS), 16, 185, 189, 190
nurse, 3, 9, 14, 18, 20–31, 36, 37, 39–42, 46, 50, 52–4, 62, 72, 75, 78, 80–6, 89, 97, 103, 110, 111, 121, 123, 125, 127, 135, 137, 139, 148, 150, 151, 152, 153, 154, 160, 163, 164, 168, 186; practical, 22, 151; registered, 18, 22, 23, 24, 27, 28, 114, 151
nursing, 3, 9, 46, 92, 94, 101, 102, 108, 110, 111, 113, 114, 119, 132, 135, 148, 151
nursing aide, 3, 14, 15, 18, 36–8, 41, 42, 113
nursing assistant, 3, 18, 37, 40, 41, 101, 111
nursing home. *See* long-term care
nutrition, 71, 79, 80

occupational and industrial segregation, 90, 95, 106, 108, 120, 121, 129
occupational categories/groups, 17, 18, 33, 183, 185–7, 189, 193
occupational health and safety, 10, 70, 73, 81, 121, 122, 123, 124, 138, 160, 168; accidents, 71; back injury, 124, 125, 131; chemicals, 70, 73, 99,

126, 127, 138; dermatitis, 126; musculoskeletal injury, 124–6, 131; needle stick injury, 127; repetitive
strain injury (RSI), 15; respiratory
disease, 123, 124; slips and falls, 15
occupational therapy, 18
office, 16, 29
'one-eyed science,' 10, 69
Ontario, 80, 90, 94, 95, 104, 113, 116,
121, 125, 128, 129, 133, 135, 147,
149, 159, 165, 168
oppression, 69
orderly, 3, 18, 36, 37, 40–2, 187
Organization for Economic Co-oper-
ation and Development (OECD),
68, 140, 141
organization of work, 6, 17, 26, 71,
72, 118, 127, 130, 132, 134, 137, 147,
155, 189
Ottawa Charter, 67
out-patient, 23
overtime, 15, 29, 42, 57, 108, 134;
unpaid, 14, 15. See also unpaid
work; wages and earnings; work
schedule

pace of work, 15, 23, 25, 72, 130, 133,
148
paid work, 15, 57, 63, 66, 69, 70–4,
78, 80, 82, 83, 85, 89, 91, 105, 107,
110, 117, 118, 119, 129, 133, 157,
184, 191, 192
palliative care, 14, 37, 39
patient, 14, 18, 20–32, 36–40, 41, 44,
46, 52, 66, 69, 71, 73, 74, 76–81, 83,
84, 86, 97–102, 105, 115–18, 123–6,
128, 130–2, 134–9, 142, 144, 145,
147, 149, 154, 160, 162–4, 166, 167,
184
pay equity, 56, 94, 95, 113

pediatrics, 20, 22, 32
pension, 59, 113, 158
personal care, 37, 38, 50, 57, 89, 91,
92, 94, 95, 101, 102, 104, 117, 123,
125, 126, 135
personal care provider, 3, 4, 22, 36,
37, 39, 40–2, 96, 97, 102, 111–13,
123, 125, 129, 135, 151, 159, 188
'personal is political,' 63
personal support worker (PSW). See
personal care provider
pharmacy, 17, 24
Philippines, 151
physician. See doctor
physiotherapy, 18
policy, 4, 5, 6, 11, 66, 67, 68, 69, 72, 81,
92, 111, 119, 120, 138, 143, 144, 161–
3, 168, 186, 188
political economy, 7, 8, 63–7, 73, 74;
feminist, 4, 7, 8, 61, 62, 63, 65, 75,
87, 88
porter, 20, 27, 96, 131, 132
postmodernism, 4
poverty, 107, 108
power, 5, 7, 63, 64, 73, 74, 76, 85, 89,
92, 93, 95, 104, 105, 109, 110, 120,
137, 145, 150, 151, 154, 157, 165
practices, 4–7, 12, 53, 68, 71, 72, 74,
81, 83, 91, 101, 108–10, 121, 127,
143, 144, 152, 156, 158, 163
precarious employment, 13, 128,
129
pre-admission (pre-operative procedures or care), 21, 22, 23, 29, 32
private agencies. See employment
agencies
private sector, 10, 11, 109, 120, 143–7,
149, 150, 156, 158
private sphere/space, 7, 63, 83
privatization, 11, 114, 115, 145, 146,

147, 148, 152, 155, 156, 157, 158, 159, 160, 163, 166, 184, 190
production, 7, 64, 146, 190
professional organizations, 9, 88, 109, 110, 111, 116, 150
professionalization, 9, 109
promotion and advancement, 15
psychiatric care, 22, 27
public administration, 112
public health, 11, 12, 71, 84, 105, 128, 152, 153, 154, 155, 167, 168, 186
public-private partnerships, 11, 145, 146, 148, 157, 158, 166
public sector, 11, 56, 111, 114, 120, 140, 141, 143–6, 148, 154, 156, 158–61, 165, 169
public sphere/space, 7, 63, 91

quarantine, 86
Quebec, 131, 134, 138, 159

race. See racialization; racism
racial harassment, 135
racialization, 4–8, 12, 14, 41, 47, 65, 69, 70, 73, 79, 82, 88, 91, 93, 95, 101, 105, 121, 137, 184, 185, 193, 194
racism, 70, 120, 135, 137, 138
receptionist, 32–6, 98
record keeping, 15, 16, 20, 21, 25, 32–6, 80, 90, 100, 167
regionalization, 11
regulation, of work/workers, 18, 102–5, 110, 147, 148, 154, 156, 160, 167
relations of ruling, 7, 63–5
reproduction, 7, 64
resistance: collective, 7, 12, 64, 88, 116, 117, 120; individual, 7, 12, 64, 88, 118, 119, 120
respect, 45, 138

restructuring, 118, 131, 134, 135, 149, 150
retraining, 115, 158. See also training; skills, upgrading of
Romanow Report, 3, 4, 13, 60, 68, 73, 79, 162

salary. See income; wages and earnings
sales and service occupations, 17, 50
sampling, of data, 19
SARS, 15, 72, 79, 124, 145, 167, 168
secretary, 112
security personnel, 4, 5, 16, 52, 123, 187, 189
segregation. See occupational and industrial segregation
self-employment, 108, 109, 191, 193
service associates: labelling as, 17, 46
service industries (services in general), 44, 87, 90, 96, 97, 100, 101, 108, 112, 115, 116, 133, 134, 136, 137, 143, 145–9, 158, 163, 166, 169, 184
sex, 68, 69, 94, 136, 137, 186. See also gender
sexual harassment, 71, 108, 135, 136, 137
sexuality, 65
shift work. See work schedule
shopping, 40, 43
sick pay, 81, 122, 129
skills, 5, 9–10, 12, 16, 20, 23, 26, 28, 30–2, 38, 47, 61, 67, 68, 72, 75, 78, 80, 83, 84, 88, 91–96, 99–105, 109, 116, 119, 120, 128, 130, 138, 145, 150–2, 186, 189; upgrading of, 15, 38 (see also retraining)
social construction, 64, 67, 68
social determinants of health, 4, 8,

10, 12, 62, 66–70, 72–5, 78, 79, 81, 82, 87, 88, 154, 169

social location, 64–6, 88, 185, 194

social status, 67, 70

social worker, 21

South Africa, 151

South America, 151

speech therapy, 18

staffing, 15, 27–9, 132, 134

state, the, 5, 7, 12, 63, 97, 143, 144, 155

statistical agencies, 19

statistics. *See under* data, numeric/ quantitative

Statistics Canada, 6, 16–19, 33–7, 44, 45, 47–9, 51, 52, 54, 55, 57–9, 90, 92, 106–8, 112, 136, 162, 183, 184, 186, 187, 189, 191, 194

stress, 14, 20, 25–7, 32, 40, 52, 71–3, 96, 127–35

supervisor, 15, 33–7, 47, 48, 51, 52, 60, 112, 137, 138, 159

support personnel, 17, 18

surgery, 20–3, 29, 31, 76, 79, 80, 97, 186

Sweden, 144

switchboard operator, 32–4, 36

team-based care or work, 11, 77, 78, 80, 82, 86, 87, 102, 137, 138, 152, 160–2, 169

technical and related occupations in health, 112, 188, 192

technology, 3, 8, 10, 26, 30, 73, 84, 100, 105, 101, 111, 131, 142, 147–9, 165

theory/theoretical framework, 6, 7, 16, 62, 66, 69, 83, 84, 109

time, of work, 6, 14, 56

toileting, 38

Toronto, 124, 127, 128, 158

training, 40, 43, 53, 61, 77, 80, 82–4,

85, 93–5, 103–5, 124, 126, 127, 130, 137, 138, 150–2, 159, 160; formal, 14, 26, 47, 62; informal, 26

tuberculosis, 123, 167

unemployment, 70. *See also* job loss

union, 9, 12–15, 88, 109, 111–16, 120, 122, 127, 137, 146, 157, 158, 167

unionization (union density/union organizing), 9, 12, 60, 109, 111–16, 120, 142, 156, 157

United Kingdom, 70, 78, 79, 81, 99, 117, 144, 150, 151, 159, 161–3, 165

United States, 123, 135, 137, 141, 143, 144, 146–8, 151

unpaid work, 14, 15, 18, 56–9, 65–7, 69, 71, 72, 74, 82, 85, 88–91, 107, 117, 119, 120, 127, 129, 130, 134, 136, 138, 144, 145, 157, 184, 191

valuation/under-valuation, of work/workers, 5, 9, 69, 70, 74, 86, 87, 88, 91, 93–6, 105, 108, 113, 119

Vancouver, 124, 160

ventilation, 71

violence, 71, 135, 136, 137

visibility/invisibility, of work/workers, 5, 7, 9, 12, 28, 29, 69, 88, 93, 95, 99, 120, 121, 122, 134, 137, 138, 152, 161, 184, 190, 192

visible minority, 19, 33, 34, 36, 41, 42, 43, 47, 50, 52, 55, 60, 115, 137, 194

wage gap, 36, 42, 43, 47, 48, 51, 52, 56, 60

wages and earnings, 10, 11, 15, 18, 19, 29, 36, 37, 39, 40, 42, 44, 47, 48, 50–2, 55–60, 65, 70, 73, 80, 81, 83, 85, 89–92, 94, 95, 107–11, 113–19, 122, 127–30, 134, 138, 142, 144, 146, 147,

150, 151, 153, 154, 156–9, 164, 166,
168, 185, 186, 189, 191, 193, 194
whiteness, 14, 194
women, 5–6, 9–12, 15, 16, 18, 28, 32,
33–7, 39, 40–4, 47–61, 67–71, 74, 77,
80, 82–91, 93–6, 99, 101, 102, 105–
13, 115–23, 125, 128–31, 133, 134,
136–8, 144, 145, 149, 150, 154, 156,
157, 164, 168, 192; women's work,
74, 85
work breaks, 15, 32
work organization. *See* organization
of work
work schedule, 14, 27, 28, 39, 86, 97,
117, 128, 131, 132, 133, 134, 138;
shift work, 15, 128, 129; weekend
work, 14, 15, 27, 28, 29, 38, 129

workers' compensation claims, 122,
125, 126, 139
working conditions, 5, 9–12, 73, 81,
85, 87, 88, 96, 102, 103, 105–7, 109,
111, 113, 114, 116, 120, 130, 131, 133,
138, 139, 144, 146, 159, 160, 161,
168, 169
workload, 30, 32, 117, 128, 129, 131,
132, 134
workplace, 6, 16, 36, 39, 71, 109–11,
116–18, 136, 137, 163
World Health Organization (WHO),
12, 18, 57, 67, 85, 105, 124, 147, 167

X-rays, 23–6, 40

yoga, 73

Great Walks of Acadia National Park & Mount Desert Island

Revised Edition

Text by Robert Gillmore
Photographs by Eileen Oktavec

To Margaret O'Reilly Oktavec and Albert William Oktavec III, who made it all possible.

Great Walks ®

No. 1 in a series of full-color, pocket-size guides to the best walks in the world published by Great Walks Inc. Other Great Walks guides: *Great Walks of Southern Arizona, Great Walks of Big Bend National Park, Great Walks of the Great Smokies, Great Walks of Yosemite National Park, Great Walks of Sequoia & Kings Canyon National Parks,* and *Great Walks of the Olympic Peninsula.* For more information on all Great Walks guides send $1 (refundable with your first order) to: Great Walks, PO Box 410, Goffstown, NH 03045.

*COVER: Surf breaks over the smooth stones on the beach at Monument Cove along the **Ocean Trail** (Walk No. 3). Otter Cliffs, the highest ocean cliffs on Mount Desert Island, are in the distance.*

CONTENTS

What Are Great Walks? 5
    What Are Great Walks Guides? 5
Foreword: New England's Natural Theme Park
   — and How to Enjoy It 7

GREAT WALKS OF
MOUNT DESERT ISLAND

  1 The Shore Path 18
  2 Dorr Point & Compass Harbor 22
  3 The Ocean Trail 28
  4 Sand Beach & Great Head 34
  5 Eagle Lake 39
  6 Bubble Pond 43
  7 Jordan Pond 47
  8 Little Long Pond 52
  9 The Asticou Terraces & the Thuya Garden ..55
10 The Asticou Azalea Garden 58
11 Gorham Mountain 60
12 Champlain Mountain 64
13 Day Mountain 70
14 Pemetic Mountain 78
15 Penobscot Mountain 84
16 Sargent Mountain 90
17 The South Bubble 94
18 The North Bubble & Conners Nubble 98
19 Cadillac Mountain Summit 105
20 South Ridge, Cadillac Mountain 111
21 Acadia Mountain 115
22 Flying Mountain 119
23 Valley Peak & St. Sauveur Mountain 125

24 Beech Mountain 130
25 Beech Cliff & Canada Cliff. 134

GREAT WALKS OF ISLE AU HAUT 139

26 The Goat Trail 140
27 The Cliff & Western Head Trails 146
28 The Eben's Head & Duck Harbor Trails . . .150
29 Duck Harbor Mountain 153

HONORABLE MENTIONS

30 Paradise Hill 158
31 Long Pond 160
32 Norumbega Mountain 162

Acknowledgments

We are grateful for the assistance of Deborah
Wade of the National Park Service, Mike Raynor of
the Acadia Corp. and Keith Miller of the Eastern
National Park and Monument Association.

What Are Great Walks?

Great Walks invariably offer beautiful and interesting world-class scenery and excellent views in the most picturesque places on earth.

Great Walks are also shorter and easier than the typical hike or climb. They're usually less than five miles long. They can be walked in a day or less. And they're usually on smooth, firm, dry and, most important, *gently graded* trails. (Long, arduous, sweaty treks up rough, steep, rocky trails are *not* Great Walks!)

What Are Great Walks Guides?

Great Walks guides carefully describe and, with beautiful full-color photographs, lavishly illustrate the world's Great Walks.

Unlike many walking guides, which describe *every* trail in a region, Great Walks describe only the *best* walks, the happy few that will especially delight you with their beauty.

Unlike many guides, which give you mainly directions, Great Walks guides carefully describe *all* the major features of every Great Walk so you can know, in advance, *precisely* what the Walk has to offer and exactly *why* it's worth your time to take it.

After all, your leisure time is valuable. In your lifetime you can walk on only a fraction of the hundreds of thousands of miles of trails in the world. Why not walk only the best?

For your convenience Great Walks guides are an easy-to-use and easy-to-carry pocket size and their covers are film laminated for extra protection against wear and tear.

Foreword:
New England's
Natural Theme Park
—and How to Enjoy It

A fortuitous combination of natural and man-made circumstances makes the walking in and around Acadia National Park among the best in the world.

The most important circumstance is that Acadia National Park is a kind of natural theme park in which the most beautiful elements of New England's landscape—ledge-topped mountains, pristine forested lakes and rockbound, island-dotted seacoast—are all gathered together, seemingly for the convenience of vacationers. In Acadia, the perennial question "Shall we go to the mountains, the lakes or the ocean?" does not apply. In Acadia you have it all.

Much of Acadia's magnificent scenery can be seen on long, glorious views from the park's mountain trails. These views are a happy result of three things: Acadia has some of the highest summits on the entire east coast of the Americas; most of the park's tallest peaks have bare, rocky summits; and most of the trees near those summits are short.

But even though Acadia's mountains are high enough and bare enough for often-nonstop views, they're low enough to be easily climbed. Cadillac Mountain, for example, is the highest peak on the North Atlantic Coast, but it's only 1,530 feet high.

What's more, most of Acadia's mountains are long ridges, so they can be ascended on gentle grades.

Although Acadia National Park is small, there are 29 Great Walks, plus three Honorable Mentions, in or around it. Almost no place else in the world offers so many Great Walks in so small an area. Moreover, all the Walks on Mount Desert Island (where most of the park is located) are just a short drive apart and few are more than 15 minutes from your hotel or campground. Almost nowhere else can you get to so many Great Walks so quickly and so easily.

Because all the Walks are in or near the national park, many of the roads you'll be driving on are well sited and landscaped and most of the scenery is otherwise unspoiled. On the Park Loop Road, for example, you'll be struck not only by its many ocean views but also by the fact that there are no telephone poles or fence posts. Wires are underground and handsome granite rocks do the work of guardrails. The only manmade thing in your view is the pavement.

Finally, Mount Desert Island's creature comforts are many and handy. Bar Harbor teems with motels, hotels, guest houses and bed-and-breakfasts—old and new, plain and very fancy. Bar Harbor also has many good restaurants and it's close to many of the island's Walks. In Acadia, a fine lunch or dinner is never more than a short drive away. In fact, the area is home to so many good things that you'd want to come here even if you never set one foot on one trail.

The Walks described below will show you the area's most beautiful scenery.

All but four Great Walks as well as all three

Honorable Mentions are on Mount Desert Island. Walks No. 1-3 take you along dramatic seacoast on level paths. Walk No. 4 goes across Sand Beach and the windswept coastal overlook known as Great Head. Walks No. 5-7 and 31 take you along the shores of lovely mountain-rimmed lakes and ponds. Walks No 8-10 are short excursions through four outstanding works of landscaping. Walks No. 11-25, 29 and 32 take you to the tops of 20 different mountains or other promontories for some of the best mountain, lake and ocean views you'll ever see.

Four of the Great Walks—Nos. 26-29—are on Isle au Haut, a hilly, spruce-covered island about 14 miles off Mount Desert Island. (Samuel de Champlain named it the *haut*, or high, island because, unlike the other, low islands in the area, Isle au Haut has a central ridge that's more than 500 feet above sea level at its highest point.) Walks No. 26-28 follow the six-mile-long island's wild southern and western coasts. Walk No. 29 takes you up Duck Harbor Mountain for a series of broad ocean views.

Unlike Mount Desert Island, which is connected to the mainland by a short bridge, Isle au Haut is accessible only by boat. From the second Monday in June to the second Saturday in September, the Isle au Haut Co. ferries passengers from Stonington, on the coast, to Duck Harbor Landing, on Isle au Haut. Duck Harbor Landing is about .2 miles from Western Head Road, where all four of the island's Great Walks begin. However, the ferry doesn't reach the landing until 11 A.M. and its last run back to Stonington leaves at 6 P.M., which gives you only seven hours on the island—not enough to do all four Walks.

If you want to spend more time on the island, you have four choices: You can keep taking the two-hour, $24-round-trip ferry ride to Duck Harbor Landing. You can camp in one of five wooden lean-tos near the landing. You can look for a house on the island to rent. Or you can stay at the island's only inn: the Keeper's House.

The inn is a rare delight. It's the handsome former residence of the "keeper" of the adjacent light-house. The lighthouse has been automated by the Coast Guard and the residence and its outbuildings are now a cozy six-bedroom inn heated with wood stoves and lit by candles and kerosene lamps. Yes, there's no electricity. But there *are* hot showers, and the inn's home-cooked breakfasts, dinners and box lunches are creative, its decor (large windows and light-filled, pastel-painted rooms with white-painted antiques) is pleasant, and the ambience is mellow. The Keeper's House also rents bicycles on which you can ride to the trailheads. For more information call 207-367-2261. For more information about the ferry call 207-367-5193. For camping information call the park headquarters at 207-288-3338.

None of these Walks is strenuous. In fact, ten of them—Nos. 1, 2, 5, 6, 8-10, 19, 25 and 31—are either easy or very easy and 11 others—Nos. 3, 4, 7, 11, 13, 17, 20, 22, 24, 27 and 30—while not exactly easy, are nevertheless undemanding. The 11 remaining Walks—Nos. 12, 14-16, 18, 21, 23, 26, 28, 29 and 32—are moderate.

Most of the Walks are on smooth or fairly smooth trails and on either level or gently graded paths. The few, brief exceptions to this rule—on Walks No. 7,

14-16, 23 and 29—are noted. The typical Walk is only about one to three miles long. (The *longest* Walk—No. 26—is only 6.6 miles long.)

How long does each Walk take? That depends, of course, on how fast you walk. But a very rough rule of thumb is: one hour per mile. If you walk faster and don't pause to enjoy the views (see below), the time per mile is less. The average Walk takes just a few hours, the longest one no more than seven or eight hours. Depending on your speed, it takes about 10 to 14 days to do all of them.

In general, the very best Walks are those that take you up mountains and along the ocean. Of these, the crème de la crème are Nos. 1, 3, 4, 11, 12, 14, 18, 19 and 24-27. Two other Walks, Nos. 9 and 10, take you to splendid gardens.

What's the best time to take these Walks? In late spring and fall the weather is usually cool—just right for walking—the park is uncrowded and hotels charge off-season rates. Fall, however, has an added bonus: the leaves are turning color and the blueberry bushes on the ledges are solid drifts of deep red. But because most park visitors seldom stray far from their cars, trails are rarely crowded at any time, even in the busy summer season. (And the blueberries, by the way, are ripe in August.)

Here are some tips to help you get the most out of these Walks:

▶ This guide tells you *exactly* what each Walk has to offer. Take advantage of it by reading it before you take *any* Walks. That way you'll be best able to select Walks that most closely suit your taste.

▶ Carry the guide on all Walks. (It'll fit easily in

any pocket.) It tells you how to reach the trailhead and gives you precise directions for each Walk, as well as detailed descriptions of what you'll see.

▶The Walks start where they start, stop where they stop and go where they go for two reasons: (1) the routes we describe provide the best walking in the area; (2) any other routes are more difficult, less scenic or both. The park has more than 100 miles of hiking trails and 50 miles of carriage roads but only the routes described below are Great Walks or Honorable Mentions.

▶Most of the park's trailhead parking areas are marked by distinctive brown signs with white letters. The beginnings of trails are signed with wooden posts with incised letters; junctions are marked by horizontal wood signs attached to wooden posts; all trail signs indicate distances (of occasionally disputable accuracy). Summits are marked by wooden signs indicating both the name of the mountain or peak and its elevation. Trails are blazed by (usually) blue paint on rocks or trees and by cairns (small rock piles) on ledges. Most trails are easy to follow and in any event we tell you everything you need to know to find your way. A map, therefore, is not necessary for *directions*. But a detailed, easy-to-read topographical map is very helpful in identifying mountains, islands, bays and other landmarks. The best topographic map of Mount Desert Island—the one that indicates the largest number of features in the clearest way—is published by DeLorme and sold for about $8 at the park Visitor Center and other outlets. The best map of Isle au Haut is published by the Park Service and is available free on the ferry to the island. Also helpful for getting around the area is the park's *Official Map and Guide*. Like all similar National Park Service publications, it clearly and attractively indicates all roads in and near the park, as well as trails and other natural and manmade features. It's yours for free at the Visitor Center and the entrance station on the Park Loop Road.

►Unless you're in excellent condition (and few people are) do your body a favor: Whenever possible, do the Walks in order of difficulty, easiest ones first. That way each Walk will help prepare you to take the harder one that follows. Ideally, you'll be able to progress from short, easy Walks to longer, harder ones with little difficulty.

►Any comfortable walking shoes are fine for Walks that follow smooth paths (Nos. 1-3, 5, 8-10, 19 and 31). For other walks we recommend the greater support and protection of above-the-ankle hiking boots. To avoid unnecessary discomfort (including blisters) make sure your footwear fits and is broken in before you start walking.

►Long-range views are clearest on sunny days, so do the mountain Walks in fair weather. Save the garden Walks (Nos. 9 and 10) and those with short-range views (Nos. 6, 7 and 31) for cloudy days.

►We suggest you carry rain gear and wear waterproof hiking boots whenever wet weather is imminent. For best protection, we recommend a lightweight waterproof hooded jacket and pants. The most comfortable rain garments are made of "breathable" Goretex fabric, which keeps rain out but also lets perspiration escape.

►Carry water on longer Walks. It will taste best if

you carry it in ceramic canteens, such as the French-made Tournus, rather than plastic or metal bottles. If you have access to a refrigerator, here's a way to keep the water cold: The night before a Walk pour just an inch or so of water in the canteen and lay it on its side in the freezer, leaving the top open to make sure the canteen doesn't crack when the water freezes and expands. Next morning fill the canteen with cold water. The ice already inside will keep the water cold.

►Never drink water from any stream or spring without filtering it or treating it with purifying tablets. The risk of an attack of *giardia lamblia* is too great to drink untreated water.

►Never urinate or defecate within 100 feet of brooks or lakes and don't wash yourself in them. (Even biodegradable soap pollutes lakes and stream if used directly in them.)

►It's obvious but it bears repeating: Binoculars enable you to see what you can't see, or see as well, without them (bald eagles, for example). A high-powered, lightweight pair is worth carrying.

►Use enough sunscreen to keep the exposed parts of your body from burning and wear something to keep the sun out of your eyes. We favor a wide-brimmed hat or a sun visor over tinted sunglasses, which substitute a tinted view of the world for the real one. A hat or visor also helps keep you cool by protecting much of your face from the sun.

►Mosquitoes and other flying insects can sometimes be a pesty problem in warmer weather. Carry some repellent, just in case.

►Be sure to begin each Walk early enough so you can finish it comfortably before dark.

►On longer Walks, carry a small flashlight in case you can't get back before dark, as well as some toilet paper and Band-Aids.

►Walks No. 5-7, 13, 15, 16, 18 and 30 are wholly or partly on carriage roads, which are popular bike routes. Most bikers will give you ample warning when they pass but some simply whizz by at astounding speeds. So it's a good idea to look out for bikes on carriage roads, especially when you're "changing lanes" (i.e., moving to the left or right).

►Remember that the world's only constant is change. The locations of the lakes and mountains on these walks won't vary from year to year but anything subject to human control—trail routes, parking lots, signs and so on—can change. Be alert for trail reroutings and follow signs.

►Above all, remember that a Great Walk is mainly an aesthetic activity, not an athletic one. Its primary purpose is not to give you exercise (although exercise you will surely get) but to expose you to exceptional natural beauty. Walk slowly enough to savor it. Most people walk too fast. Don't make their mistake. You no more want to rush through these Walks than you want to rush through the Louvre.

Great Walks of
Mount Desert Island

1 The Shore Path

This .5-mile round trip is a leisurely prom-
enade on a wide, smooth, gravelly path along
the top of seawalls at the very edge of Frenchman Bay in Bar Harbor. On its shore side the
Walk offers intimate looks at the inns and summer homes for which Bar Harbor is famous.
On its ocean side the Walk provides uninterrupted vistas of the blue waters of the bay,
dotted by the unspoiled rockbound, spruce-
topped Porcupine Islands.

The Shore Path begins at the town pier at the end
of Main Street. The path isn't marked but it's easy to
find. Face the handsome, gray-shingled Bar Harbor
Inn, just east of the pier. To your left is a stony
beach. To your right is the lawn of tiny Agamont
Park. Between the beach and the park is an asphalt
sidewalk heading toward the ocean side of the inn.
The sidewalk is the beginning of the Walk.

The path curves along the beach, past a long
wooden pier at which excursion boats dock. Red
geraniums grow in boxes on the pier railings. The
island off to your left and closest to shore is Bar
Island. To the right of Bar Island is Sheep Porcupine
Island.

The pier is the first and last thing on the Shore
Path that stands between you and the ocean. From
here until the end of the Walk, the only things to the

left of the path will be rocky shores and blue ocean. On your right you'll pass the rolling lawn of the Bar Harbor Inn and then the yellow-and-white umbrellas shading the tables of Gatsby's Terrace, the inn's outdoor dining area. The inn's large, bow-fronted dining room is above the terrace.

The path changes from asphalt to gravel and quickly bends around a small point. Now you'll be able to see all four Porcupine Islands: from left to right, Sheep Porcupine; Burnt Porcupine, farther offshore; Long Porcupine, even farther offshore — its long side is perpendicular to you, so it'll look larger but not much longer than the others — and Bald Porcupine, nearer to shore, at the eastern end of a long, low rock breakwater. The islands were named Porcupine not because porcupines lived on them but because — with their low, slightly humpy shapes, their covering of pointy quill-like spruce trees, and the granite rock at the ends of the islands that resembles noses — they *look* like porcupines. Or at least to some people they do.

Still more islands, and Schoodic Peninsula behind them, are visible on the other side of Frenchman Bay. Almost straight ahead of you, over the breakwater, you can make out the white-and-orange lighthouse on Egg Rock, nearly two miles away.

After leaving the last gray-shingled building of the Bar Harbor Inn, the path passes Grant Park (also known as Albert Meadow), a tiny, grassy public park outfitted with benches and picnic tables and shaded by a huge birch tree. A sign at the southern edge of the park explains that the Shore Path was created more than 100 years ago "by the original owners of the private properties on which it is located" and that the present owners "are pleased to continue this tradition."

Next you'll see Balance Rock Inn on your right. A sign beside the trail explains that the inn was built in 1903 as a summer residence "for Scottish railroad magnate Alexander Maitland and his family and servants." The pleasing neoclassical revival building overlooks a wide lawn and its namesake, Balance Rock, a 6-foot-wide, 15-foot-high boulder that seems to rest precariously on the stony beach. Like Bubble Rock (Walk No. 17), its uncertain position is an illusion: No one has come close to pushing it over.

After passing an apple tree on your left and patches of Queen Anne's lace on your right, the Walk runs along the left of a picturesque weathered board fence. To the right of the fence are the back yards of private homes.

The path then passes a Tudor revival mansion. A discreet sign on a white arbor identifies the imposing structure as the Breakwater. Like the Balance Rock Inn, which was built one year earlier, the Breakwater was originally a summer "cottage" for a wealthy family. Now it's a sumptuously appointed bed-and-breakfast.

After crossing a short wooden bridge, the Shore Path ends abruptly at a chain-link fence. Turn

---

White sailboats and rocky, spruce-tipped islands in the blue waters of Frenchman Bay, seen from the **Shore Path** *(Walk No. 1) in Bar Harbor. Bar Island is on the left.* ▶

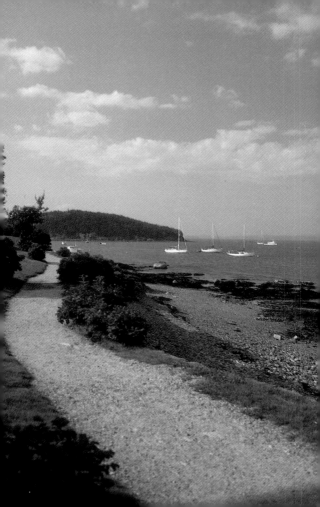

around here and enjoy the views again as you retrace your steps to the beginning of the Walk.

If, perchance, you want to get to Main Street from the Shore Path, you can do so from three places. At the end of the path you can take a right and follow the short unpaved road to Wayman Lane, which leads to Main Street. Or you can leave the path at the southern end of the weathered board fence (not far from the Breakwater) and follow a short path to Hancock Street, which also leads to Main Street. Or you can cross Albert Meadow and follow a short street to Main Street.

Travel Tip: You can make the Walk's views last even longer if you stop for lunch or a drink at Gatsby's Terrace, which we think has the best sea view of any restaurant on the island. From your table you can gaze at the flotilla of white boats in the harbor and the islands beyond them.

2 Dorr Point & Compass Harbor

This easy one-mile Walk takes you to the end of a long, narrow point with a sweeping ocean view that ranges from secluded Compass Harbor to Odgen Point to the Porcupine Islands to Schoodic Peninsula to the Egg Rock lighthouse. You'll also explore some quiet pebble beaches and the intriguing remains of the estate of George B. Dorr, a founder of Acadia National Park and its first superintendent.

This Walk begins at an unmarked parking area on Route 3, exactly one mile south of the intersection of Main and Mount Desert streets in downtown Bar Harbor. As you drive out of Bar Harbor, the ledgy face of Champlain Mountain (Walk No. 12) rises directly ahead of you. You'll pass the stone walls, gates and gatehouses of present and former oceanfront mansions on your left. About .5 miles after passing Cromwell Harbor Road on your right, you'll reach the small gravel trailhead parking area, on your left. (If you pass the Ocean Drive Motor Court, also on the left, you've gone a couple of hundred feet too far.)

The trail is an old road. A brown-and-white park service sign on the gate says "Fire Road/Do Not Block." Large granite rocks stand on either side of the gate and a nine-foot-tall rhododendron, the vestige of old landscaping, grows on the right.

The level road passes through an open, sunny grove of large maples, oaks and other hardwoods. You're now walking on the grounds of what was George Dorr's estate; try to imagine what these woods were like when he lived here.

In about 100 feet you'll cross a small brook; note the ruined walls along the stream on your left.

About 300 feet from the parking area the road forks. Go left and follow a slightly narrower road as it gently curves to the right, around low ledges on the right of the path. You'll soon start glimpsing the ocean through the trees.

About .2 miles from the parking lot you'll pass paths going to the left and right. Keep going straight ahead. You'll then see the round, 1,000-foot-wide Compass Harbor on your left.

The road narrows to a trail as it curves around the southern edge of the harbor and passes through a grassy clearing with an enormous, multi-trunked white pine on the right.

Then the path runs along the top of the narrow peninsula known as Dorr Point. In one place the steep slopes of the 50-foot-long point have been so eroded that the top of the peninsula is only six feet wide.

The path ends at jagged ledges at the end of the point. Now you're in the very center of a horseshoe-shaped band of water that stretches from Compass Harbor on your far left to the mouth of Frenchman Bay on your far right. Your vista, seen from left to right, begins at your left rear: that is, along Dorr Point, which is the southern arm of the shallow, usually placid harbor; then it runs along the concave rocky shore of the harbor to Ogden Point, which is the harbor's northern arm. Grassy, parklike Ogden Point is dotted with clumps of spruces and hardwood trees. Behind the point you can see the high eastern end of Bar Island. To the right of Bar Island and behind the *end* of Ogden Point is Sheep Porcupine Island; note the high granite "nose" on its eastern

---

The pebbly beach of **Compass Harbor** *(Walk No. 2). Spruce-topped Ogden Point is on the horizon on the left. Bald Porcupine Island is on the right.* ▶

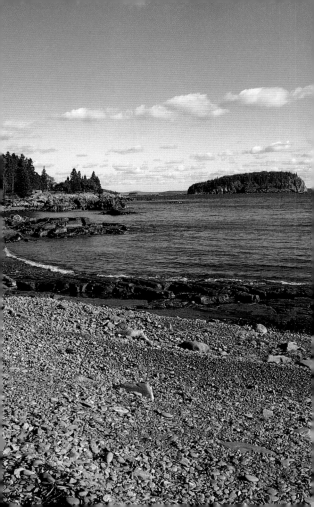

end. To the right of Sheep Porcupine, and much farther away, is Burnt Porcupine Island. To the right of Burnt Porcupine, and less than a mile away, is Bald Porcupine Island, its steep, bare rock sides echoed by the tall pointed spruces above them. A long, rocky breakwater extends from Bald Porcupine Island almost all the way to the mouth of Cromwell Cove, which is just on the other side of Ogden Point. The tiny island of Rumkey is between Burnt and Bald Porcupine islands; Long Porcupine Island is hidden behind Bald Porcupine. Six miles away, across Frenchman Bay, is Schoodic Peninsula (note the water tower). To the right of the peninsula, at the mouth of Frenchman Bay, is Egg Rock lighthouse. Far to your right and just a couple of hundred feet away is a tiny pebble beach.

When you're ready, retrace your steps to the clearing with the big white pine. From there you can make three side trips: to the pebble beach farther south, to the head of Compass Harbor and to the ruins of Dorr's mansion.

If you want to go to the beach, simply walk through the trees along the shore; you'll reach the beach in a minute.

To get to the head of the harbor, start walking back to the parking area. Less than 100 feet from the clearing you'll come to the trails you passed on your way in. Follow the path on the right through the woods at the edge of the harbor. Between the trees on your right you'll see the harbor's gray ledges and rocky beaches. On the horizon you'll see Ogden Point and Burnt and Bald Porcupine islands.

The path ends at a granite bench beside a small

grassy clearing. You're now on the grounds of Nannau, a handsome, weathered brown-shingled mansion built as a summer "cottage" for a wealthy family in 1904. The mansion, a couple of hundred feet from the shore, is now a bed-and-breakfast inn.

Because the inn is private, turn around here and retrace your steps to the clearing.

To reach the ruins of the Dorr estate, follow the faint path to the right of the big pine. You'll walk barely 150 feet before the trail curves to the right.

Suddenly, in the middle of the woods, you'll see a long flight of granite steps dead ahead. Follow the 42 steps up the slope to a brick-and-stone ruin. At the top of the steps are the remains of a terrace, its brick floor laid in a handsome herringbone pattern. When the trees were smaller you could see Frenchman Bay from here. Note the large rhododendrons—more remains of the original landscaping—on the south side of the ruin.

When you're ready to continue, find the path on the southwest side of the former terrace and follow it through the woods. In a few hundred feet the trail splits. Take the righthand fork and follow the path as it curves to the right.

You'll quickly come to the junction, about 300 feet from the parking area, that you passed on your way to Compass Harbor. Take a left and retrace your steps to your car.

3 The Ocean Trail

This undemanding four-mile round trip follows perhaps the most interesting two miles of seashore in Acadia National Park. Its almost uninterrupted views include Sand Beach, Great Head, Schoodic Peninsula, Western Point, Newport and Otter coves, the 30-foot-high sea stack in Monument Cove, the Beehive and Gorham, Dorr, Champlain and Cadillac mountains. You'll walk along the top of Otter Cliffs — the highest ocean-edge cliffs in the park — and pass the well-named Thunder Hole, where the surf booms as it crashes into a narrow tunnel in the coast ledge.

To get to the trailhead, take the Park Loop Road to Sand Beach, which is about nine miles south of the park Visitor Center in Hulls Cove (where the Loop Road starts) and about three miles south of the intersection of the Loop Road and Route 3 south of Bar Harbor. The path begins at the southern end of the parking lot closest to the Loop Road.

The first half of the Ocean Trail follows the shore side of the Loop Road. If you're in a hurry you can drive along this part of the shore and pick up the path

*Otter Cliffs at sunrise, seen from the **Ocean Trail** (Walk No. 3).* ▶

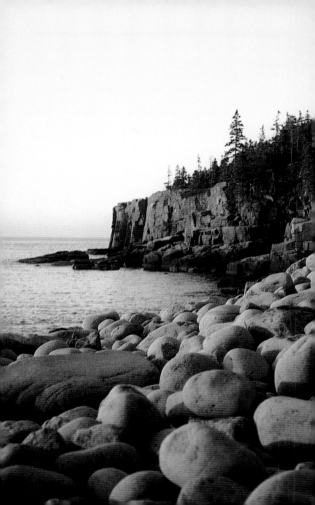

farther down the road. However, the sights, sounds and smells of the park are better on foot. One day we saw a deer in the spruce-and-pine woods on the other side of the road; no one in the passing cars seemed to notice it.

The path here is smooth gravel, mostly level and often just a few feet from the ocean. Short, well-worn side paths take you over the rough-chiseled ledges that are even closer to the sea. Low pitch pines and bayberry bushes grow between the ledges and, in the fall, dozens of eider ducks float on the swells below.

To your left you have long views of Sand Beach and the rockbound, evergreen-covered Great Head (Walk No. 4) on the other side of Newport Cove. Off the mouth of the cove is the low, wave-washed rock islet known (appropriately) as Old Soaker. To your right is 525-foot Gorham Mountain (Walk No. 11).

About .5 miles from Sand Beach you'll come to Thunder Hole. As a sign at the site explains, the thunderlike "boom" you hear is caused when waves rush into a long, narrow tunnel in the rock, sealing off and compressing the air inside. Thunder Hole makes the most noise on an incoming tide, about three hours after low tide. Check local newspapers for the tide schedule. Cement steps take you not only to the top of Thunder Hole but also to a waterside, observation platform from which you can see Sand Beach on your left, Otter Cliffs on your right and Schoodic Peninsula straight ahead.

In another 1,000 feet or so the trail passes tiny Monument Cove. Follow the very short side path to the overlook on the left of the trail. The beach below is composed of thousands of the smoothest rocks you'll ever see. Many look like huge eggs or giant peas. Also on the beach is a remarkable 30-foot-high column of rock, known as a sea stack, after which the cove is named. Sea stacks are carved by the surf from much larger pieces of rock and eventually they'll be worn away too.

Be alert for patches of poison ivy beside the trail as you approach another cove. When you reach this little bay, follow another very short side path to an overlook where you'll have a close view of Otter Cliffs.

About a mile from the trailhead the Loop Road moves slightly away from both the path and the shore and the trail heads into a cool, lush, shady spruce-and-fir grove. Ahead of you, on your left, Otter Cliffs loom 100 feet above the water. As you approach the cliffs, you can hear the crackle of waves breaking over stony beaches beneath you. As you get closer to the crest of the cliffs, very short side trails let you get close to the edge. (Approach carefully; there's no railing.) Peer cautiously over the edge of the cliffs (lying on your stomach) and you'll see stone beaches and white surf below. From this spot you can also see, to your far left, the ridges of Cadillac and Dorr mountains (Walk No. 19), the south ridge of Champlain Mountain (Walk No. 12), Gorham Mountain and the bare rock of the 520-foot Beehive. You can also look back to Sand Beach and Old Soaker and across to Great Head.

Now the path quickly reaches a small asphalt observation platform at the foot of a short flight of granite steps. After ascending the steps the trail passes between two low, concentric granite walls.

You're now about 120 feet above sea level, the highest point of the Walk. You can sometimes see ducks and cormorants diving in the ocean far below you and you'll hear the pleasant clang of a bell on a green buoy offshore. Turn around and you'll see Gorham and Champlain mountains and the Beehive.

The trail then switches back and forth down stone steps, closer to the ocean. Soon you'll pass, on your right, a bronze plaque that says: "These groves of spruce and fir, these granite ledges, the magnificent window on the sea, were given to the United States by John D. Rockefeller, Jr." (Actually you'll probably notice the plaque only on your return trip because it's easy to miss when you're walking the trail from north to south.)

The path quickly reaches Otter Point, a pleasant, grassy, spruce-shaded headland, just a few feet above the ocean, that seems to be made for picnicking, dawdling and nature watching. About 4.5 miles to the south is the half-mile-wide, 92-foot-high Baker Island. To the right of Baker are the flatter Cranberry Isles.

A vertical wooden post sign marks a short dirt road that connects the Ocean Trail to the Loop Road. Keep left at this junction and follow the path around the point to the narrow, mile-long Otter Cove. Here your view includes not only Baker and the Cranberry Isles but also Western Point, on the

A dusting of early morning snow on the Otter Cliffs and on the smooth stones of a beach along the **Ocean Trail** *(Walk No. 3).* ▶

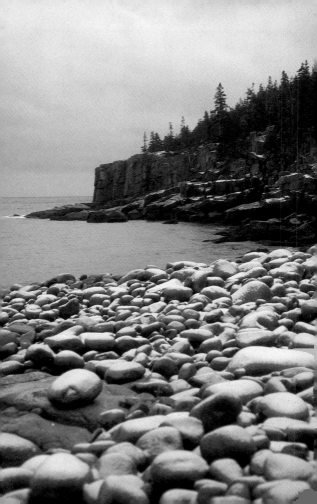

western shore of Otter Cove, and, on your right, the low triple-arched bridge on which the Loop Road crosses Otter Cove about .7 miles to the north. The Ocean Trail ends where stone steps go up to the Loop Road opposite the western entrance to the Otter Point parking area. From here you retrace your steps to your car. On your return trip, the light, the tide and especially your views will be different. You won't be seeing quite the same thing twice.

4 Sand Beach & Great Head

This undemanding Walk, barely a mile and a quarter long, offers stirring ocean and mountain views. You'll see the Beehive, Otter and Cadillac cliffs and Gorham Mountain across Newport Cove, Schoodic Peninsula across Frenchman Bay, the Egg Rock lighthouse, and Baker Island and Little Cranberry Island five miles offshore.

Sand Beach is often separated from Great Head peninsula by a tiny channel that links Newport Cove to the lagoon behind the beach. At high tide, this channel is usually too deep to cross without getting your feet wet. For the driest crossing, take this Walk when the tide is lowest. (Local newspapers publish tide tables.)

Like Walk No. 3, this outing begins at Sand Beach, which is on the Park Loop Road, about nine miles south of the park Visitor Center and about three miles south of the intersection of the Loop Road and Route 3, just south of Bar Harbor.

Park in the lower lot, the one closest to the ocean. Look back toward the Loop Road and you'll see the pink granite cliff of the Beehive rising above a forest of white birches. The steep eastern slope of Champlain Mountain (Walk No. 12) is to the right.

Walk to the southern end of the parking lot—the end closest to the sea—and start descending the granite steps to Sand Beach. A plaque near the top of the steps explains how the park's only sand beach was formed—it's a mixture of finely ground rock and a "high percentage of shell fragments and other remains of marine animals." The beach is popular for strolling, sunning, picnicking and sea watching but not for swimming: the water is *cold,* even in the summer.

The granite steps take you down to the western end of the 1,000-foot-long beach. From here you walk toward the Great Head peninsula, at the eastern end of the beach. You'll pass sand dunes and a rustic rail fence on your left. On your right is Newport Cove. On your far right are the Otter Cliffs on Otter Point (Walk No. 3). Just to the left of the point is Baker Island. At the mouth of the cove is the tiny rock island known as Old Soaker. Look behind you occasionally as you walk across the beach and you'll see, from left to right, Gorham Mountain (Walk No. 11) and Cadillac Cliffs on its lower slope; the Beehive and the near vertical east wall of Champlain Mountain.

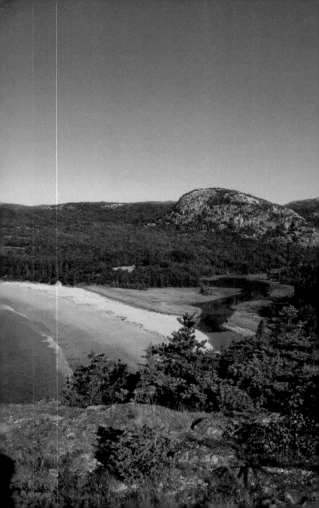

Soon you'll come to the channel separating the beach and the dunes from the Great Head peninsula. On your left you'll see up the narrow, sinuous, 1,000-foot-long lagoon, surrounded by marshes. On the other side of the channel is the post marking the Great Head Trail.

Cross the channel at its shallowest point. (If you can't cross without soaking your shoes and socks, take them off and cross barefoot. You don't want to walk in wet footwear.) Now walk up the granite steps behind the trail post and you'll come to a small grassy clearing. On your left you'll see a six-foot-wide mill-stone flat on the ground. On your right you'll see the beginnings of three trails.

The Great Head Trail is on the far right. It switches back and forth up the ledgy slope, through spruces and dwarf white birches. There's more ledge than bare earth here, so follow the discreet blue blazes to keep on the path.

After a few hundred feet the Great Head Trail splits. Follow the right fork (you'll return on the left one) and you'll quickly reach the top of the Great Head ridge. Here you'll have exhilarating views of the ocean on both sides of the trail. To your left (east) is Frenchman Bay and Schoodic Peninsula. On your right is a bird's-eye view of Sand Beach, the lagoon and Newport Cove. Opposite the cove are Gorham Mountain and the tall, ledgy hump of the Beehive.

Sand Beach, the lagoon and the steep, 520-foot hump known as the Beehive seen from **Great Head** *(Walk No. 4).*
◀

Frenchman Bay drops from sight as the trail leads to the southern edge of the peninsula, but there are uninterrupted views of Newport Cove, Gorham Mountain and Otter Point. The essence of the relentless beauty of this coast is its almost gross simplicity. This part of Mount Desert Island is neither delicate nor subtle. It's a rough, wild place where steep, bare granite rock and dark evergreen forests rise steeply out of a frothy sea.

As you reach the southern edge of Great Head, the surf gets rougher and higher. Waves turn to foam as they crash into the immense, jagged rock headlands and the pure white froth contrasts powerfully with the gray ledges. In the fall, flocks of eider ducks drift up and down on the swells.

Soon the trail reaches the highest point on Great Head, a 145-foot pinnacle near its southeastern shore. Here, on the stone ruins of a teahouse built by the wealthy Satterlee family, you can see the ocean in three directions. To the east, five miles across Frenchman Bay, is Schoodic Peninsula. In the mouth of the bay is Egg Rock lighthouse. To the north, on the edge of the bay, is Oak Hill Cliff; north of the cliff is Schooner Head. Still farther north are the Porcupine Islands off Bar Harbor. To the west, over low spruces, you can see, from right to left: Champlain Mountain, the Beehive, Gorham Mountain and Otter Point. The top of the long ridge of Cadillac Mountain (Walks No. 19 and 20) is on the horizon. To the south is Baker Island and, to the right of Baker, the eastern end of Little Cranberry Island.

From the teahouse ruins the path heads north,

away from the ocean and through scrub spruces and an elegant beech grove. In about 300 yards, when you just begin to glimpse the ocean again on your right, the trail splits. Take a left.

In another 300 yards or so the trail quickly climbs to the wide, flat top of the magnificent Great Head ridge. As you ascend the ridge, look behind you; you'll start to get wide views of Frenchman Bay. On the ridge itself you'll have exhilarating views of *both* sides of the peninsula. Stroll slowly through the scrub pines on this wonderful viewpoint. Make the experience last. If you have time, have a picnic.

As you start descending the west side of the peninsula, the path will rejoin the trail on which you climbed up the ridge. From here, retrace your steps to the parking area and enjoy the views of—and from—Sand Beach again.

5 Eagle Lake

This very easy 1.3-mile round trip presents a series of dramatic lake-and-mountain vistas from a smooth, nearly level carriage road. Across Eagle Lake—Mount Desert Island's second-largest body of fresh water after Long Pond (Walk No. 31)—you'll have continuing views of some of the island's highest peaks—Cadillac, Pemetic, Penobscot and Sargent mountains—as well as Conners Nubble and the North and South Bubbles.

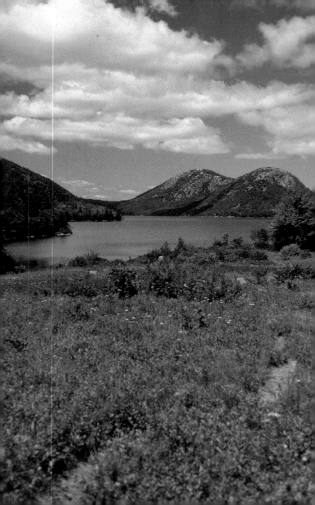

Carriage roads are popular bike routes and some cyclists will pass you at amazing speeds. Most will give you warning but it's still a good idea to look behind you before "changing lanes" (i. e., moving to the left or right).

The Walk begins at a parking area on the north side of Route 233, 2.3 miles west of the intersection of Routes 3 and 233 in Bar Harbor.

From the parking area you'll see, on the other side of Route 233, a tiny inlet in the northwestern end of Eagle Lake. On the horizon, across the two-mile-long lake, is a dramatic mountainscape. In the center is the haystack-shaped hump of 1,247-foot Pemetic Mountain (Walk No. 14), the park's fourth-highest peak. Left of Pemetic is the low valley of Bubble Pond (Walk No. 6) and rising steeply to the left of the valley is the western slope of 1,530-foot Cadillac Mountain (Walks No. 19 and 20), the park's highest summit. To the right of Pemetic is another low valley, Jordan Carry; to the right of the valley are the steep eastern slopes of the Bubbles (Walks No. 17 and 18).

From the west side of the parking area a short path takes you immediately to a carriage road, which crosses Route 233 under a large, handsome stone-arch bridge, one of 17 such structures on the carriage

The twin peaks of the **Bubbles** *(Walks No. 17 and 18) seen from the blueberry fields on the southern end of* **Jordan Pond** *(Walk No. 7).*
◄

roads. Follow the carriage road under Route 233. On the other side of the highway take a left onto another carriage road and you'll immediately come to the head of the inlet you saw from the parking area. Now you'll have a closer view of the peaks and valleys you saw earlier.

Walk past the inlet and the wooded point to the east of it and you'll quickly come to a boat-launch area. Here your view is even wider. You can see everything you saw before, plus the tops of the 766-foot South Bubble and the wider, higher 872-foot North Bubble; 1,194-foot Penobscot Mountain (Walk No. 15), the park's fifth-highest peak, behind the Bubbles; and the higher, longer ridge of 1,373-foot Sargent Mountain (Walk No. 16), the park's second-highest summit, on the right. If the light is right, you'll also see the ledgy knob of the 588-foot Conners Nubble (Walk No. 18), whose steep sides appear to rise almost straight out of the lake below Penobscot Mountain. You may also see Bubble Rock on the horizon, just left of the summit of the South Bubble, and you'll probably see cars going up the road to the top of Cadillac Mountain.

The road passes through trees and quickly comes to a third viewpoint. Then it runs through still more trees before coming to a fourth clearing, where you can see even more of Sargent Mountain, on the right.

After passing through more woods the road reaches yet another clearing. Here a side road goes to the right and in about 100 feet brings you to a small brick building beside a dam at the edge of Eagle Lake. The lake is Bar Harbor's water supply; the brick building is the Bar Harbor Water Company's pumping station. The wide stream that begins at the dam is Duck Brook; it flows into Frenchman Bay just north of Bar Harbor.

After you've enjoyed the view from this spot, go back to the carriage road and follow it again into the woods. You'll cross Duck Brook almost immediately and catch still more views of the mountains through the trees.

Then the road curves to the right, around the northeast corner of the lake, and you'll have another vista across the water. But now you can see only Sargent Mountain to the east, the low, rounded 724-foot McFarland Mountain, northwest of the lake, and the brick pumping station on your right.

Turn around here and head back toward your car. When you reach the boat-launch area, you can keep following the road back to your car or you can follow the well-worn .1-mile path that runs along the shore toward the inlet at the northwestern end of the lake. The trail runs over wide, flat waterside ledges that are ideal for resting, sunning, picnicking and view gazing. Then it reenters the woods and rejoins the carriage road just east of the inlet. From there you can take a left and follow the road back to your car.

6 Bubble Pond

This very easy and dramatic 1.6-mile round trip follows a nearly level carriage road along the shore of Bubble Pond, which lies at the bottom of a long, narrow gorge. It provides uninterrupted views of the pond and the precipitous slopes of Cadillac and Pemetic mountains, which rise steeply from its shores. You'll also see surging cascades and a placid, gardenlike pool in the pond's outlet.

Like all carriage roads, this route is used by bicyclists. Remember to keep alert for them when they pass.

The Walk begins at the Bubble Pond parking area, on the east side of the Park Loop Road, about 2.5 miles south of the intersection of the Loop Road and Route 233 and about 2.5 miles north of the Jordan Pond parking area.

From the southern end of the parking lot, follow the short asphalt path that curves down to the northern tip of the pond. Here you'll have a dramatic view: On your left, the steep side of Cadillac Mountain (Walks No. 19 and 20) plunges into the pond's east shore. On your right, the even steeper slope of Pemetic Mountain (Walk No. 14) rises abruptly from the west shore. Straight ahead, at the southern end of the pond, is the deep, narrow notch formed by both peaks.

Little Long Pond *(Walk No. 8) is framed by carefully mowed fields, by the south ridge of* **Penobscot Mountain** *(Walk No. 15) and by the top of the* **Bubbles** *(Walks No. 17 and 18) (rear). David Rockefeller's boathouse (right) is a focal point.* ▶

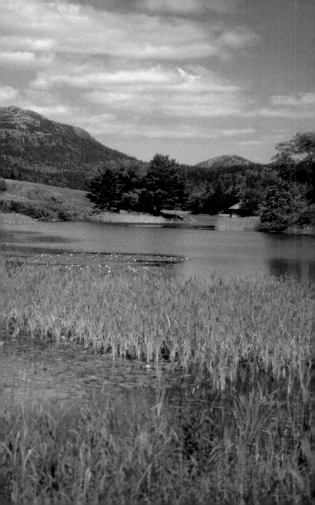

After you've savored this view, start walking to your right, along the shore. You'll immediately pass a post marking the Pemetic Mountain Trail.

Keep following the path along the pond. Less than .1 miles from the post the path joins the carriage road, which you'll follow along the entire length of the .7-mile-long tarn.

So close do the slopes of Pemetic Mountain come to the pond that the road has no choice but to hug the water. Sometimes your feet are only inches from the gently lapping waves. So smooth and level is the road, so soothing are the sounds of the pond that the Walk is one of the most relaxing in the park.

As the road ever so gradually bends to the right, past cedars growing on the shore, more and more of the pond slowly comes into view. On your right, through the trees, you can see some of the thousands of rocks that have tumbled down Pemetic Mountain. On your left, across the 500-foot-wide pond, you can see the precipitous lower slopes of Cadillac, so steep that rock slides have covered some of the ledge.

About .7 miles from the parking area, near the southern end of the pond, the road starts to climb away from the tarn. At this point look for an unmarked path on the left that takes you along the pond's flat, grassy southern shore. Start following the path and you'll quickly cross several tiny brooks flowing into the pond. Soon after that you'll have a close view of the pink granite boulders in a large landslide on the eastern shore. You'll also see a dramatic view up the pond: the ledges and cliffs of the almost-vertical-looking slope of Pemetic Mountain on the left, the steep face of Cadillac on the right and, in between, the low notch between the two summits at the northern end of the tarn.

When you're ready, turn around and walk back toward the parking area. When you reach the northern end of the pond, keep walking toward Cadillac Mountain and you'll immediately come to the outlet of the tarn—at this point a long, placid, gardenlike pool dotted with low, wide, smooth rocks.

Cross the pool on the wooden footbridge and follow the outlet downstream. You'll quickly come to a handsome dam made of huge granite blocks. The brook plunges over the dam in a frothy fall, four feet wide and three feet high. Then it surges between craggy ledges and rushes down a steep glen before disappearing under a bridge on the Loop Road.

After you've enjoyed this entertaining water show, follow the path back to your car. On your way, take another look at the view from the northern edge of Bubble Pond.

7 Jordan Pond

Probably the best pond-side Walk in the park is the undemanding, mostly level 3.6-mile path that takes you all around the unspoiled 1.3-mile-long Jordan Pond. The trail is always close to, if not actually on, the very edge of the water and the pond is surrounded by the steep slopes of five different promontories: the twin peaks of the Bubbles and the long ridges of

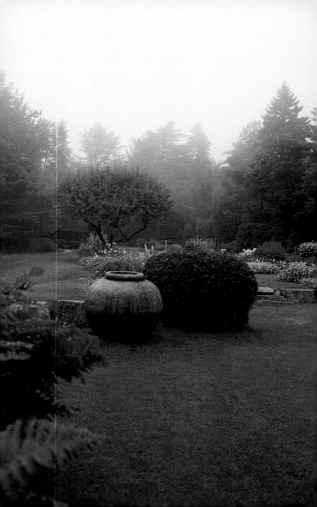

Pemetic, Penobscot and Sargent mountains. You'll also have close views of Jordan Cliffs and the rock slide known as the Tumbledown.

Parts of the trail go over rock slides and tree roots. This excursion is still a Great Walk, however, because the rocky and rooty sections are neither long nor strenuous—just slow and sometimes picky—and they're outweighed by the otherwise pleasant trail and fine views.

The Walk begins at the Jordan Pond parking area, which is on the west side of the Park Loop Road, eight miles from the park Visitor Center at Hulls Cove, five miles from Bar Harbor, and just north of Jordan Pond House (see below). The Loop Road has several good views of Jordan Pond and Eagle Lake (Walk No. 5), both of which are below and just to the west of the road.

The trailhead is on the western side of the second (westernmost) parking lot. A trail sign here says the "boat ramp" is straight ahead. Go straight and in about 200 yards you'll come to Jordan Pond.

At the shore you'll see the flat, steep face of Penobscot Mountain (Walk No. 15) directly ahead of you, on the west side of the pond. To your right, at

*A cement urn created by the sculptor Eric Soderholtz is a focal point in the **Thuya Garden** seen on a misty day. The garden and the adjacent **Asticou Terraces** are on Walk No. 9.*
◀

the northern end of the pond, you'll see one of Acadia's most famous views: the twin rounded peaks of the Bubbles (Walks No. 17 and 18). Legend has it that the Bubbles were named by a fellow who thought they reminded him of his girlfriend Bubbles; because this is a family publication, we'll leave it at that. You'll keep seeing these steep, miniature mountains after you take the path to your right, which goes counterclockwise around the pond. From here until the end of the Walk, your directions are the same (and rather what you might expect): *Take a left at every trail junction.*

You'll come to your first junction in less than .2 miles and very soon after that you'll cross a marshy cove on a low stone causeway. On the other side of the causeway the trail splits again (remember: go left).

Now the trail is at its best. It hugs the edge of the pond, so you'll enjoy constant views of the water and the pleasant sound of tiny waves lapping the rocky shore. The path is smooth, and carefully placed rocks and log cribs keep the trail level and your feet dry.

Soon you'll be able to see Jordan Pond House, at the southern end of the pond. On the west side you can see the rock slide known as the Tumbledown on the slope of Penobscot Mountain and the carriage road that runs through it. Above the Tumbledown are Jordan Cliffs.

After slightly more than a mile of easy walking you'll come to yet another intersection. Then you'll pass under the steep slopes and cliffs of the Bubbles, on your right. The young white birches here are lovely (but watch out for poison ivy on your right).

Next the trail crosses a rock slide. For the easiest passage, step carefully from one rock to another.

Then, to the right of Penobscot Mountain, you'll see the steep slope of Sargent Mountain (Walk No. 16) rising from the northwestern edge of the pond. (Keep an eye out for another patch of poison ivy on your left.)

In a few minutes more you'll be at the pond's northernmost point. After passing another trail junction (keep left, as usual), turn around for a view of the evergreen-festooned rock cliffs of the Bubbles on your left and behind you, and the steep slopes of Penobscot and Sargent mountains on your right.

The trail then passes a long beach and crosses a marshy cove on handsome log bridges. Look for the beaver lodge on your right.

After reaching the west side of the pond you'll pass yet another trail junction (keep left). On the opposite side of the pond you'll see the Bubbles. To the right of the Bubbles and above the Loop Road are the cliffs of Pemetic Mountain (Walk No. 14).

Now the trail becomes less easy. First it will be rocky in places, then it will cross the rocks of the Tumbledown. As you cross the rocks, look to your right, high above the carriage road, and you'll see Jordan Cliffs.

After passing better and better views of the Bubbles rising dramatically out of the pond, the trail runs through a shady grove of young and old spruce trees. You'll be stepping over roots here for a bit but soon you'll be walking on a smooth boardwalk made of parallel pairs of split logs, flat sides up. The boardwalk will take you over both roots and wet areas almost all the way back to the southern end of the pond.

After rounding a bend, you'll see the gray Jordan Pond House on a small hill.

In a few more minutes you'll pass a concrete dam and spillway on the southern end of the pond. Here the trail crosses a carriage road. Take a left on the road and cross an imposing stone-arch bridge over the spillway, which is the beginning of Jordan Stream. (As on all carriage roads, keep an eye out for bicyclists.) On the other side of the bridge, follow the path that leaves the carriage road on the left and curves along the south shore of the pond. You'll have another view of the Bubbles on your left and you'll see Jordan Pond House on your right. In another couple of hundred feet ahead the path returns to the boat ramp, where the Walk began.

Travel Tip: Instead of returning to your starting point, walk up to Jordan Pond House and, depending on the time of day, enjoy either lunch, "afternoon tea" or dinner at one of the island's best restaurants. Afternoon tea—which, like all Jordan Pond House meals, features its renowned trademark hot popovers—is served on green-topped wooden tables on the lawn, where you can enjoy the classic view of the pond and the Bubbles behind it. A National Park concession operated by the Acadia Corporation, Jordan Pond House also has public restrooms, a snack shop and an excellent gift shop.

8 Little Long Pond

This very easy one-mile round trip, over an

unusually pleasant, wide grassy path, offers a look at landscaping in the grand manner. You can also visit David Rockefeller's boathouse and picnic on the mowed fields beside the pond.

Little Long Pond is on the north side of Route 3 in Seal Harbor, exactly .7 miles west of the intersection of Route 3 and the park road to Jordan Pond. The pond isn't marked but you can see it from Route 3. It's separated from Bracy Cove by a narrow neck of land that's traversed by Route 3 and by a stone seawall on the south side of the highway. There's no parking area—you have to park beside the pond.

Seen from the highway, the pond site is a lovely pastoral composition. In the center is the .6-mile-long pond, its long axis perpendicular to the road and its shoreline accented by reeds and trees as it undulates into the distance. The pond is framed by mowed fields sloping down to the water. Surrounding the fields are dark green forests. In the distance, looming over the entire scene, are, from left to right, the southern slope of Penobscot Mountain (Walk No. 15), the two smaller round humps of the Bubbles (Walks No. 17 and 18) and the equally curvy southern ridge of Pemetic Mountain (Walk No. 14). Tucked into the eastern shore of the pond is a focal point: Rockefeller's simple brown-shingled boathouse.

On the north side of the road, near the southwest corner of the pond, you'll see a row of widely spaced boulders beside the road. On the other side of the rocks is a wide path. Start following the path and you'll quickly come to a red-and-white painted metal sign. The sign omits the name Rockefeller, saying instead that the "owner" has allowed public access to the property only for quiet sorts of recreation (such as walking) and that camping, fires and noisier means of transportation are prohibited without his consent. The Rockefellers, who donated about a third of what is now Acadia National Park, no longer use the property and are happy to have the public benefit from it instead. David Rockefeller is preserving the character of the site by maintaining the boathouse and by keeping the fields mowed.

From the sign you can see a carriage path on your left, one of many built by David Rockefeller's father, John D., Jr. Notice its substantial granite abutment and imagine how much money John D. must have lavished on the more than 50 miles of these roads.

You may also see a path leading toward the western shore of the pond. Don't take either the path or the carriage road to the left. Instead, follow the carriage road across the southern end of the pond (parallel to Route 3), then follow a grassy path curving to the left, through the field along the southeastern shore. The path quickly joins a grassy road, which soon takes you to the boathouse.

The doors are locked but you can peer through the windows at the changing rooms and the small, well-built wooden rowboat inside. Gaze over the pond at the fields and forests beyond and at the small beaches on both sides of the boathouse and imagine: You're walking on the Rockefellers' private porch beside their private pond. In fact, you're welcome to do exactly that and to picnic as well. Just be sure to clean up when you're done. Little Long Pond is little known (except by people who've lived in the area for a while) so you'll usually find hardly anyone here. On some days you'll be all alone and it will be *your* private beach and picnic spot.

You can follow the smooth, level, mown-grass road for another quarter-mile before it ends at a carriage road. The pond will be close on your left and the woods will be on your right as you enjoy one of the softest, gentlest paths on all of Mount Desert Island.

When you reach the carriage road, turn around and retrace your steps to your car.

9 The Asticou Terraces & the Thuya Garden

This easy mile-long round trip takes you to two adjacent but very different works of landscape design: the naturalistic Asticou Terraces, created by the Boston landscape architect Joseph Henry Curtis, and the Thuya Garden, designed by the businessman and talented amateur landscape designer Charles K. Savage.

The Walk begins on Route 3 in Northeast Harbor, less than .5 miles southeast of the junction of Route 3 and Route 3 and 198. A red-lettered sign marks a parking lot on the west (ocean) side of Route 3. On the other side of the road a discreet carved wood-and-stone sign says "Asticou Terraces." The

sign marks the beginning of a very smooth stone-
and-gravel path that gently switches back and forth
100 feet up the steep slope of the spruce-forested
hillside.

The Terraces are a near masterpiece of naturalistic landscaping, moving in both their simplicity and
their subtlety. The simplicity results from the use of
just a few materials: granite stones for the steps and
paths, native shrubs such as blueberries and sheep
laurel for understory plants and spruce trees for the
rest. The Terraces are subtle not only because all the
materials are natural to the site but, more important,
because the line between the natural and the man-
made is invisible. You may wonder: Was the site
originally all spruce? It could easily have been. Or
did Curtis have to take out some other species to
create the unity of the tree monoculture? Were these
ferns here or did Curtis move them? On some pav-
ings you're not sure which stones were already in
place, which are part of the ledge and which were
added. So delicate were Curtis's additions that it's
hard to tell. The Terraces are woodland landscaping
at its best: not the creation of a garden from scratch
but the subtle amending of an existing natural site to
improve it, transforming it from mere woods into a
woodland garden.

You'll barely start your walk when you'll see a path
on your left marked by a sign saying "Curtis Memorial." The path takes you to a 30-by-60-foot oval
terrace paved with granite fieldstones and ringed
with blueberries and sheep laurel. On the ocean side
of the terrace you can see the sailboat-filled Northeast Harbor. On your left, on the face of a 20-foot-

high cliff, is a bronze memorial to Curtis, with his bearded profile in relief and the notation that these terraces "are his gift for the quiet recreation of the people of this town and their summer guests."

Walking past the memorial, take a left at two intersections and you'll quickly climb to a handsome fieldstone gazebo. Inside you'll find three rustic wooden benches from which you can enjoy a view of Northeast Harbor. Like everything else on the Terraces, the gazebo honors the principle of unity in design. It blends into its site because it's made of the same granite fieldstones as the paths leading to it, and its pleasing hip roof appears to be made of the same wood as the benches beneath it. The gazebo also honors Frank Lloyd Wright's commandment that a building be not only *on* a site but *of* it.

Retrace your steps to where you took your second left and continue straight ahead. The path quickly takes you to a smaller, rustic, all-wood gazebo near the crest of the hill, which also overlooks the harbor.

From here the path leads you over a charming, moss-banked streamlet on a low rock bridge, over gray granite ledges, past juniper and blueberry bushes, then over a series of low steps made of wooden cribs filled with crushed pink granite. Behind you, through the trees, you'll have more views of Northeast Harbor.

The path ends at Thuya Lodge, Joseph Curtis's blue-gray, wood-framed summer home. (Thuya is the phonetic spelling of *thuja,* the scientific name for cedar, which grows abundantly on Mount Desert Island.) Like the Terraces and the Thuya Garden, the Lodge is now the property of the town of Mount

Desert. Inside you'll find a large horticultural library, a bathroom and a solicitous guide who'll cheerfully answer your questions. The building is open July 1 through Labor Day. Admission is free.

The Thuya Garden, which is open July through September, is next to the Lodge. Unlike the Terraces, the one-acre garden is rather formal: a rolling, well-manicured lawn is the setting for large, straight-sided beds of mostly perennial flowers. Along the edges of the garden, which is surrounded by forest, are informal settings of trees, shrubs and shade-loving ground covers.

After you've toured the garden, retrace your steps down the Terraces and back to your car. For the shortest route stay left at all trail intersections: don't go right to the gazebos or the Curtis Memorial.

If, perchance, you'd like to *drive* to the Thuya Garden, head south on Route 3 from the Terraces parking area and take the first road on your left, about .2 miles from the parking area. The road will bring you to the Thuya Lodge in about .3 miles.

10 The Asticou Azalea Garden

This quarter-mile stroll—easily the shortest, gentlest Great Walk on Mount Desert Island—follows smooth, level paths through a well-designed 2.3-acre naturalistic garden. The paths wind along and across a brook, past Japanese-style sand gardens, around a wide pond, beneath evergreen trees and through about 50 varieties of azaleas, 20 types of rhododendrons, a large number of ferns and mosses, and other trees, shrubs and ground covers.

The garden entrance is about 100 yards north of the intersection of Route 3 and Route 3 and 198 in Northeast Harbor, and about .5 miles from the Asticou Terraces and the Thuya Garden (Walk No. 9). You can see the garden on the north side of Route 3.

Although Charles K. Savage designed both the Thuya Garden and this one, the two designs are quite different. Unlike the more formal Thuya Garden, the Azalea Garden has no flowerbeds and very little lawn.

The azaleas and rhododendrons in the garden were taken from Reef Point in Bar Harbor, the former estate of the landscape architect Beatrix Farrand. The Azalea Garden began in the mid-1950s when, with financial help from John D. Rockefeller, Jr., Savage acquired and graded the site, purchased the shrubs and replanted them here.

Today the garden is maintained by the Island Foundation. It's open during daylight hours from April 1 to October 1 and admission is free. Many of its species are discreetly labeled and knowledgeable guides can answer your questions.

The best time to see the azaleas bloom is usually the last two weeks of June. The peak rhododendron and mountain laurel bloom is usually in early July.

Travel Tip: The Azalea Garden is only about 200 feet west of the Asticou Inn, on Route 3. The inn is a well-appointed turn-of-the-century accommodation made even more elegant by its age. The Asticou deck, which provides a fine view of Northeast Harbor, is a good place for an alfresco lunch, a la carte or a well-presented buffet complete with squid salad and opulent desserts.

11 Gorham Mountain

This undemanding 1.8-mile round trip is the quickest and easiest way to see how glorious an Acadian mountain walk can be. After just a few minutes of gentle walking, you'll reach open ledges, where you'll have close, continuous views of the southeastern coast of Mount Desert Island. You'll see Otter Cove and Otter Cliffs on Otter Point, Western Point, the Cranberry Isles, Sand Beach, Great Head, Newport Cove, Old Soaker, Frenchman Bay, Schoodic Peninsula, the Egg Rock lighthouse, Schooner Head, Otter Creek, the Tarn, the Beehive, Huguenot Head and Cadillac, Dorr and Champlain mountains.

The Walk begins in the southwest corner of the Gorham Mountain parking area, which is on the right (west) side of the one-way Park Loop Road, about one mile south of Sand Beach and about five miles south of the intersection of the Loop Road and Route 3 south of Bar Harbor.

The trail climbs gently past white birches and low spruces and pitch pines and over smooth ledges ringed with blueberry, sheep laurel and bayberry bushes. Some of these ledges are as pretty as rock gardens.

Less than .2 miles from the trailhead you'll start glimpsing the ocean through the trees on your right.

A few hundred feet farther the trail reaches a huge pink granite boulder. Attached to the rock is a handsome bronze plaque saying: "Waldron Bates/pathmaker/1856-1909." The plaque honors the man who built many of Mount Desert Island's trails.

At this point the trail splits. The right fork goes to the bottom of Cadillac Cliffs, on the east slope of the mountain (a rough trail with no views). The left fork heads to the summit.

Go left. Almost immediately after the trail junction, and only a few minutes from the trailhead, you'll reach open ledges with wide views. To the south is Otter Cove (Walk No. 3). On the west side of the cove is Western Point; on the east side is Otter Point. Farther to the south, across Eastern Way, are the Cranberry Isles. To the east is the broad Frenchman Bay.

Walk just a few feet more and you'll see Schoodic Peninsula across Frenchman Bay and more of the ocean behind you. Then, on your right, you'll see Sand Beach and, to the right of the beach, the ledge-tipped peninsula of Great Head (Walk No. 4). Beyond Great Head, in Frenchman Bay, is the orange-and-white lighthouse on Egg Rock.

A few feet ahead you'll see the rock island known as Old Soaker in the mouth of Newport Cove. Behind Old Soaker is the water tower on Schoodic Peninsula. To your rear are Otter Cliffs on the east side of Otter Point (Walk No. 3).

The trail now runs along the top of Cadillac Cliffs. You're about 400 feet above the ocean but less than 1,500 feet from it and you have a 180-degree view — from Otter Point to upper Frenchman Bay. You also have near-bird's-eye vistas of the sea undulating in and out of an unspoiled spruce-and-rock covered coast. You can hear the ringing of the bell on the green buoy off Otter Point and you can see flocks of eider ducks riding the swells. Ahead of you is Gorham's ledgy summit.

About .5 miles from the trailhead, the path to Cadillac Cliffs returns to the Gorham Mountain trail on your right. Go straight ahead toward the summit.

In another .1 miles you'll climb up a ledge with another ocean view. Now you'll see the ocean on both sides of Otter Point and the low Cranberry Isles beyond it. On your left you'll have your first look at the long south ridge of Cadillac Mountain (Walk No. 20).

As you climb farther up the wide, open ledge your views get better and better. In the valley between Gorham and Cadillac mountains, on your left, you'll see houses in the village of Otter Creek. Above the village, on the steep east face of Cadillac, is the cliff known as Eagles Crag. To the right of Cadillac is the lower, 1,270-foot Dorr Mountain, the island's third-highest peak. On your right you'll see surf crashing against the ledges on the east side of the Loop Road, almost 500 feet below. Behind you are Cadillac

Cliffs. In the south, to the right of Otter Point, you again see Otter Cove.

As you climb easily toward the summit, past shrub-size evergreens, you'll see the ledgy hump of the 520-foot Beehive rising just to the left of Frenchman Bay. To the left of the Beehive is the south ridge of 1,058-foot Champlain Mountain (Walk No. 12). To the right of the Beehive are large, handsome houses on Schooner Head (which is outside the park) and surf crashing against the rocky point. You'll also have a 200-degree ocean view, stretching from the west, to the Cranberry Isles, to the northern reaches of Frenchman Bay.

About .9 miles from the trailhead you'll reach the summit. Except for blueberry bushes and low evergreens, it's a bare, flat ledge with views in every direction. Now you can see the triple-arch bridge over Otter Cove and the tiny pond known as the Tarn in the long valley between Dorr and Champlain mountains. To the right of the Tarn, 731-foot Huguenot Head peeks above the western slope of Champlain.

Walk past the summit and you'll have even closer views of Cadillac, Dorr and Champlain mountains, as well as the creased ledges of the Beehive and the valley to the south of it.

When you're ready, turn around and follow the path back to your car—and enjoy Gorham's remarkable views again as you walk "into" many of them on your way down the mountain.

12
Champlain Mountain

This moderate three-mile round trip up Mount Desert Island's easternmost major summit offers close, almost continuous views of coastal landmarks. You'll see Bar Harbor, Beaver Dam Pond, Frenchman Bay, the Porcupine Islands, the Egg Rock lighthouse, the Thrumcap, Schoodic Peninsula, Great Head, Sand Beach, the Beehive, Otter Point, Otter Cove and Southwest Harbor. You'll also see five mountains — Dorr, Cadillac, Kebo, Gorham and Halfway — as well as Huguenot Head and two little lakes, the Tarn and the Bowl.

Champlain Mountain is named for the man who named Mount Desert Island: the French explorer Samuel de Champlain (see pages 71-72).

The easiest way up its 1,058-foot summit is via the scenic Bear Brook Trail, which gently ascends Champlain's north ridge. The trail begins on the Park Loop Road, about .5 miles east of where it runs under Route 3 about two miles south of downtown Bar Harbor. Almost immediately after going under

The pond's mirror-smooth surface reflects the evergreens in the **Asticou Azalea Garden** *(Walk No. 10).* ▶

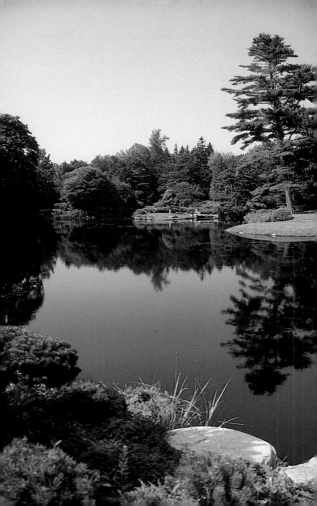

Route 3 you'll pass the Bear Brook Picnic Area on your left, then Beaver Dam Pond on your right (yes, there usually *is* a beaver dam here—right beside the road). Then, just before an overlook of Frenchman Bay on your left, you'll see the small brown-and-white Bear Brook Trail sign on your right. Park at the overlook, cross the road (keeping an eye out for traffic) and begin the Walk.

The smooth path, marked with blazes and cairns, immediately climbs over sunny granite ledges fringed with low birches and pines. Right away you'll get your first view: the steep, ledgy west slope of 1,270-foot Dorr Mountain, the park's third-highest summit, on your right, and, left of Dorr, the rounded summit of 731-foot Huguenot Head, actually a shoulder of Champlain. Just a little bit farther ahead on the path you'll see Frenchman Bay.

As you climb higher and higher your vistas get better and better. Soon you'll see the rocky, spruce-coated humps of the Porcupine Islands off Bar Harbor (Walk No. 1); then Bar Island; then Schoodic Peninsula, on the other side of Frenchman Bay; then the low, 407-foot Kebo Mountain, to the right of Dorr; Great Meadow, below Dorr and Kebo; Beaver Dam Pond and more and more of Bar Harbor. (The only flaws in this otherwise wonderful view are the boxy beige buildings of the Jackson Laboratories, south of Bar Harbor. Try to look the other way and pretend the buildings aren't there.)

The trail is now very pleasant, alternating between smooth gravel paths and wide, smooth ledges as it passes blueberry bushes, pitch pines and spruces.

Very soon you'll come to a ledgy outcrop, where you have an even better view of the ocean. Now you can see more of both Frenchman Bay and the eastern coast of Mount Desert Island, including Schooner Head, to the south; the lighthouse on Egg Rock; the tiny, grass-topped rock island known as the Thrumcap, just offshore, and dozens of white boats dotting the bay.

About halfway up the mountain you'll reach a trail junction. The left fork goes down the steep eastern side of the mountain. The right fork goes to the summit. Take a right—but before you do, turn around and savor the more-than-200-degree panorama, which ranges from Dorr Mountain on your left to the long, slender Schoodic Peninsula and the low islands around it.

As you gradually ascend the spine of the ridge, you'll be climbing farther and farther above the islands and boats in Frenchman Bay. Soon you'll be able to see right up the middle of Main Street in Bar Harbor.

After passing through birches and pines, you'll emerge on sweeping ledges, bare except for a low decoration of handsome scrub pines, sheep laurel, blueberry bushes and other low shrubs. Large two- and three-foot-high cairns now guide your way. Here you'll have a continuous vista of nearly 270 degrees that extends from the summit of Cadillac Mountain (Walk No. 19), west of Dorr, to the mouth of Frenchman Bay. At least 180 degrees of the view is blue ocean.

About a mile from the Loop Road you reach the bare summit, where the ocean view alone is 270

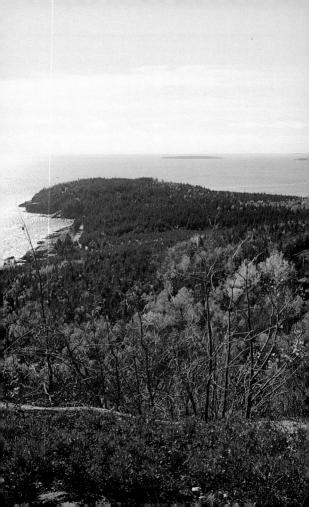

degrees—from Eastern Bay, on the north side of the island, down the eastern shore of the island, past the mansions on Schooner Head Road, to Southwest Harbor and the long, low islands off the southern coast. To the west is the long green ridge of Cadillac Mountain and the more ledgy slope of Dorr. Look carefully and you can see tiny people on top of Cadillac.

After you've enjoyed this remarkable view, take the trail to the Bowl, which goes along the top of Champlain's south ridge.

As you amble across the long, wide, flat ledge of the ridge, more and more landmarks will come into view. Soon, to the left of the trail and about a mile away, you'll see the bare 546-foot-high rock hump of the Beehive. Left of the Beehive is the peninsula of Great Head (Walk No. 4). Right of the Beehive, and almost straight ahead, is Otter Cove (Walk No. 3). Otter Point is on the left side of the cove, Western Point on the right. Then you'll see 525-foot Gorham Mountain (Walk No. 11), north of Otter Point, and Halfway Mountain, north of Gorham and just to the right of the Beehive.

As you walk farther among the low pitch pines, which turn the ledges into a natural rock garden, you'll also see Sand Beach (Walk No. 4) and the

---

Otter Point seen from **Gorham Mountain** *(Walk No. 11). Otter Cliffs are to the left of the point. Baker Island is in the distance; Little Cranberry Island is to the right. In the fall, blueberry bushes on the sunny ledges are bright red.*
◄

sinuous, grassy banks of the mirror-smooth lagoon behind it.

After passing through more pines, you'll get your first look at the Bowl, a tiny tarn in a hollow between the Beehive and Champlain and Halfway mountains.

Keep following the trail down a small dip and back up to a shoulder of the ridge. Now take a few steps to your right, to the western edge of the ridge, and look north. You'll see up the long, steep pass that separates Dorr and Champlain mountains and the narrow little sheet of water in the bottom of the valley called (appropriately) the Tarn. You'll also see the flanks of Huguenot Head to the right of the Tarn. Now walk to the other (east) side of the ridge and you'll see the Egg Rock lighthouse and Schoodic Peninsula.

By now you've walked about .5 miles from the summit and you've enjoyed the best views Champlain has to offer. Turn around here, retrace your steps to your car and enjoy these remarkable vistas again on your way back.

13 Day Mountain

This undemanding 1.8-mile round trip, up one of Mount Desert Island's lowest mountains, offers sweeping views in every direction. You'll see many landmarks, including the Triad, the Beehive, Jordan Cliffs, Frenchman

Bay, Schoodic Peninsula, the Cranberry Isles, Seal Harbor and Somes Sound, as well as Gorham, Champlain, Cadillac, Pemetic, Penobscot, Cedar Swamp, Norumbega, Eliot and Western mountains.

The Walk begins in a parking area on the south side of Route 3, about a mile east of Seal Harbor and about 1.5 miles west of Otter Creek. The parking area has no sign, but it's on the ocean side of the road, about 50 feet east of the height of land, or divide, on the south slope of Day Mountain. From the parking area you can look east and see the Beehive, on the left, the ridge of Gorham Mountain (Walk No. 11) and the mouth of Frenchman Bay.

The trail is on the north side of the road; it's marked by a wooden post indicating that Day's summit is .8 miles away and that the Champlain Monument is to the right.

Take the 100-foot path to the monument and you'll quickly come to a four-foot-high granite rock set on a wide, blueberry-festooned ledge about 20 feet above Route 3. You can see the ocean, nearly 200 feet below and about half a mile away. A plaque on the rock explains that the monument was created "in honor of Samuel de Champlain," the French explorer "who gave the island its name." Another plaque, on the back of the rock, quotes a passage from Champlain's journal. On September 5, 1604, he wrote that his ship "passed...near an island" that was "very high" and "notched in places, so as to appear from the sea like a range of seven or eight mountains close together. The summits of most of them are bare of trees for they are nothing but rock.... I named it the island of the desert mountains." A third plaque says the memorial was erected by the Seal Harbor Village Improvement Society in 1904—the 300th anniversary of both Champlain's voyage and the naming of *L'Isle de Mont-deserts,* or Mount Desert Island.

When you're ready, walk back to the Day Mountain trail and follow the nearly level, slightly rooty path toward the summit. In a few hundred feet you'll come to a trail junction. The short trail on the left (marked by a sign saying "Icy Hill") comes out on Route 3 just west of the height of land. Keep going straight on the Day Mountain trail, which starts climbing very gently, mostly over smooth ledges.

About .2 miles from Route 3 the path reaches the junction of two broad gravel carriage roads. Go right on the first one you come to (it's perpendicular to the trail). Then take an immediate left onto another, 50-foot-long road, which links the first carriage road to the second. Follow the short road to the second carriage road and take a right. Almost immediately you'll see the trail on the left, about 70 feet from

The four Porcupine Islands in Frenchman Bay seen from the north ridge of **Champlain Mountain** *(Walk No. 12), Mount Desert's closest major summit to the ocean. From left to right: Sheep Porcupine Island, Burnt Porcupine, Bald Porcupine (in front of Burnt Porcupine) and Long Porcupine. The tiny island beyond Long Porcupine, at the righthand edge of the photograph, is Stave Island, which is off Schoodic Peninsula, on the other side of Frenchman Bay.* ▶

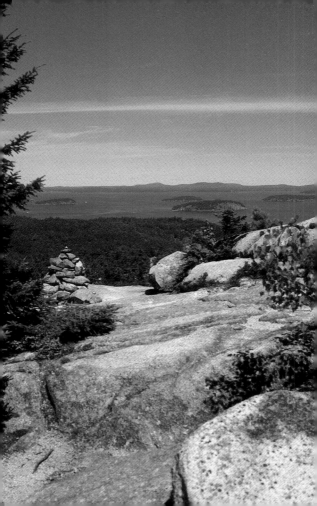

where the path ended at the first carriage road. Beside the trail is a white birch tree with a diamond-shaped piece of blue metal stuck into it; also attached to the tree is a sign saying "Summit."

The trail continues gently up the mountain. Through the trees on your left you'll have occasional glimpses of Mount Desert Island's island-dotted southern coast.

About .4 miles from Route 3 the trail crosses a carriage road again. (This time the trail goes directly across the road.) Remember what this spot looks like because you'll be walking on the *road* on your way back down the mountain and you'll pick up the trail here to go back to your car. There's no sign by the trail, so you'll have to look for other landmarks.

Now you'll climb up and across handsome broad ledges fringed with blueberry bushes, sheep laurel and low spruces. There are no trees here to block your view so you begin to see mountains to the west and the Beehive, Gorham Mountain and Frenchman Bay to the east.

The vistas widen and deepen with almost every step you take. Gradually you see more and more of Frenchman Bay, then Schoodic Peninsula, on the other side of the bay, then Champlain Mountain (Walk No. 12), to the left of Gorham. Behind you the Cranberry Isles appear and, beyond them, the wide blue sweep of the ocean. Then you can see Seal Harbor, less than a mile away. To your left are long, parallel north-south mountain ridges. The modest 422-foot Eliot Mountain is two miles west of Seal Harbor. On the western horizon is the long massif of 1,071-foot Western Mountain, the park's sixth-highest summit. To the right of Western is 839-foot Beech Mountain (Walk No. 24); note the fire tower near its summit. To the right of Beech Mountain is 1,194-foot Penobscot Mountain (Walk No. 15), the park's fifth-highest peak. Behind Penobscot is 942-foot Cedar Swamp Mountain; behind Cedar Swamp is 852-foot Norumbega (Walk No. 32). Beyond Norumbega is Somes Sound.

About .6 miles from Route 3 the trail again crosses a carriage road and then runs across more ledges. Now you have a 180-degree ocean view—from Frenchman Bay in the east to the mouth of Somes Sound in the west and the archipelago of low, sprawling offshore islands in between. You can also see the mountains in the west.

Then the trail goes into the woods and climbs briefly up to the carriage road that curves around the top of Day. Cross the road and walk up to the post in the middle of the ledgy summit, where you'll have a 130-degree view of mountains and a 70-degree vista of the ocean. In the heart of the mountain panorama are three summits dramatically separated by deep valleys. To the northwest is the long, high ridge of Penobscot Mountain; on its steep eastern slope are Jordan Cliffs. East of Penobscot and almost 1,000 feet below its summit is the long valley of Jordan Stream, which flows from Jordan Pond (Walk No. 7) to Little Long Pond (Walk No. 8). Rising from the valley are the ledgy summits of the Triad, almost 700 feet high and less than a mile away. Immediately behind the Triad is 1,247-foot Pemetic Mountain (Walk No. 14), the park's fourth-highest mountain. Right of the Triad is the long valley of Hunters

Brook. To the right of the valley is the southern ridge of Cadillac Mountain (Walk No. 20). Farther to the east is Champlain Mountain. On the western horizon is (appropriately) Western Mountain. To the south are Seal Harbor and the offshore islands.

After savoring this view, follow the carriage road around the east side of the mountain. (Remember to stay alert for bicycles whizzing by.) Here the road is a corniche curving along the top of the cliffs known as The Cleft. As you stroll easily along the wide, smooth, almost level road, you'll have continuous views to your left. You'll see, from left to right: Champlain Mountain, the Beehive, Gorham Mountain, Schoodic Peninsula across Frenchman Bay and the Cranberry Isles to the south.

The road curves around the south slope of the mountain, crosses the trail you walked on earlier, then winds along the west side of the mountain. Now, on your left, you'll see houses in Seal Harbor, islands to the south and mountains to the west.

Then the road switches back to the left and you'll have more views of ocean and mountains through the trees on your right.

Next the trail curves back around the south slope of the mountain and, about .5 miles from the summit, crosses the trail again. From here you follow the path back to your car. If you happen to miss the trail when you come by, don't worry. Just follow the

The archipelago of low, sprawling offshore islands seen from ledges on **Pemetic Mountain** *(Walk No. 14) in the fall. Note the bright red blueberry bushes in the foreground.* ►

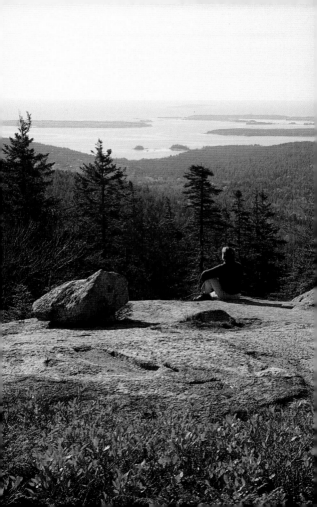

carriage road to the next trail crossing — the one where two carriage roads join — pick up the trail there and follow it back down the mountain.

14 Pemetic Mountain

This moderate 3.2-mile round trip to the top of Mount Desert Island's fourth-highest peak offers continuing views of more than two dozen Acadian landmarks, including Schoodic Peninsula, Frenchman Bay, Eastern Bay, Otter Point, Otter Cove, Seal Harbor, Northeast Harbor, Southwest Harbor, the Cranberry Isles, the mouth of Somes Sound, Little Long Pond, Jordan Pond, Jordan Cliffs, Eagle Lake, the Bubbles, the Triad, and Cadillac, Champlain, Day, Norumbega, Penobscot and Sargent mountains.

Although this Walk is the gentlest and most scenic ascent of Pemetic, the middle part of the trail requires some steep climbing over rocks and ledges. This outing is nevertheless a Great Walk because the climbs are brief and the extraordinary views are more than worth the effort.

The Walk begins in a parking area on the west side of the Park Loop Road, about .5 miles north of Jordan Pond House and about 4.8 miles south of the junction of the Loop Road and Route 233, west of Bar Harbor.

The trail is across the road, beside a rushing brook. A post between the brook and the trail indicates that the summit of Pemetic Mountain is 1.6 miles away.

The path follows the brook briefly upstream, then crosses it on a wooden bridge and climbs almost imperceptibly through a damp, moss-carpeted evergreen forest. As you gradually ascend the lower slope of the mountain you'll hear, and occasionally glimpse, another brook on your right.

About .2 miles from the trailhead, near low ledges to the right of the path, you'll reach a trail junction. The path to the Triad goes straight ahead; the trail up Pemetic makes a sharp left. Go left.

The trail now climbs more steeply, sometimes over sunny ledges and sometimes over rocks and the roots of evergreen.

About .3 miles from the trailhead you'll climb up a steep rock outcrop and get your first views: the Cranberry Isles to the south and, through the trees, Jordan Pond (Walk No. 7), Jordan Pond House and Jordan Cliffs on the eastern slope of Penobscot Mountain (Walk No. 15).

The views get broader as you climb. Look behind you and you'll see, from left to right, Seal Harbor, the fields around Little Long Pond (Walk No. 8) and Northeast Harbor. Then, through the trees on your right, you'll see the wooded slopes of the 698-foot Triad, less than half a mile away, and the south ridge of Cadillac Mountain (Walk No. 20) beyond it.

The trail curves to the right side of Pemetic's

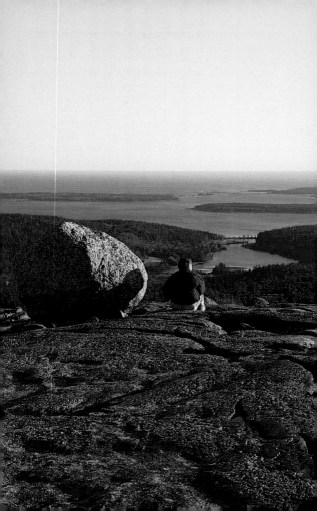

north-south ridge and you'll have another view to the east. On the horizon is the long, ledgy ridge of Cadillac; in front of Cadillac is the Triad; to the right of the Triad, and less than 1.5 miles away, is the bare summit of Day Mountain (Walk No. 13).

The trail then descends briefly into a spruce grove and climbs up another ledge. Here you can see Jordan Pond, Jordan Pond House, Southwest Harbor and the mouth of Somes Sound, Norumbega Mountain (Walk No. 32), on the east side of the sound, and the bare top of Penobscot Mountain.

At the top of the next ledge you'll be able to see the carriage road on top of Day Mountain. You'll also have your first view of Little Long Pond and the valley of Jordan Stream, which flows from Jordan Pond to Little Long Pond. Here, too, the Cranberry Isles will be in full view. Sutton Island is the long island, closest to the shore, Great Cranberry Island is beyond Sutton and Little Cranberry is to the left of Great Cranberry. Closer to the shore is Bear Island.

Now the trail levels off and, about a mile from the trailhead, emerges onto a very broad sloping ledge. In a few yards you'll come to another trail junction, marked by a wooden sign in a cairn. The right path

The view from the wide ledges on **Penobscot Mountain** *(Walks No. 15 and 16):* **Little Long Pond** *(Walk No. 8) and the narrow causeway separating it from the ocean. Sutton Island is the long island nearest shore; Little Cranberry Island is on the left; Great Cranberry Island is on the right, beyond Sutton Island.*
◄

goes to the Triad, the left to the top of Pemetic. (The sign is incorrect—the summit is about .6 miles away, not .9.)

The junction marks a fundamental change in the Walk. From here to the summit there are virtually no more large trees, only tiny, wind-battered spruces scattered across the wide ledges. From now on your views are continuous.

At the junction you already have a 180-degree vista. On the horizon, but less than a mile away, is the long, steep, mostly bare ridge of Cadillac. To the northeast is a notch in the ridge where the exquisite pond known as the Featherbed is found (see Walk No. 20). Between Pemetic and Cadillac is the long, deep valley drained by Hunters Brook and the tributaries of Bubble Pond (Walk No. 6). To the right of Cadillac is Otter Point (Walk No. 3). To the right of Otter Point is the Triad. South of the Triad is Day Mountain.

Watch for blazes and cairns as you follow the trail up windswept ledges. On your left you'll see Penobscot Mountain again, as well as 1,373-foot Sargent Mountain (Walk No. 16), the park's second-highest peak, to the right of Penobscot, and 1,071-foot Western Mountain on the horizon behind it. Then you'll start seeing Otter Cove to the right of Otter Point, then Champlain Mountain (Walk No. 12) through the notch on Cadillac and Schoodic Peninsula over Cadillac's south ridge.

The trail crosses a tiny stream trickling down from a cedar swamp in a depression to the right of the trail. Then the path curves to the left of the ridge, where you'll have another view of Jordan Pond, now more than 1,000 feet below you but less than half a mile away. Walk a bit to the left of the trail and you'll also see the carriage road and the rock slide known as the Tumbledown on the lower slope of Penobscot Mountain, which rises from the west side of Jordan Pond. You'll also see Jordan Pond House, on the southern end of the pond, and you'll have bird's-eye views of the nearly bare tops of the South and North Bubbles (Walks No. 17 and 18), on the northern end of the pond. Farther to your right is the long north ridge of the North Bubble. About 1.5 miles beyond the ridge is Aunt Betty Pond. Seven miles to the north, between Mount Desert Island and the mainland, is Eastern Bay.

By now the trail has nearly leveled off and you're beginning to cross the mountain's rolling, .2-mile-long summit ledge. Soon you'll see the bare top of Conners Nubble (Walk No. 18), to the right of the North Bubble, and Eagle Lake (Walk No. 5), to the right of the Nubble. Hundreds of feet below, between Eagle Lake and Jordan Pond, is the valley known as Jordan Carry.

Less than .2 miles from the top of Pemetic you'll start seeing a tiny "peak" ahead of you. That's the huge cairn built against a quilted boulder on the summit.

When you reach this granite monument you'll be higher than only three other places on the island — the summits of Dorr, Sargent and Cadillac mountains — and, not surprisingly, you'll have panoramic views. To the northeast you'll see tiny cars on the road to the top of Cadillac. Beyond Cadillac you'll see the ridge of Champlain Mountain. To your left you'll have a 180-degree view that runs from the south end of Mount Desert Island to the north: from the offshore islands, to the valley of Jordan Stream, to Jordan Pond and past the Bubbles to Jordan Carry, then to Eagle Lake and Frenchman Bay. To the south you'll have a 180-degree vista of the Atlantic Ocean: from Schoodic Peninsula in the east to Blue Hill Bay in the west. Take time to wander around the summit and savor the views from different spots.

The summit is also a fine place for a long lunch. (If it happens to be too windy for your taste, find the lee side of the summit cairn and take a seat out of the wind.)

When you're ready to return to your car, retrace your steps to the parking area and enjoy the views again from another perspective.

15
Penobscot Mountain

This moderate 3.3-mile round trip takes you gently to the top of Acadia's fifth-highest mountain and provides frequent views of more than two dozen landmarks, including Frenchman Bay, Seal Harbor, Southwest Harbor, Somes Sound, Bear and Greening islands, the Cranberry Isles, Eagle Lake, Jordan Pond, Little Long Pond and Sargent Mountain Pond; Jordan Cliffs, Jordan Stream, the Amphitheater, the Bubbles, Conners Nubble, the Triad and nine different mountains: Acadia, Cadillac, Cedar Swamp, Day, Eliot, Norumbega, Pemetic, St. Sauveur and Sargent.

This Walk also requires a brief (.1-mile) climb up the cliffs on the east side of Penobscot Mountain. In some places you'll be on your hands and knees on the way *up* the mountain and on your hands, knees and fanny on your way *down*. The trip is still a Great Walk, however, because the climb isn't arduous, just slow, and the outstanding views and gentle grades on the rest of the outing far outweigh the extra effort.

Note: The entire route of this Walk is included in the longer Walk No. 16 (Sargent Mountain).

Like Walk No. 7 (Jordan Pond), this Walk begins in the Jordan Pond parking area, on the west side of the Park Loop Road, about .1 miles north of Jordan Pond House and about five miles south of the intersection of the Loop Road and Route 233, west of Bar Harbor.*

*If you want to begin the Walk at Jordan Pond House, follow these directions to the trail: Walk to the lawn next to the public restrooms, which are underneath the gift shop on the back (west) side of Jordan Pond House. Go west, across the lawn, to the woods. At the edge of the woods you'll see a path and a sign beside it saying that the trail leads to the Sargent and Penobscot mountain trails. The path goes down a steep slope via log steps and in about 50 feet reaches the intersection of two carriage roads on the east side of Jordan Stream. Cross the brook on the foot bridge to the right of the intersection.

From the west side of the westernmost parking lot (the one farthest from the Loop Road and closest to the pond), follow the wide path to the boat ramp on Jordan Pond. In about 200 feet you'll come to the pond, where you'll see the steep eastern slope of Penobscot Mountain on the west side of the tarn and the twin peaks of the Bubbles (Walks No. 17 and 18) on the northern end.

Follow the path to the left, along the south shore of the pond. Almost immediately you'll see, on your left, the long clearing in front of Jordan Pond House, covered with blueberry bushes.

After passing the clearing, the path curves to the left, into the woods and away from the pond. About .1 miles from the trailhead it runs into a carriage road just east of where the road crosses Jordan Stream on a handsome stone-arch bridge.

Take a left on the carriage road and follow it along the east bank of Jordan Stream. The stream, the outlet of Jordan Pond, is one of the largest and fastest brooks on Mount Desert Island. (As on all carriage roads, remember to watch out for bicycles going by.)

You'll walk on the carriage road for just a few hundred feet before it intersects another carriage road. Just before the intersection, take a right and cross Jordan Stream on a foot bridge. A signpost to the left of the bridge says the path on the other side of the stream leads to the "Sargent and Penobscot trails."

On the other side of Jordan Stream the path splits. The trail on the right follows Jordan Stream back to Jordan Pond; the other path goes straight ahead to Penobscot and Sargent mountains.

Go straight and follow the trail through evergreen woods. The path is level at first, then climbs gently before descending gradually to a small brook.

Cross the brook (on stones) and start climbing the lower slope of Penobscot Mountain. On your left a tiny stream tumbles down the steep hill parallel to the trail.

Just a couple of hundred feet from the brook (and about .5 miles from Jordan Pond) you'll climb up rock steps to a charming brook, with small rock-bottomed pools, just below another carriage road. Here the trail to Jordan Cliffs goes to the right, the Penobscot-Sargent mountain trail to the left.

Take a left and climb up the stone steps to the carriage road. As you cross the road, look to your left. You'll see Southwest Harbor and the low islands offshore.

Now climb up the stone steps on the other side of the carriage road and begin the slow climb of the cliffs and boulders on the slope of Penobscot Mountain. (Follow the blue blazes on the rocks.) Almost immediately you'll see three peaks behind you: the long ridge of Pemetic Mountain (Walk No. 14), on the west side of Jordan Pond; the Triad, to the right of Pemetic and above Jordan Pond House, and Day Mountain (Walk No. 13), to the right of the Triad.

The well-built trail switches back to the left, then back to the right. Then it runs along a shelf in the ledge, below a 30-foot-high cliff to the left of the path and beside a wooden fence on the top of a cliff to the right. Next you'll cross a short foot bridge over a chasm and get your first view of Jordan Pond.

Then the trail switches back to the left again and

climbs up a crack in the ledge. Here you'll see the South Bubble (Walk No. 17), on the southern end of the pond. As you climb you'll have wider and wider views of the mile-long tarn. Then you'll catch a glimpse of the North Bubble (Walk No. 18).

About .1 miles from the (second) carriage road you'll reach the top of the cliffs. Then the trail ascends a steep slope but soon levels off on a ledge. (Note the ocean and the islands to your left as you climb.) The path then bends to the right to begin its gentle ascent of the wide, open, ledgy ridge of Penobscot. From here to the summit—about .9 miles away—there are no large trees. Your views will be restricted only by the mass of the ridge itself.

Soon you'll have a 270-degree view, sweeping from the North and South Bubbles, in the north; to Pemetic and Day mountains, the Triad, Jordan Pond and Jordan Pond House, in the east; to Little Long Pond (Walk No. 8), less than 1.5 miles behind you; to the mouth of Somes Sound and Southwest Harbor, in the south. So close is Little Long Pond to the ocean that from here it looks like a tiny arm of the sea. Greening Island is off the mouth of Somes Sound. The .2-mile-wide Bear Island is to the left of Greening and the Cranberry Isles are beyond Bear Island.

As you climb the nearly treeless ridge you'll notice the south ridge of Cadillac Mountain (Walk No. 20) in the notch between Pemetic Mountain and the Triad. You'll also spot the Park Loop Road above Jordan Pond and the low (422-foot) Eliot Mountain to the right of Little Long Pond. Then you'll see more of Northeast Harbor, southwest of Eliot

Mountain. If there are clouds in the south and the light is right, the clouds will cast shadows on the ocean that look like low, dark islands.

The trail then curves to the left (west) side of the ridge, where you'll look into the deep gulch known as the Amphitheater. A carriage road curves along the lower slope of 942-foot Cedar Swamp Mountain, which forms the steep west wall of the ravine.

As you climb, more and more landmarks will come into view: Seal Harbor, to the left of Little Long Pond; 1,071-foot Western Mountain, Acadia's sixth-highest summit, on the horizon beyond Cedar Swamp Mountain; the mountains on the mainland (beyond the Bubbles); Acadia, St. Sauveur and Norumbega mountains (Walk Nos. 21, 23 and 32) between Cedar Swamp and Western mountains; and the summit of Cadillac Mountain to the north of Pemetic Mountain.

Then the trail descends slightly, crosses a tiny marsh and resumes its gradual climb. You're now more than 1,000 feet high and your view expands to include Eagle Lake (Walk No. 5) and Frenchman Bay, to the north.

You'll pass a tiny, picturesque 50-foot-long pond to the left of the trail. Then you'll see the ledgy top of Conners Nubble (Walk No. 18) above Eagle Lake and you'll have another view of the Bubbles.

About 1.5 miles from Jordan Stream you'll come to the six-foot-high cairn on Penobscot's summit. From here you can see Sargent Mountain Pond in the spruce trees in the bottom of the draw between Penobscot and Sargent mountains. To the right of Sargent Mountain are Eagle Lake and, in the distance, Frenchman Bay. Enjoy the view and, when you're ready, retrace your steps to your car.

16 Sargent Mountain

This moderate 5.2-mile round trip is a grand tour. It takes you to the top of both Penobscot Mountain and Sargent Mountain—Acadia's second-highest summit—and offers often continuous views of more than 50 Acadian landmarks, including the Porcupine Islands; Eastern, Western, Blue Hill and Frenchman bays; Bear and Greening islands and the Cranberry Isles; Echo and Eagle lakes; Long, Little Long, Jordan, Sargent Mountain and Upper and Lower Hadlock ponds; the towns of Seal Harbor, Northeast Harbor and Southwest Harbor; Schoodic Peninsula, Somes Sound, Jordan Cliffs, Jordan Stream, the Amphitheater, the Bubbles, Conners Nubble, the Triad, Bald and Gilmore peaks and Acadia, Beech, Cadillac, Cedar Swamp, Champlain, Day, Eliot, Norumbega, Parkman, Pemetic, Penobscot, St. Sauveur and Western mountains.

The first 1.6 miles of this Walk follow the route of Walk No. 15 (Penobscot Mountain) and require some climbing over ledges. See page 84 for a description of Walk No. 15 and directions to the trailhead.

When you reach the summit of Penobscot—the destination of Walk No. 15—the trail splits. The righthand path goes down the east side of Penobscot toward the Jordan Cliffs Trail. The lefthand trail goes straight ahead toward Sargent Mountain.

Follow the Sargent Mountain trail down the ledge north of the summit and into the spruces beyond. For the next third of a mile or so you'll have a brief change of scene: Instead of wide, open granite ledges, you'll be walking on dirt paths through thick stands of evergreens.

The path keeps dropping down a rocky, rooty trail and, about .1 miles from the Penobscot summit, reaches another trail junction in the bottom of the narrow, shady ravine between Penobscot and Sargent mountains. The righthand path goes to Jordan Pond; the trail to Sargent Mountain goes straight ahead.

Follow the Sargent Mountain trail up the ledge on the opposite side of the ravine. Almost immediately the path curves to the left and becomes nearly level as it runs along a low shoulder above the draw. On your left, above the ravine, you'll see cliffs on the north slope of Penobscot and, to the right of the mountain, the ocean and the offshore islands to the south.

In another couple of hundred feet you'll reach the south shore of Sargent Mountain Pond, a tiny (100-foot-wide) lake surrounded by spruce trees.

Bending away from the pond, the trail quickly climbs to the top of a ledge with a splendid 120-degree view. On your left you can see cars on the road on Cadillac Mountain (Walks No. 19 and 20). To the right of Cadillac is Pemetic Mountain (Walk No. 14). To the right of Pemetic is Penobscot; look carefully and you'll see the cairn on its very tip. Down the valley between Penobscot Mountain, on the left, and Cedar Swamp Mountain, on the right, are Little Long Pond (Walk No. 8) and Seal Harbor. Offshore are Sutton and Great Cranberry islands. Through the spruces on your right you can see a bit of Southwest Harbor.

At this point the trail splits again. The left fork goes south toward Birch Spring; the right fork heads north toward Sargent Mountain, now less than .9 miles away.

Take the righthand trail, which quickly takes you out of the trees and up the broad, rolling, lichen-covered ledge on Sargent's south slope. Now you're more than 1,100 feet high—higher than the summits of all but five peaks on the island—and you again have continuous unobstructed views in all directions. To your left is the north-south ridge of 852-foot Norumbega Mountain (Walk No. 32), on the east side of Somes Sound. Across the sound are 679-foot St. Sauveur Mountain (Walk No. 23) and, north of St. Sauveur, 681-foot Acadia Mountain (Walk No. 21). Western Mountain is on the horizon. To the right of Norumbega and less than a mile away is a cluster of three summits: 974-foot Bald Mountain, farthest to the left; 941-foot Parkman Mountain, in the middle, and 1,036-foot Gilmore Peak, on the right. About five miles beyond them is Western Bay, which separates Mount Desert Island from the mainland. Straight ahead is the treeless slope of Sargent. On your right are Cadillac and Pemetic mountains and Frenchman Bay behind them. Penobscot rises to your rear.

The trail runs briefly through spruces again, then reemerges on the ledges. Now you can see Upper Hadlock Pond, to your left rear.

About .5 miles from the summit you come to another trail junction. The path on the left goes to Upper Hadlock Pond; the trail to the top of Sargent goes straight ahead. Here you can also see Lower Hadlock Pond, south of Upper Hadlock, as well as Southwest Harbor, Greening Island, off the mouth of Somes Sound, and other islands farther offshore.

Now you walk across almost level ledge. In about .3 miles you'll reach yet another trail junction. The left path goes to Parkman Mountain; the summit of Sargent is .2 miles straight ahead.

When you reach the massive, 7-foot-high, 20-foot-wide cairn at the summit, you're higher than any other place on Mount Desert Island except the top of Cadillac. No wonder the views are awesome! Almost 1,400 feet below you and less than two miles away is the northern end of Somes Sound. You'll see Somes Harbor and Bar Island, in the mouth of the harbor, the white houses in the village of Somesville and several ponds around the village. Beyond the sound is Echo Lake and beyond the lake is Beech Mountain (Walk No. 24). Long Pond (Walk No. 31), the island's largest body of fresh water, is west of Beech Mountain and Western Mountain is on the horizon. You'll also have a 180-degree view — to the west, north and east — of the narrow bays that separate Mount Desert Island from the mainland.

Walk a couple of hundred feet to the east and you'll see Conners Nubble (Walk No. 18) over Eagle Lake (Walk No. 5) and the North and South Bubbles

(Walks No. 17 and 18) to the right of the Nubble. You'll also see the Porcupine Islands in Frenchman Bay.

Take the time to savor these extraordinary views over a long lunch. When you're ready, turn around and enjoy the vistas again as you walk back to your car.

17 The South Bubble

This undemanding one-mile round trip takes you easily to the top of one of Acadia's most photographed promontories, where you'll have close views of lakes and mountains all around you, including Jordan Pond, Echo Lake, the bare eminences of the North Bubble and Conners Nubble and the dramatic steep slopes of Cadillac, Pemetic, Penobscot and Sargent mountains. You'll also see the ocean and the offshore islands and you'll come face to face with the massive Bubble Rock.

The Walk to the South Bubble can be reduced to a .7-mile round trip if you climb it on Walk No. 18 (the North Bubble & Conners Nubble). If you plan to ascend the South Bubble on that Walk, you may want to skip this one.

Walks No. 17 and 18 both begin at the Bubble Rock parking area, on the west side of the Park Loop

Road, about 1.8 miles north of Jordan Pond House and about five miles south of the intersection of the Loop Road and Route 233, west of Bar Harbor. Just south of the parking area, on the west side of the road, is a viewpoint from which you can see Bubble Rock, high up on the South Bubble. The rock appears to rest precariously on the edge of a cliff, ready to tumble over the edge at any moment. A park sign here explains that the boulder is an "erratic," one of many rocks deposited by the glacier that carved Acadia's valleys and Somes Sound thousands of years ago.

Starting in the middle of the west side of the parking lot, the trail climbs gently through a beech grove for a couple of hundred feet, then turns sharply right.

In another 50 feet it crosses another trail. The path to the right goes to the North Bubble and Conners Nubble (Walk No. 18). The South Bubble is straight ahead. Go straight and follow the smooth path as it rises gently up the South Bubble's lower slope.

In another .1 mile or so the trail turns left and immediately starts ascending steps made from rocks in log cribs.

In another 50 feet the steep trail to the North Bubble splits off on the right. Keep going straight up the steps, past young beeches and white birches.

In yet another 50 feet or so the trail levels off. You're now in the saddle, or col, between the North and South Bubbles.

A few yards ahead, the trail divides again. The path straight ahead goes down to Jordan Pond (Walk No. 7). The trail to the left goes to the South Bubble. Take a left and follow the path over ledges toward the summit. As you near the top, look behind you; you'll see the North Bubble and even the wooden sign at its summit. To your left you'll see the north-south ridge of Pemetic Mountain (Walk No. 14). To the left of Pemetic is the north-south ridge of Cadillac (Walks No. 19 and 20). To your right is the steep slope of Sargent Mountain (Walk No. 16). Left of Sargent, on the precipitous face of Penobscot Mountain (Walk No. 15), are Jordan Cliffs.

Very soon you'll reach the South Bubble's broad, nearly bare summit ledge. On your right is a large cairn marking the promontory's highest point. To the north is a 180-degree view that includes, from left to right: Sargent Mountain, the 872-foot North Bubble, 588-foot Conners Nubble, Eagle Lake (Walk No. 5) and Cadillac Mountain.

A couple of hundred feet east of the sign at the summit is Bubble Rock, an 18-foot-long, 10-foot-high boulder resting on the very edge of the ledge. You wonder how many pranksters have tried to push the rock over the cliff—and how much power would be needed even to budge this multiton monolith. Near the rock you can enjoy another northern vista that stretches from the North Bubble to Cadillac Mountain.

Walk back to the trail near the summit of the South Bubble and follow the blue blazes past blueberry bushes and sheep laurel to the southern edge of

---

Jordan Pond *(Walk No. 7) seen from the* **South Bubble** *(Walk No. 17). Jordan Pond House is at the southern end of the pond.* **Penobscot Mountain** *(Walks No. 15 and 16) rises from the pond on the right.* ▶

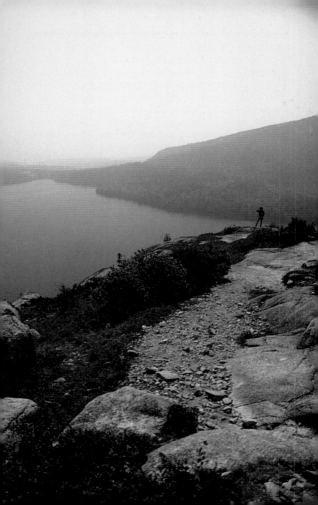

the summit ledge. Here you have one of the South Bubble's grandest views. Below you is almost all of Jordan Pond. At its southern end is Jordan Pond House. South of the pond, beyond the low valley of Jordan Stream, is the Atlantic Ocean, with the Cranberry Isles just off shore. The valley is more than two miles long but from here it looks like a tiny neck of flat land between the pond and the sea. To the left of the pond are the steep faces of Cadillac and Pemetic mountains. To the right of the pond, and rising even more sharply, are Penobscot and Sargent mountains. At the edge of the pond and on the lower slope of Penobscot is the rock slide known as the Tumbledown; if you look carefully you can see the carriage road running through it.

Keep following the trail blazes down several tiers of ledge and you'll have even closer views of Jordan Pond. Walk to your right and you'll be able to see the marshes and wooden bridges at the northern end of the pond, as well as Jordan Carry, the low pass that separates the Bubbles from Sargent Mountain.

If it's not too windy the summit is a fine place to tarry awhile before retracing your steps to your car. During much of the first half of your return trip, you'll be walking "into" the views of the evergreen-festooned ledges of the North Bubble. Enjoy them.

18 The North Bubble & Conners Nubble

This moderate three-mile loop takes you

gradually up two bare summits that offer close, dramatic views of Jordan Pond and Echo Lake and Cadillac, Pemetic, Penobscot and Sargent mountains. Farther away you'll see Frenchman Bay, Western Bay and Schoodic Peninsula.

On your return trip you can make an easy ascent of the South Bubble (Walk No. 17).

Like No. 17, this Walk begins at the Bubble Rock parking area, on the west side of the Park Loop Road, about 1.8 miles north of Jordan Pond House and about five miles south of the intersection of Route 233 and the Park Loop Road, west of Bar Harbor.

At first the Walk follows the route of Walk No. 17 (described on page 94). It climbs gently through a beech grove for a couple of hundred feet, then turns sharply right and, in another 50 feet, crosses another path. The trail to the South Bubble goes straight ahead; the path on the right—to Eagle Lake (Walk No. 5)—takes you to the North Bubble and Conners Nubble.

Follow the righthand trail as it descends almost imperceptibly through moist woods and crosses sluggish brooks on wooden bridges or carefully placed rocks. After passing through hemlock groves and ferns the trail crosses a carriage road about .6 miles from the parking area and just a few hundred feet south of Eagle Lake.

Take a left on the carriage road (and, as on all carriage roads, stay alert for bicycles whizzing by). Almost immediately you'll cross a tepid stream that runs into Eagle Lake and you'll see the cliffs of the North Bubble ahead. As the road gently climbs the North Bubble's steep slope, you'll pass cliffs and huge boulders of talus on your left.

You'll walk about .5 miles on the carriage road before it curves left to cross the saddle between the North Bubble and Conners Nubble. At the crest of the saddle, a trail crosses the road. The trail on the left goes to the North Bubble; you'll follow it later. The trail on the right goes to the top of Conners Nubble in less than .2 miles.

Follow the righthand trail through some pleasant birches and quaking aspens. Then climb briefly up to the Nubble's flat, bare summit ledge and *voila!* Suddenly you have a stunning 360-degree view of forest-fringed Eagle Lake, Frenchman Bay and five of the major promontories of Mount Desert Island.

The Nubble is only 588 feet high but it's the highest point between the Bubbles, to the south, and Frenchman Bay, to the northeast. It's also more than 300 feet above, but less than 500 feet from, Eagle Lake, which extends to the north and east. You therefore have a water-filled view to the northeast: You can gaze up the length of the Eagle Lake, over what looks like a very narrow neck of flat land separating the two-mile-long lake from the ocean, and out over Frenchman Bay, which stretches across to

---

*Bubble Rock, an 18-foot-long, 10-foot-high glacial "erratic," seems to rest precariously on the edge of the **South Bubble** (Walk No. 17). The steep slope of **Pemetic Mountain** (Walk No. 14) is on the left.* ▶

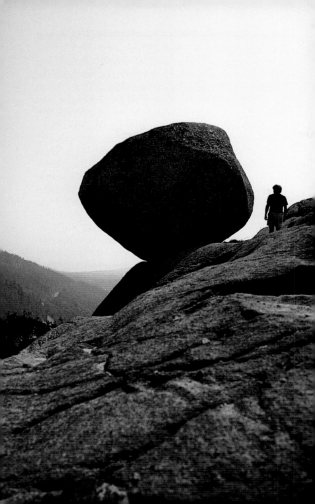

Schoodic Peninsula. And that's just a part of the vista. Clockwise, from north to south, you see not only Frenchman Bay and Eagle Lake but also the long ridge of Cadillac Mountain (Walks No. 19 and 20), which parallels the eastern shore of the lake, and the northern slopes of Pemetic Mountain (Walk No. 14). Both mountains are less than a mile away. Continuing clockwise, you see, from south to north, the northern slopes of the Bubbles and the long, steep eastern ridge of Sargent Mountain (Walk No. 16)—all less than a mile away—and across the northwestern lowlands of Mount Desert Island to Western Bay and the mainland beyond. Walk around the wide, smooth granite summit, covered with yellow lichen, blueberries and scrub birches, and you'll enjoy even closer views of the lofty peaks around you.

After savoring one of the best views on Mount Desert Island, retrace your steps down the Nubble to the carriage road and take the trail to the North Bubble, on the other side of the road.

The mossy path runs through a grove of young beeches, then climbs briefly through birches and spruces, which get shorter as you climb higher and the ground gets ledgier.

Soon you'll see your first views. Behind you is Conners Nubble, its cliffs plunging into Eagle Lake and its bands of ledge looking like a rough fortress. If the light is right you'll see the wooden marker on its summit. To the right of the Nubble is another water-filled view over Eagle Lake and Frenchman Bay. Farther to the right is Cadillac Mountain.

Soon the trail levels off and you walk from cairn to cairn on smooth, open ledge, past blueberries, sheep laurel and low spruces. Now your views are almost continuous. Soon you'll see Pemetic Mountain across Jordan Carry, the valley on your left. Beyond the Southwest Pass, the valley to your right, is Sargent Mountain, now less than a quarter-mile away.

The trail goes in and out of stands of low trees as it winds gently for more than half a mile toward the top of the North Bubble. The walking here is superb: an effortless stroll from view to view on a high rock perch.

After passing through low birches and spruces the trail suddenly emerges on the 872-foot summit of the North Bubble. Walk farther out on the ledge and enjoy its 300-degree view. On your left you'll see the stone massifs of Cadillac and Pemetic mountains. Ahead is the evergreen-bedecked rock of the South Bubble. Behind the Bubble is Jordan Pond (Walk No. 7) and behind the pond are the ocean and the long, low islands offshore. To your right are the northern end of the pond and the slopes of Sargent Mountain and Penobscot Mountain (Walk No. 15) rising steeply from the west shore.

After enjoying the view, follow the trail down the southern face of the North Bubble. At first the path is steep; but the steep section is brief (less than 500 feet); it's downhill, so it's not tiring; and it passes overlooks with still more views. You'll see everything you saw from the top of the North Bubble plus Eagle Lake and Frenchman Bay to your left.

The trail soon descends to the saddle between the North and South Bubbles and meets the path to the South Bubble, on the right. From here you can ei-

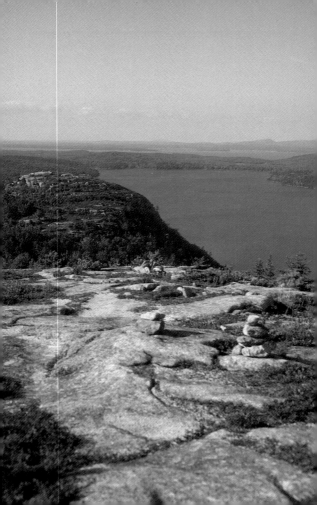

ther climb to the top of the South Bubble — now just about .3 miles away — or retrace the route of Walk No. 17 (the South Bubble) back to your car.

If you want to climb the South Bubble, follow the description on pages 95-98.

If you want to go back to your car, follow the beginning of Walk No. 17 in reverse: Go straight ahead, down a 50-foot flight of steps made of rocks and log cribs. At the foot of the steps the trail turns right and becomes a wide, smooth track through a beech forest. About .1 miles from the intersection of the North and South Bubble trails, you'll cross the path you followed to the carriage road south of Eagle Lake. From there you return to the parking area, just a couple of hundred feet away.

19 Cadillac Mountain Summit

This very easy, quarter-mile paved Walk around Cadillac's summit offers a 270-degree ocean-and-mountain view from the highest

---

Conners Nubble *(Walk No. 18) rises more than 300 feet above unspoiled* **Eagle Lake** *(Walk No. 5). Frenchman Bay and the mainland are in the distance. The view is from the long, ledgy north ridge of the* **North Bubble** *(Walk No. 18). Note the cairns marking the trail.*

◀

point on Mount Desert Island—indeed, the highest point on the east coast of the Americas between Canada and Rio de Janiero. The panorama sweeps from Southwest Harbor to the northern reaches of Frenchman Bay and includes a view *down* onto the summit of Acadia's third-highest peak, Dorr Mountain.

These views are rivaled by those from the paved road to Cadillac's summit, one of the most scenic drives in the world. From overlooks along the 3.5-mile highway you'll see Bar Island and the Porcupine Islands off Bar Harbor, the lighthouse on Egg Rock, Schoodic Peninsula, Otter Point, Seal Harbor, Little Long Pond, the Cranberry Isles and other offshore islands, Somes Sound, Eagle Lake, Conners Nubble, the Bubbles, the Beehive, and Gorham, Pemetic, Penobscot and Sargent mountains. Some of these vistas are stunning.

The Cadillac Mountain Road begins on the Park Loop Road, on the west side of the mountain, about 3.5 miles south of the park Visitor Center in Hulls Cove and about a mile south of the intersection of the Loop Road and Route 233, west of Bar Harbor.

You drive barely .7 miles up the road before you come to the first overlook, on the left side of the highway. (Be careful driving across the road.) You're 700 feet above sea level here and Frenchman Bay is spread out below you. You can see Bar Island and the Porcupine Islands around Bar Harbor (Walk

No. 1), the lighthouse on Egg Rock and Schoodic Peninsula, on the other side of the bay.

Drive another mile and you'll come to the second overlook, on your right. You're now 1,000 feet above sea level, higher than most other places on the island. More than 700 feet below, but less than a mile away, is the unspoiled, forest-ringed, two-mile-long Eagle Lake (Walk No. 5). From right to left, you can also see Western Bay, which separates the west side of Mount Desert Island from the mainland; Somes Sound; the cliffs of Conners Nubble (Walk No. 18), on the southwestern shore of Eagle Lake; the steep, ledgy slopes of Sargent and Penobscot mountains (Walks No. 15 and 16); the double humps of the Bubbles (Walks No. 17 and 18); the south coast of Mount Desert Island and the north ridge of Pemetic Mountain (Walk No. 14).

Just .2 miles ahead is the third outlook, on your left. Here, 1,100 feet above sea level, you have a 180-degree panorama that sweeps from Western Bay and Mount Desert Narrows — two straits between the island and the mainland — to Schoodic Peninsula in the southeast and includes almost all the islands in Frenchman Bay in between.

A half-mile farther, on the right, is another 180-degree view. You're now more than 1,400 feet above sea level and you can see, from south to north: the Atlantic Ocean off Seal Harbor; Pemetic Mountain and the low valley to the west of it; Penobscot and Sargent mountains; the North and South Bubbles — long ridges from this vantage point — in front of Sargent and Penobscot, respectively; Eagle Lake and

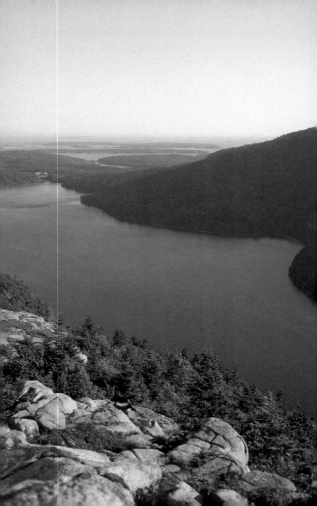

the entire northern tip of the island, including the northern reaches of Frenchman Bay.

In another .3 miles you come to yet another outlook, on the right. Here, 1,460 feet above sea level, you look down Cadillac's two-mile-long south ridge to some prominent coastal landmarks, including, from left to right: Schoodic Peninsula, the ledgy hump of the Beehive, Gorham Mountain (Walk No. 11), tiny, spruce-tipped Otter Point, Seal Harbor and Little Long Pond (Walk No. 8). Farther away is the sprawling archipelago of low, dark green offshore islands. Beyond the islands is the long ocean horizon. To the right of Little Long Pond you can also see Pemetic, Penobscot and Sargent mountains, the Bubbles, the mouth of Somes Sound and, ten miles away, the mainland. It's a view you can contemplate for a long time.

Just a few feet ahead, on the left, is the Blue Hill Overlook. Turn into the parking lot, walk west on the ledge and experience what may be the mountain's most moving vista. From here the Bubbles and Penobscot and Sargent mountains look like a massive gray monolith festooned with evergreens. You're now so high—more than 1,500 feet—that practically everything else you can see—Eagle Lake, the ocean,

---

Jordan Pond *(Walk No. 7), almost 600 feet below the* **North Bubble** *(Walk No. 18). Jordan Pond House is at the southern end of the pond.* **Little Long Pond** *(Walk No. 8) is to the right of the Jordan Pond House. The ocean and the long, low Cranberry Isles are in the distance.*
◄

the offshore islands and the lakes and lowlands between the mountains — seems like a low, flat, delicate, blue-green, land-and-water membrane. The lowland makes the massif look more massive; the massif, in turn, makes everything else look more fragile. On a slightly misty day, the mountains look like a giant, mossy boulder surrounded by a giant cranberry bog.

Your next stop, just a couple of hundred feet away, is Cadillac's 1,530-foot summit. You'll pass a building on your right that houses restrooms and a gift-and-snack shop. About 200 feet beyond it, at the southern edge of the parking area, is the beginning of the paved summit path. About 100 feet to the left of the walkway, two Park Service plaques identify the landmarks you'll look down on. End to end, the nearly level Walk provides an uninterrupted 270-degree view to the north, east and south. The ocean-and-mountain panorama includes, counterclockwise from the southwest: Southwest Harbor, Seal Harbor, the coastal islands, Otter Cove and the arched bridge over it, Otter Point, the Beehive, Schoodic Peninsula, the long, parallel ridges of Dorr and Champlain mountains (Walk No. 12), the Porcupines and other islands in Frenchman Bay, Bar Harbor and the mainland to the north. Dorr's bare, ledgy 1,270-foot summit is less than half a mile away; you'll be able to see the huge cairn holding up its wooden summit post. Dorr is Acadia's third-highest mountain but now it's more than 200 feet below you.

You'll also pass two interesting Park Service signs. One explains Bar Harbor's very social history; the other describes the granite of which much of Mount Desert Island is made.

The path returns to the parking area a couple of hundred feet north of where you began the Walk.

20 South Ridge, Cadillac Mountain

This undemanding two-mile round trip is a stroll along the crest of Cadillac Mountain's long, treeless south ridge. En route you'll have uninterrupted views of Gorham, Pemetic, Penobscot and Sargent mountains and the Bubbles. You'll also see Seal Harbor, Otter Cove, Schoodic Point, the offshore islands, Little Long Pond, the Beehive, the tiny tarn known as the Bowl and the exquisite pond called the Featherbed. Moreover, like Walk No. 19, you reach the trailhead via the Cadillac Mountain Road, which provides multidirectional views as good as those on the Walk.

Cadillac is the only mountain on Mount Desert Island with an auto road to its summit. Thanks to the road, you can drive up Cadillac and walk down. Because you don't have to walk up the mountain, you can avoid its often rough and viewless lower trails, which run through woods. Instead you can walk on a trail with constant views.

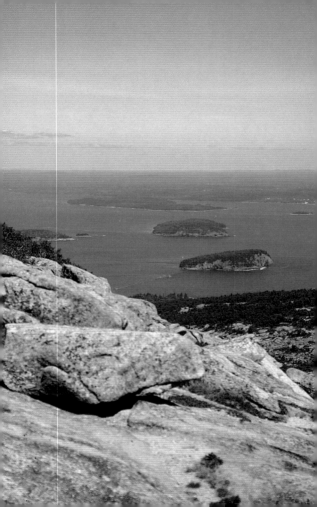

This Walk begins in the Blue Hill Overlook, on the Cadillac Mountain Road, just west of the summit. See Walk No. 19 for directions to the turnoff as well as a description of the extraordinary views along the road.

Leave your car in the overlook parking area and walk just a few feet down the road (away from the summit). Almost immediately you'll come to the bend in the road where you can see over Cadillac's two-mile-long south ridge (described on page 109). Watch out for cars as you cross the road and start walking south along the crest of the ledgy ridge, toward any of the cairns marking the path. (You'll see several on the open ledge, especially with binoculars.)

Your view here is continuous. It includes, from left to right, Schoodic Peninsula, on the east side of Frenchman Bay, the rocky hump of the Beehive, Gorham Mountain (Walk No. 11), tiny, spruce-covered Otter Point, Seal Harbor and Little Long Pond (Walk No. 8). Straight ahead are the low, sprawling offshore islands. Sutton Island is closest to the mainland. Little Cranberry Island is beyond Sutton and to the left. Great Cranberry is behind Sutton and to the right. The much smaller Baker Island is on the

The Porcupine Islands in Frenchman Bay are only some of the landmarks you can see from the quarter-mile long summit walk on **Cadillac Mountain** *(Walk No. 19), the highest peak on the eastern shore of the Americas from Canada to Rio de Janeiro.*
◄

left. To the right of Little Long Pond are (from left to right) Pemetic Mountain, Penobscot and Sargent mountains (Walks No. 14-16). In front of Penobscot and Sargent are the twin peaks of the Bubbles (Walks No. 17 and 18). Behind Pemetic is the mouth of Somes Sound.

As you walk easily across the ledge, past blueberries, huckleberries and other low shrubs, Sargent, Penobscot and Pemetic mountains and the Bubbles will look like a single ridge about a mile to your right. As you approach the southern coast of Mount Desert Island, you'll have closer and closer views of the elegant sweep of offshore islands.

About .1 miles from the road you'll come to a trail junction. The righthand path goes down the west side of the mountain to Bubble Pond (Walk No. 6). The lefthand path goes straight ahead, almost due south on the ridge, toward Blackwoods Campground. Keep going straight.

As you gradually descend the ridge you'll have better and better views of the Beehive, the bay of Seal Harbor, the mile-long Otter Cove and the bridge across it. You'll also see, in a line between you and the Beehive, a tiny pond in the hollow to your left. In the same line, just in front of the Beehive, is a larger pond known as the Bowl.

About .7 miles from the summit road, you'll come to a dip, or hollow, in the ridge. Nestled in the hollow about 100 feet below you is the exquisite pond known as the Featherbed, so called because it's filled with tall, soft-looking lime-green rushes.

The path makes a steep but very short descent to the Featherbed. On the shore of the pond you'll come to another trail junction. The trail on the right goes down the west side of the mountain; the path on the left descends the east side; the middle path stays on the crest of the ridge.

Follow the middle path past the Featherbed and back up to the top of the ridge. Soon you'll see a grass- and moss-lined pool, about 50 feet long and six feet wide, nestled elegantly in the solid ledge. You're now about a mile from the road and you've enjoyed the best views on the south ridge. Turn around here and retrace your steps to your car.

21 Acadia Mountain

This moderate two-mile round trip is a dramatic excursion. As you climb the 681-foot summit, your views will get better and better until they climax with a wide vista up and down Somes Sound — the only fjord on the East Coast of the United States — and over the islands off the southern coast of Mount Desert Island. Your views will also include Echo Lake, Valley Peak and six mountains: Beech, Flying, Norumbega, Sargent, St. Sauveur and Western.

The Walk begins in a parking area on the west side of Route 102, about three miles south of the charming village of Somesville. The trail starts on the other side of the road.

The path climbs up a short flight of stone steps, then over granite ledges dotted with cairns and deco-

rated with blueberries, huckleberries and fragrant scrub pines.

In .1 miles the trail forks. The right fork goes up St. Sauveur Mountain (Walk No. 23), the left to the top of Acadia. Go left.

The trail now runs through open spruce and cedar woods and crosses a brook flowing over mossy ledges.

About .1 miles after the trail junction you'll cross a gravel road and, just a few feet farther on, climb up the cleft of a massive ledge. Then you'll walk on a needle-carpeted path, past tall evergreens, and climb through the cleft of another massive ledge.

Now the trail switches back and forth over more ledges and past pitch pines and blueberries growing in the thin, sun-dappled, needle-covered soil. Here, just a few minutes into your Walk, you can turn around and catch your first views of the two-mile-long Echo Lake and the forested hills behind it.

Climb higher, over more ledges, and turn around again to see not only Echo Lake but also the fire tower on Beech Mountain (Walk No. 24), to the left. On the horizon are the steep, forested slopes of 1,071-foot Western Mountain. To the right of the mountain is Blue Hill Bay, the arm of the ocean between Mount Desert Island and the mainland.

As you keep climbing you'll get an even better

Late-afternoon sun blazes on the long ribbons of Echo Lake and Blue Hill Bay (rear), seen from **Acadia Mountain** *(Walk No. 21).*
◀

view of Echo Lake as well as your first glimpses of the mouth of Somes Sound, the offshore islands and white boats dotting the blue ocean.

Then you'll crest the western edge of Acadia's east-west summit ridge. As the trail levels off you'll walk through more of the pleasant, open, ledgy woods so typical of Mount Desert Island mountains and you'll enjoy better and better views of Somes Sound. Behind you lie the long, blue ribbons of Echo Lake and Blue Hill Bay.

Soon you'll reach the nearly bare ledge of Acadia's 681-foot western summit. Here you'll enjoy even longer and broader views of the ocean. Walk a couple of hundred feet to the northern edge of the summit ledge and you'll see the northern end of Somes Sound, the white buildings of Somesville and Somes Harbor. Walk another 100 feet or so to the eastern edge of the ledge and you'll see the steep, north-south ridge of 852-foot Norumbega Mountain (Walk No. 32), which forms the eastern wall of Somes Sound at its narrow midsection. (Acadia Mountain forms the western wall.)

Return to the trail and walk through the low woods on the saddle between Acadia's east and west peaks. In a few minutes the Walk will culminate in one of the best views on the entire island. At the top of the cliffs of Acadia's eastern summit—only 1,500 feet from the sound but nearly 700 feet above it—you'll have a 180-degree view up and down the fjord and out into the Atlantic. You'll see past Northeast Harbor, on the east side of the Sound; Southwest Harbor, south of the Sound; Greening Island, just beyond the Narrows at the mouth of the Sound; and the low, elegant sprawl of a half-dozen other offshore islands. To the right of the islands you can see still another 90 degrees. From left to right, the landmarks are the low (284-foot) Flying Mountain (Walk No. 22), on a point of land near the southwestern end of the Sound; the graceful curve of Valley Cove, on the northern edge of the point; 521-foot Valley Peak and the long ridge of St. Sauveur Mountain (both Walk No. 23); and, far to your right, the fire tower atop 839-foot Beech Mountain. In the summer the blue water below you is dotted with a flotilla of white sailboats.

From this vantage point the long, narrow sound looks more like a blue river than an arm of the ocean. But the steep slope of Norumbega on the opposite shore and the even higher ridge of 1,373-foot Sargent Mountain (Walk No. 16) beyond it are reminders that the Sound is geologically a fjord: a deep, narrow ocean bay carved by glaciers and surrounded by mountains.

This ledgy perch is a superb place for a picnic, or at least a long rest. Whatever you do, take time to appreciate the surpassing panorama before following the trail back to your car.

22 Flying Mountain

This undemanding 1.1-mile loop takes you up Acadia's lowest and gentlest mountain, where you'll enjoy panoramic views of Somes Sound, the mountains around the fjord, and

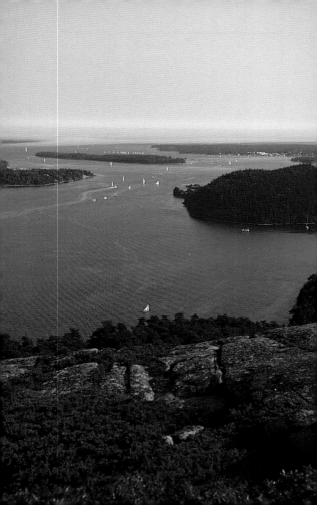

the south coast of Mount Desert Island. You'll see Fernald Cove, Southwest Harbor, Greening Island, the Cranberry Isles, Northeast Harbor, Valley Cove, Valley Peak and Norumbega, Acadia, St. Sauveur, Beech and Western mountains.

The Walk involves some *very* brief climbing up and down ledges. The trip is still a Great Walk, however, because the climbing is neither difficult nor tedious and it's vastly outweighed by the Walk's many excellent views and otherwise undemanding trail.

The Walk begins at a parking area near the end of Fernald Cove Road, near the mouth of Somes Sound. Fernald Cove Road goes east from Route 102, which runs along the west side of Somes Sound; the intersection is about a mile north of Southwest Harbor and exactly 5.5 miles south of the junction of Route 102 and Route 3 and 198 in Somesville.

The mouth of Somes Sound — the only fjord on the east coast of the United States — seen from the ledges on the eastern summit of **Acadia Mountain** *(Walk No. 21). The bay to the right is Valley Cove. The thickly forested point at the edge of the cove is* **Flying Mountain** *(Walk No. 22). Northeast Harbor is on the left; Southwest Harbor is near the horizon on the right. Greening Island is between Northeast Harbor and Southwest Harbor; Great Cranberry Island is on the horizon to the left.*

◄

Fernald Cove Road crosses the northwestern edge of Fernald Cove about .8 miles from Route 102. Just a few hundred feet past the cove, on the left, is the pleasingly landscaped Valley Cove parking area.

The trail begins at an opening in the stone wall on the east side of the parking area. Walk up the stone steps and follow a rooty trail through spruce woods.

Soon you'll see a trail branching off to the left. Ignore it and keep going straight. You'll climb gently over ledges and quickly see a large mound of ledge looming across the trail. Climb to the top of the ledge (with a couple of assists from your hands and knees) and *voila!* After walking less than ten minutes and less than 1,000 feet, you're at the top of Flying Mountain—and the views are terrific. About 284 feet below you and less than 1,000 feet away is Somes Sound. Directly across the long, narrow fjord, impressive residences dot the grassy eastern shore. Rising to the left of the mansions are the steep slopes of 852-foot Norumbega Mountain (Walk No. 32). To the right are the houses of Northeast Harbor. Farther to the right, in the mouth of the sound, is Greening Island. To the left of Greening and farther away are the low Cranberry Isles. Directly below you on your right, and less than 1,500 feet away, is Fernald Cove. On the south side of the cove is Connor Point. Farther away is Southwest Harbor. Less than 1,000 feet to the west are the cliffs of Valley Peak (Walk No. 23). Beyond Valley Peak is Beech Mountain (Walk No. 24); you can see the fire tower on its summit. On the horizon is 1,071-foot Western Mountain.

The views continue as the trail curves across the

open ledge to the east side of the mountain, bringing you even closer to the sound. Now you can see, directly below, the flat mowed fields along the undulating western shore of the sound north of Fernald Cove.

The trail now climbs off the summit ledge and heads north along the nearly level, ledgy spruce-covered spine of the Flying Mountain ridge.

Less than .2 miles from the summit you reach a junction. The trail to the right, marked by a sign saying "Overlook," takes you, in just a couple of hundred feet, to another ledge above Somes Sound. From here you can see far up the curving walls of the steep-sided fjord. To the left, the nearly vertical face of 681-foot Acadia Mountain (Walk No. 21) springs straight out of the water. On the opposite shore, Norumbega rises even higher.

Go back to the main trail and keep following it to the northern shoulder of Flying Mountain. In just a few feet you'll reach a ledge where you'll have a view, above the spruces, of Valley Peak, on the left; St. Sauveur Mountain (Walk No. 23), to the right of Valley Peak, and Acadia Mountain, straight ahead. Below Acadia Mountain is the cliff-walled bay on the west side of Somes Sound known as Valley Cove.

Then you'll immediately come to another ledge, where the view is even better. You'll see the nearly vertical Eagle Cliffs—among the steepest on the island—on St. Sauveur Mountain as well as sailboats in Valley Cove, Norumbega Mountain to the east and the northern reaches of the five-mile-long Somes Sound.

Now you'll climb down the steep ledge (occasion-

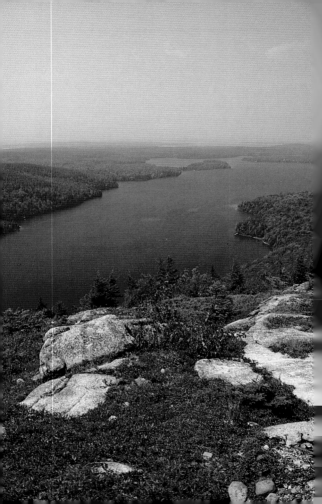

ally on your fanny), then down rough talus through open spruce woods. (This section is brief and not difficult; you just have to take your time negotiating the rocks in the trail.)

Then the trail runs through the spruces and, about .5 miles from the trailhead, reaches the shore of Valley Cove, a small, graceful inlet ringed by mountain walls that look even taller than the cove is wide. Just a few hundred feet away, on the western edge of the cove, is the talus of the rock slide below Eagle Cliffs. Across the cove is Acadia Mountain. Opposite the sound is Norumbega Mountain.

After crossing several brooks running into the cove, you'll walk up log steps and then up a wide, rooty path to a loop at the end of the Valley Cove Road.

Follow the smooth, level, half-mile-long gravel road back to the parking area. As you walk through the spruce woods, you'll have glimpses, through the trees, of the steep slopes of Flying Mountain, on your left, and the cliffs of Valley Peak, on your right.

23 Valley Peak & St. Sauveur Mountain

This moderate 1.4-mile round trip presents a

*The sinuous shore of **Long Pond** (Walk No. 31), Mount Desert Island's largest body of fresh water, seen from **Beech Mountain** (Walk No. 24).*
◀

gallery of vistas of Somes Sound from ledgy overlooks on two different summits near its western shore. You'll see Fernald and Norwood coves, Southwest Harbor, Baker and Greening islands, the Cranberry Isles, Northeast Harbor, Valley Peak (from St. Sauveur), as well as Acadia, Eliot, Day, Norumbega, Penobscot, Sargent and Flying mountains.

The first part of the Walk is a steep, rocky, rooty trail. It's still a Great Walk, however, because the section is only a quarter-mile long—too short to be tedious—and the views easily outweigh the brief inconvenience.

Like Walk No. 22 (Flying Mountain), this excursion begins near the end of Fernald Point Road. To reach the trailhead, follow the directions to Walk No. 22 on page 119. When you reach the Valley Cove parking area, follow the gravel Valley Cove Road, which begins on the north side of the parking area. The Walk begins at the Valley Peak trailhead, which is on the left (west) side of the road, .1 miles beyond the parking area. You can park at the trailhead if there's room; otherwise leave your car at the Valley Cove parking area.

The trail immediately descends through a spruce forest and quickly reaches a brook that flows into Fernald Cove. The rooty path crosses the stream on a log bridge, then recrosses it on stones and another log bridge.

Then the trail becomes rooty *and* rocky as it starts climbing the east slope of Valley Peak, and it gets steeper as it climbs higher up the mountain. Through the trees behind you you'll have glimpses of the west slope of Flying Mountain. Then you'll see Somes Sound and Northeast Harbor.

About .3 miles from the trailhead the trail begins to level off. Instead of passing through spruces, it now runs over smooth granite ledges fringed with junipers, low pitch pines and cedars.

As you approach the summit of Valley Peak, your view expands with each step. You'll see Northeast Harbor on the east side of Somes Sound, Southwest Harbor on the west side, Greening Island at the mouth of the sound and the Cranberry Isles beyond. Then you'll see the narrow Fernald Cove, less than a quarter of a mile away, on the west side of the sound, then Bear Island off Northeast Harbor.

About .4 miles from the trailhead you'll reach the summit ledge. Walk to the right of the summit marker — a wooden sign in a cairn — and follow the ledge to the north, parallel to Somes Sound. Here you'll have a 200-degree view of water that stretches from the northern reaches of the sound all the way to Southwest Harbor. The vista includes the long ridge of 1,373-foot Sargent Mountain, the park's second-highest peak, on the horizon on the other side of the sound. In front of Sargent is 852-foot Norumbega Mountain, rising from the east side of the fjord. On the flat shore to the right of Norumbega are a score of large, handsome residences. To the right of the houses you can see, from left to right, Northeast Harbor; Greening Island, in the mouth of the sound, the Cranberry Isles beyond it, and Southwest Harbor, on the other side of the sound. North of South-

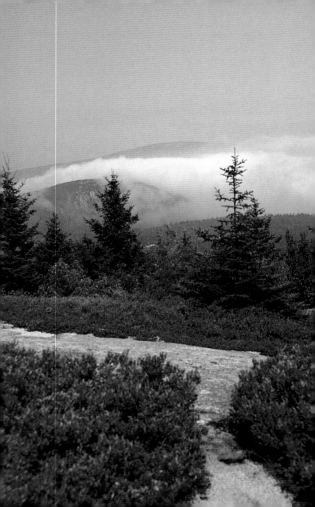

west Harbor is Norwood Cove. Directly below is the placid green Fernald Cove. North of the cove is the low, grass-covered Fernald Point; south of the cove is Connor Point.

Follow the path farther along the ledge (it's marked with cairns and blue blazes), then into the woods. You'll soon start climbing gently up St. Sauveur Mountain and catching glimpses of the sound through the trees on your right.

About .2 miles from Valley Peak you'll emerge onto the eastern ledges of St. Sauveur. As you walk north along the clifftop you'll enjoy unobstructed views up and down Somes Sound.

About .3 miles from Valley Peak you'll reach an overlook on the northeast shoulder of St. Sauveur. Now you'll see Acadia Mountain (Walk No. 21) rising out of the deep waters of the sound to your left. You'll also see Day Mountain (Walk No. 13) and Eliot Mountain beyond Northeast Harbor. Directly below, on the curving wall of Valley Cove, are the awesome 600-foot-high Eagle Cliffs. To your right is Valley Peak. Left of the peak is Flying Mountain.

You're now about 650 feet above the sound — high

Clouds fill Somes Sound and dramatically encircle mountains east of **Beech Mountain** *(Walk No. 24).* **Sargent Mountain** *(Walk No. 16), the second-highest peak on Mount Desert Island, is on the horizon. The precipitous ledgy face of* **Acadia Mountain** *(Walk No. 21) is on the left. The low, forested ridge of* **St. Sauveur Mountain** *(Walk No. 23) is on the right.*

◄

enough to see the massive cairns on the summits of Sargent and Penobscot mountains on the horizon on the far side of the sound. From this altitude, Northeast Harbor, Southwest Harbor and the offshore islands look so low and flat that, in a big storm, the sea might wash right over them.

From here the path heads west, away from the ledges and toward the summit of St. Sauveur. The summit, however, has no views at all—let alone one as spendid as the one you're watching now. So after you've enjoyed the panorama, follow the trail back to your car.

24 Beech Mountain

This undemanding 2.2-mile round trip provides lofty but intimate views of Long Pond, Mount Desert Island's largest lake. It also offers panoramic views of more than a dozen island landmarks, including Beech Cliff, Echo Lake, Somes Sound, Southwest Harbor and the offshore islands, Bartlett Island, Western Bay and Acadia, St. Sauveur, Flying, Sargent, Norumbega, Cadillac, Day and Western mountains.

The Walk begins in a parking area at the end of Beech Hill Road, about four miles south of Somesville. To reach the trailhead, turn west off Route 102 about .2 miles south of Higgins' store in the center of Somesville; there's a park sign at the junction. In another .2 miles turn left onto Beech Hill Road, which will take you gradually up the long ridge that separates Echo Lake from Long Pond (Walk No. 31). Across mowed fields you'll see mountains on both sides of the road. Straight ahead is the fire tower on Beech Mountain. On your right is 1,071-foot Western Mountain, the sixth-highest summit on Mount Desert Island. On your left is the long north-south ridge of 1,373-foot Sargent Mountain (Walk No. 16), the island's second-highest peak, on the horizon. To the right of Sargent, and almost a mile closer, is another north-south ridge: 852-foot Norumbega Mountain (Walk No. 32). To the right of Norumbega, and closer still, is 681-foot Acadia Mountain (Walk No. 21). Acadia's ridge runs east-west, perpendicular to the road, so from here the mountain looks much more compact than either Norumbega or Sargent.

About 3.5 miles from Higgins' store the paved road dead-ends alongside the parking area, which nestles against cliffs and a large boulder on the lower slope of Beech Mountain. The trail to the summit begins in the northwest corner of the parking lot.

After running along a brook for a couple of hundred feet, the path splits. Both forks will take you to the summit but the righthand trail is gentler and its views are much better. Go right.

The trail is a wide, smooth, gravelly path through a mixed forest. Very soon you'll see Long Pond below on your right, set in the middle of forest. Its thinly developed wooded shoreline (much of which is outside the national park) twists in and out of coves. The long, pointed Northern Neck extends into the center of the pond from the north; the smaller Southern Neck reaches toward the Northern Neck from the west side of the pond. The two peninsulas are only about 700 feet apart; together they almost divide the pond in two.

As you gently climb the mountain, the views of the pond through the trees get better and better and you'll see 480-foot Carter Nubble behind you, on the east side of the pond.

As you near the top of the mountain, you're almost 800 feet above Long Pond but only about 1,500 feet away from it, so you have glorious bird's-eye views. Over low evergreens and ledges thick with blueberries, you can see almost the entire length of the four-mile-long pond. Directly across the water, the steep, ledgy slopes of Western Mountain spring up from the shore. In the distance is the long, narrow Western Bay, which separates Mount Desert Island from the mainland. You'll be able to see this vista almost all the way to the top of the mountain.

Near the summit, the trail intersects two paths that go down to Long Pond. Go straight ahead—i.e., take the left fork—at each junction. Immediately after the intersections you'll climb a flight of log steps. At the top of the steps, look to your right. On top of a wide, bare ledge you'll see a 30-foot-high steel observation tower. It's occasionally manned by national park volunteers.

Sailboats skim across Echo Lake below the 600-foot-high **Beech Cliff** *(Walk No. 25). The forested slopes of* **Acadia Mountain** *(Walk No. 21) rise steeply on the right.* ▶

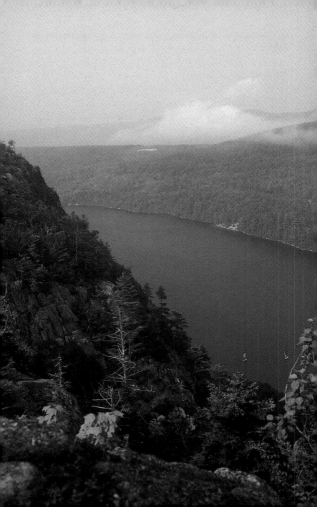

Climb up the tower and enjoy its 360-degree views of landmarks in the heart of Mount Desert Island. To the northeast you can see Beech Cliff (Walk No. 25) above Echo Lake, as well as Somesville and the northern end of Somes Sound. East of Echo Lake is Acadia Mountain. South of Acadia, and almost due east, is St. Sauveur Mountain (Walk No. 23). South of St. Sauveur is Flying Mountain (Walk No. 22). Behind Acadia is Sargent Mountain and behind St. Sauveur is Norumbega. In the distance, to the right, is the long south ridge of Cadillac Mountain, the park's highest summit (Walks No. 19 and 20). To the right of Cadillac is Day Mountain (Walk No. 13). To the south is Southwest Harbor and Greening Island, off the mouth of Somes Sound. To the southeast are the Cranberry Isles. To the west is the long blue ribbon of Long Pond and, beyond the pond, the steep slopes of Western Mountain. To the northwest are Bartlett Island and Western Bay.

You can also see many of these landmarks from the broad ledge beneath the tower, making it a fine place for lunch.

When you're ready, follow the path back to your car—and enjoy the views of Long Pond again.

25 Beech Cliff & Canada Cliff

This easy one-mile round trip brings you to

the top of the Beech and Canada cliffs, where you'll have exhilarating bird's-eye views of Echo Lake, more than 500 feet below. You'll also see Acadia, St. Sauveur, Norumbega and Sargent mountains, on the far side of the lake, as well as Somes Sound, Somesville, Southwest Harbor, Greening Island and the Cranberry Isles. No other Walk on Mount Desert Island offers such grand views for so little effort.

Like Walk No. 24, this trip begins in a parking area at the end of Beech Hill Road, about 3.5 miles south of Somesville. See pages 130-131 for a description of the route to the trailhead.

The path to the cliffs begins on the east side of Beech Hill Road, opposite the northeast corner of the parking lot, and rises very gently as it passes through a moist evergreen grove.

In about .3 miles the path crosses two trails: an unmarked path on the left and a trail on the right that goes to Echo Lake. Walk straight ahead. Almost immediately you'll come to the top of Beech Cliff.

Be careful here—there's nothing between you and a long fall but air. Follow the faint path along the top of the cliff. You'll see—and hear—people on the beach in the cove at the southern end of Echo Lake, almost directly below you. You'll also have a bird's-eye view of sailboats tacking back and forth on the two-mile-long lake, more than 500 feet below. Since you're almost on top of the lake, you'll actually be able to see its bottom through the shallow green water near the shore.

On the other side of the lake are the overlapping ridges of four mountains. Rising dramatically from the opposite shore of the lake is St. Sauveur Mountain (Walk No. 23). Beyond and to the left of St. Sauveur is Acadia (Walk No. 21). Behind both Acadia and St. Sauveur is Norumbega (Walk No. 32) and behind both Acadia and Norumbega is Sargent (Walk No. 16). In the distance to the right is Greening Island, in the mouth of Somes Sound; the Cranberry Isles, beyond Greening Island; and Southwest Harbor, to the right of Greening. On your far right is Canada Cliff.

As you walk north along the top of the cliff you'll see the northern end of Echo Lake and, farther away, the village of Somesville and the northern end of Somes Sound.

Soon the path bends away from the cliff and into the woods. Turn around here and walk back to the path to Echo Lake.

Follow the Echo Lake trail for about 300 feet and you'll come to the top of Canada Cliff, which also overlooks Echo Lake. Walk (carefully!) along the edge of the precipice. The view here rivals the one you just saw. The near-vertical Beech Cliff, now on your left, sweeps dramatically up from the lake. On the other side of the long lake are the knitted ridges of St. Sauveur, Acadia, Norumbega and Sargent mountains. Somesville lies off the northern end of the lake; the mouth of Somes Sound is to your right. These views continue until the path curves away from the cliff in another couple of hundred feet and reenters the woods.

The vistas from Beech and Canada cliffs capture

the essence of Mount Desert Island: a landscape made of steep mountains surrounded by some kind of water—a lake, a pond, a fjord or the ocean.

Obviously, these ledges are wonderful picnic spots. Tarry long enough and you'll probably see a bald eagle soaring above the lake.

After enjoying the view, turn around and retrace your steps to your car.

Great Walks
of Isle au Haut

See pages 9 and 10 for information on how to get to the island and where to stay.

All four of the island's Great Walks begin at the junction of Western Head Road and the path from the ferry landing. To reach the junction, take a left when you walk off the landing and follow the narrow, evergreen-shaded path along the south shore of Duck Harbor. You'll cross, on large stones, a brook flowing into the harbor and, about .2 miles from the landing, come to Western Head Road. You'll see a picnic table and a portable toilet near the intersection.

The routes of Walks No. 26, 27 and 28 overlap in places. If you take the Walks separately you'll be walking some trails—particularly Western Head Road—at least three times. If you have enough time and energy, you can avoid the repetition by combining parts of two, or even all three Walks in one outing. For example, instead of taking Western Head Road to the Goat Trail (Walk No. 26), you could take either the Cliff and Western Head trails (Walk No. 27) or the Duck Harbor Mountain Trail (Walk No. 29). Or you could take the Cliff and Western Head trails to the Goat Trail and the Duck Harbor Mountain Trail back to Duck Harbor, or vice versa, and thereby do all three Walks in one outing. (That combined Walk, however, would be about 8.2 miles, leaving you little time to linger at beautiful places.) Consult the park map of Isle au Haut and create your own combinations.

26 The Goat Trail

This moderate 6.6-mile round trip is the most exhilarating walk on Isle au Haut and the most exciting *ocean shore* walk in Acadia National Park. It takes you down to the beaches of five often-deserted coves and up bare, wind-blown headlands, where you have continuous bird's-eye vistas of waves crashing against the island's wild and rugged southern coast.

From the intersection of Western Head Road and the trail to the ferry landing, follow the grassy road as it rises gently through a clearing, past blueberry bushes and spruces, and past the trail to Duck Harbor Mountain (Walk No. 29), on the left. After less than a quarter of a mile the road levels off and runs through lush spruce woods. Through the trees on your left you'll see granite cliffs on the lower slopes of Duck Harbor Mountain.

After about 1.3 miles of very pleasant, nearly level walking, you'll reach the Goat Trail, on your left.

Start walking on the Goat Trail and you'll immediately see Deep Cove on your right. You'll also see

Ledgy, surf-washed headlands on Isle au Haut, seen from the **Goat Trail** *(Walk No. 26). Eastern Head is in the distance, on the left. In the fall, blueberry bushes (lower right) are bright red.* ▶

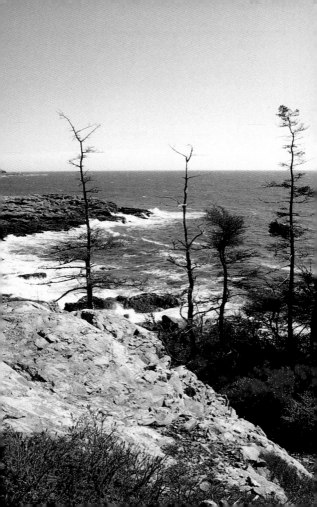

surf breaking on tiny rock islands offshore, on the ledge walls of the cove, and on Eastern Head, almost two miles to the east.

The path runs through grassy spruce woods, close to the rocky beach of the cove, and quickly crosses a stream flowing into the ocean.

Then the nearly level trail passes through thick, damp spruce woods until, about .4 miles from Western Head Road, it reaches a junction with the Duck Harbor Mountain Trail at Squeaker Cove. The tiny cove, just a couple of hundred feet wide, is framed by granite cliffs. Waves rush through the rock walls and crash on the rocky beach. The surf grinds the stones against each other, gradually wearing them down, making them smoother and rounder. The "squeaking" sound of rocks scraping against rocks gives the cove its name.

The Goat Trail now climbs quickly back into deep, moss-floored spruce woods and soon approaches a narrow stream rushing into a tiny, 25-foot-wide cove. The trail bends back from the brook and climbs away from the ocean before crossing the creek farther upstream.

Then the trail quickly climbs up to a ledge knob with the best view of the entire Walk. Here you're 100 feet above the ocean — about the highest point on the Goat Trail. Squeaker Cove is directly below and barely a few hundred feet away. The finely textured stony beach at the head of the cove is a pleasant contrast with the solid, massive headlands on either side of it. The concavity of Squeaker Cove is gracefully echoed by Deep Cove, just beyond it, and by another cove farther away. The rock point on the west side of Squeaker Cove is echoed by another point on the west wall of Deep Cove and by Western Head, on the end of the island. This elegant undulating rock sculpture is dramatically defined by a long, unbroken fringe of white surf at its base. High above the surf, north of Squeaker Cove, are the southern ledges of Duck Harbor Mountain.

This vantage point is a pleasant aerie—a sunny, lichen-covered ledge landscaped by nature with low spruces and thick, neat clumps of even lower blueberry bushes. It's perfect for lunch, or at least a long pause.

The bird's-eye vistas continue as the trail curves along the top of more headlands, high above the ocean. Now you'll have 180-degree views of the entire south coast of the island, from Eastern Head to Western Head. You'll see miles of surf crashing against head walls and over tiny rock islands, and flocks of white-and-black eider ducks bobbing on the rocking sea.

Then the path winds down from the headlands and back into the woods. Soon, through the spruces, you'll catch glimpses of Barred (not Bar) Harbor; if the tide isn't too high you'll see the sandbar at its mouth that gives the cove its name. Then the trail curves along the head of the harbor, close to its rocky beach, affording continuous views of the most beautiful cove on the Walk. The two long, elegant arms of the harbor curve like the pincers of a crab, embracing the shallow water of the cove in a graceful circle.

About .9 miles from Squeaker Cove the Median Ridge Trail joins the Goat Trail on the left. Go

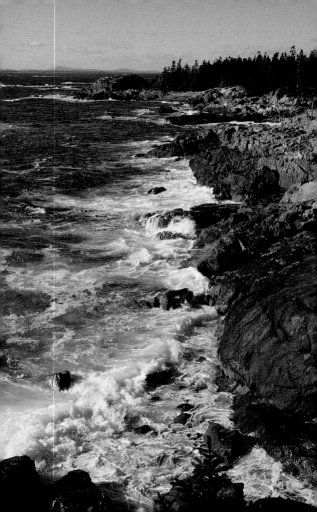

straight ahead. Right after the intersection you'll cross a small brook on stones just before it flows into Barred Harbor.

Next the trail curves around the east side of the harbor, where you'll have another view of Western Head. Then it reenters the woods, where you'll have more views of the harbor through the trees on your right.

The path soon emerges on ledges, with a wide view that includes both Eastern and Western heads. Then it crosses a rock beach at the head of a small, unnamed cove. The last time we were here—a bright, windy fall day—the green-tinted blue sea was dotted with white caps and surf was leaping up the ledges below us.

The ocean views continue as the path winds through sunny, grassy spruce woods to the western side of Merchant Cove, a large bay on the west side of Head Harbor. On the opposite shore, about half a mile away, is the long, low, surf-washed peninsula of Eastern Head, the eastern arm of Head Harbor.

The Goat Trail curves along the grassy shore of Merchant Cove, offering uninterrupted views of the cove and Eastern Head. After passing long drifts of beach peas (which look like sweet peas) on the left, you'll reach the head of the cove. The wooden sign identifying the cove is about .6 miles from the Me-

Surf crashes on the rough rocky coast of Isle au Haut, seen from the **Western Head Trail** *(Walk No. 27). In the distance are the Camden Hills, on the mainland.*
◀

dian Ridge Trail and about two miles from Western Head Road.

From here you can return to Duck Harbor in one of three ways: by retracing your route in its entirety (making the Walk a 6.6-mile round trip), by taking the Cliff and Western Head trails (Walk No. 27) or — if you have a lot of time and energy — by taking the Duck Harbor Mountain Trail (Walk No. 29).

27 The Cliff & Western Head Trails

This moderate excursion — 4.3 or 5.2 miles, depending on how you return to the trailhead — is one of the most exciting shore walks in the park. It offers both cliff-top and beachside views of the dramatic coast on both sides of the long point known as Western Head.

Like the other Great Walks on Isle au Haut, this one begins on Western Head Road in Duck Harbor. See the second paragraph of Walk No. 26 on page 140 for a description of the road.

After about .6 miles of easy, pleasant walking on Western Head Road you'll reach the northern end of the Western Head Trail, which joins the road on your right.

The sometimes rooty trail passes through a moist spruce forest and crosses wet areas on boardwalks made of two half-logs placed side by side. The path descends gradually, almost imperceptibly, to the shore.

About a quarter-mile from the road you'll reach a ledgy headland, where you'll have a 180-degree view up and down the rocky west coast of Western Head. The Saddleback Ledge lighthouse is about three miles offshore.

The ocean views continue as the path crosses a stony 200-foot-long beach, traverses a grassy area above a large headland, and crosses one small and one large (300-foot-long) pebbly beach. A tranquil marsh, protected from the sea by a rock berm, lies just to the left of the second beach.

Then the trail goes through a short tunnel of spruces, skirts a tiny rock beach and enters grassy woods, where you have a 150-degree view of the coast.

After crossing a tiny pebble beach, the path reenters the woods, crosses a slightly larger pebble beach, then reenters the open woods and climbs up a grassy headland, where you'll have the best view of the Walk. This overlook is well situated: It's as far west as, and about 50 feet above, the beaches you just walked along, so you can look north and see, straight ahead, a half-mile of milk-white surf crashing against a half-mile of rockbound coast.

Climbing down from the headland, the path runs through more sunny spruce woodlands. Now nearly level, the trail hugs the shore, often only a few feet above the water, so you'll have many views of the ocean.

About a mile from Western Head Road you'll start to see the Western Ear, the southernmost point on Isle au Haut, ahead on your right.

THE CLIFF & WESTERN HEAD TRAILS   147

About 1.3 miles from the road, you'll come to the junction of the southern end of the Western Head Trail and the western end of the Cliff Trail.

Before taking a left on the Cliff Trail, go right and follow a very faint unmarked trail down a tiny ravine. In just a couple of hundred feet you'll reach the ocean. Walk to the left along the ledges and you'll have a close view of the spruce-topped Western Ear. At high tide the Ear is a quarter-mile-wide island. At low tide, it's a knob at the end of a peninsula linked to Isle au Haut by a low, pebbly beach. At that time you can walk across the beach to the Ear and enjoy panoramic views—the west coast of Isle au Haut, where you just walked, the tiny rock islands offshore, the hills of the mainland, and the island's entire southern coast, which stretches from the Western Ear to Eastern Head. If you do cross to the Western Ear, be sure to come back before the tide covers up the beach.

When you're ready, retrace your steps to the Cliff Trail and follow it through a tunnel of young spruces and past rocks and ledges to a tiny, pebbly beach at the head of a little cove.

From there you'll climb back into the woods, go through another spruce tunnel, skirt the bottom of a 20-foot-high ledge, cross a small stream (where you'll have more ocean views) and climb down more ledge to a stream flowing across a rocky beach.

Cross both the stream and the beach and you'll soon come to a ledge with a wide vista—all the way from Eastern Head on your left to Western Head on your right.

Next the trail skirts a tiny cove with foaming surf,

then rolls along the top of a bluff, nearly 100 feet above the ocean. This is the most exciting part of the Cliff Trail. You can see steep cliffs ahead of you, surf crashing on the rocks below them, and Eastern Head, two miles away. The views become wider and more dramatic as you descend into a ravine, then climb back onto the headland. On no other ocean walk in Acadia are you so high above the ocean, yet so close to it, for so long.

About .7 miles from the Western Head Trail the path bends away from the headlands and runs along several 15-foot-high boulders on your right. Also on the right, just after the rocks, is a series of charming pools in a narrow cleft in the ledge.

In just a few feet more, at the base of 20-foot cliffs, the eastern end of the Cliff Trail joins the southern end of Western Head Road.

If you're short of time, you can follow the wide, nearly level road back to Duck Harbor, making this Walk a 4.3-mile loop. Soon after its intersection with the Cliff Trail, the Western Head Road curves along the west shore of Deep Cove, where you'll have another view of Eastern Head. The road reaches Duck Harbor about 1.7 miles from the Cliff Trail.

If you have more time (and stamina) you can turn around and retrace your steps to Duck Harbor. That would make the Walk a 5.2-mile round trip — .9 miles longer than taking Western Head Road all the way back to Duck Harbor but immeasurably more scenic.

28 The Eben's Head & Duck Harbor Trails

This undemanding five-mile round trip highlights the west coast of Isle au Haut. You'll have views of Duck Harbor, Moore's Harbor, the Seal Trap and Isle au Haut Bay, and you'll see a picturesque log cabin beside one of the island's largest cascading creeks.

Like the other Great Walks on Isle au Haut, this one begins in Duck Harbor, at the intersection of Western Head Road and the short trail to the ferry landing.

Follow Western Head Road north toward Duck Harbor, which from here looks more like a mountain lake than an arm of the ocean. The road gradually winds around the head of the harbor, passing a spring on the right and crossing a large, pretty stream cascading into the bay.

On the north side of the harbor, Western Head Road ends at the island loop road. Go left at the intersection and follow the loop road along the north side of the narrow, half-mile-long harbor.

About a quarter-mile from the intersection you'll pass the southern end of the Duck Harbor Trail, on your right. In another 100 feet you'll see the southern end of the Eben's Head Trail in a grassy area on your left.

Follow the nearly level Eben's Head Trail and you'll immediately see Duck Harbor and the ferry landing, on your left, as well as the rock islands in Isle au Haut Bay, which separates Isle au Haut from Vinalhaven Island, to the northwest.

Your wide view of the ocean continues as the trail runs through sunny, grassy spruce woods along the headland. Soon you'll come to an unmarked path that leaves the trail on the left and takes you quickly to a rock promontory at the mouth of Duck Harbor. Here you'll have a sweeping water view up the narrow harbor to your left and across Isle au Haut Bay to your right.

Then the Eben's Head Trail descends to a beach of smooth pebbles, crosses the beach and ascends the ledges on the other side (watch for cairns marking the route).

Now the nearly level trail winds along the tops of low cliffs, where you have continuing ocean views. Three miles offshore is the lighthouse on Saddleback Ledge. Ahead of you is the mouth of Moore's Harbor. In the middle of the large western arm of the harbor is the narrow bay known as the Seal Trap.

About .5 miles from the loop road you'll start to cross another pebble beach. In about 100 feet a cairn marks the spot where the trail turns right. Then the path reenters the woods, curves through a dense stand of small spruce trees and quickly returns to the loop road.

Just a few hundred feet farther, the road comes to the edge of a rocky beach at the edge of a small cove. Across the cove is the Seal Trap; Moore's Harbor is to the right.

Then the road curves to the right and gradually climbs uphill, away from the coast. About .5 miles from the end of the Eben's Head Trail, the road levels off and crosses the Duck Harbor Trail.

Go left on the Duck Harbor Trail, which slowly descends the lower slope of Wentworth Mountain. You'll cross a wet area, then a brook, on half-log boardwalks. Then you'll climb up sunny, picturesque ledges decorated with drifts of small pitch pines and thick clusters of blueberry bushes. In the fall, when the blueberry bushes are deep red, these natural rock gardens are stunning.

About .3 miles from the loop road, the .2-mile-long side trail to Deep Cove leaves the Duck Harbor Trail on the left. If you want to see a small, pleasant spruce-ringed bay, follow the smooth trail as it gently descends to the ocean. As it approaches the cove, it passes through a tunnel of thick, young spruces. Then it crosses, on logs, a stream flowing into the cove and emerges on a rocky beach at the head of the bay.

When you're ready, return to the Duck Harbor Trail, which now runs over rocks and roots as it passes through deep spruce woods.

About .4 miles from the Deep Cove Trail you'll begin to see, through the trees on your left, a tiny inlet on the southern edge of Moore's Harbor.

Then you'll cross the large, cascading Eli's Creek where it rushes around a tiny island. On the south side of the island you'll cross the creek — carefully — on ledges. On the north side you'll cross it on a 20-foot-long wooden bridge.

Follow the north bank of the creek upstream for

about a hundred feet as it cascades down the steep hillside. Almost immediately you'll see a picturesque log cabin beside a large pool in the brook.

After exploring this lovely place, return to the Duck Harbor Trail and follow it over a wet, grassy area on half-log boardwalks. Through the trees on your left you'll see the mile-long Moore's Harbor, the largest harbor on Isle au Haut.

Soon the trail takes you to a pebbly beach where you'll have a 180-degree view, including the long, spruce-covered arms of the harbor, its surf-washed rock islands, and Saddleback Ledge lighthouse in the distance.

After you've enjoyed this view, turn around and follow the trail back to Duck Harbor.

29
Duck Harbor Mountain

This moderate excursion — a 2.4-mile round trip or a 3.2-mile loop, depending on how you return to the trailhead — is a classic Acadian mountain walk. You quickly ascend a low (309-foot) mountain whose ledgy knobs offer continuing panoramic views of the magnificent west and south coasts of Isle au Haut.

Unlike most Great Walks, this one requires bits of steep climbing and occasional hands-and-feet ascents of ledges (and one or two hands-feet-and-fanny descents). But the climbing and scrambling are brief exceptions to an otherwise moderate walk and the extraordinary views justify the periodic inconvenience. This Walk will be most enjoyable if you take it slowly, both to make the climbing easier and to appreciate the views longer.

Like all Great Walks on Isle au Haut, this one begins at the intersection of Western Head Road and the trail to the ferry landing at Duck Harbor.

Follow the grassy Western Head Road as it rises gently through a clearing, past blueberry bushes and spruces. In just a few hundred feet you'll reach the Duck Harbor Mountain Trail, on the left.

The narrow trail immediately starts climbing, over steplike roots and rocks, up the steep slope of the mountain. After just a couple of hundred feet the trail levels off on a wide granite ledge, where you'll enjoy your first views. One hundred feet below you is Isle au Haut Bay. Farther away is Vinalhaven and other islands in Penobscot Bay. In the distance, on the horizon, is the mainland.

Take a right where the trail forks and keep climbing over gray ledges bordered by low spruces, juniper and thick clumps of sheep laurel and blueberries. (Blue blazes and cairns mark the trail.) Your panorama will get longer and wider with almost every step. Soon you'll have a 150-degree view that includes the tree-covered hilly spine of Isle au Haut to the north, the narrow, half-mile-long Duck Harbor below you and some of the many dark green, spruce-covered islands in Isle au Haut Bay.

In just a few minutes you'll reach a granite knob on a shoulder of the mountain, where the view widens to 180 degrees. Now you can also see the ocean on the *east* side of the island, as well as the Camden Hills and other low mountains on the mainland and the buildings around the harbor in Stonington.

The trail leaves the ledge and runs briefly through shady, moss-floored spruce woods before climbing onto a second ledgy knob with even wider views. Now you can see the round-topped, 934-foot monadnock of Blue Hill on the mainland, to the right (east) of Stonington.

Then the trail runs over a series of ledge knobs before reaching the summit, marked by a small, round metal Geodetic Survey marker embedded in the rock. Here you'll see even more of the ocean to the east.

The trail again passes through spruce woods and soon brings you to the first Pudding, one of a half-dozen or so low ledge knobs separated by spruce forest on the southeast ridge of the mountain. Each Pudding has a slightly different ocean view.

The first Pudding offers a 180-degree vista to the west, over Penobscot Bay. From the second you can see the south coast of Isle au Haut, which stretches from Western Head, in the southwestern corner of the island, to Eastern Head, a peninsula in the southeastern end of the island. Just west of Eastern Head is Head Harbor. On the southern horizon is the crisp horizon of an open, islandless sea.

After sliding down the second Pudding on your hands, feet and fanny, you'll pass between large mossy boulders and spruces. Then, on hands and knees, you'll clamber up the third Pudding, where you'll see Western Head; Deep Cove, to the south; and a wide sheet of blue ocean.

At the next Pudding you'll have another view to the south and east and, at the last Pudding, a sweeping, 240-degree view running from the south coast of Isle au Haut all the way to the mainland.

You'll have still more views to the south as the trail descends long, steep ledges. Then you'll pass through nearly level spruce woods and quickly come to the Goat Trail (Walk No. 26) at Squeaker Cove.

If you want to return to the ferry landing, the easiest and probably quickest way is to take the Goat Trail to Western Head Road and, from there, the pleasant (but viewless) Western Head Road back to Duck Harbor. That route would make this Walk a 3.2-mile loop.

A shorter but more difficult route would be simply to go back over Duck Harbor Mountain. That would make the Walk a 2.4-mile round trip. The route would also be much more scenic, though rather more strenuous, than returning by the Goat Trail and Western Head Road.

Honorable Mentions

30 Paradise Hill

This undemanding 1.5-mile round trip takes you to a carriage road 260 feet above Frenchman Bay, where you'll have a view of Hulls Cove, the Porcupine Islands and Schoodic Peninsula. En route you'll see a 50-foot-long beaver dam and two beaver lodges in a pond off the trail.

This short trip is not a Great Walk because it offers only one view along its entire length. We describe it, however, because the view is excellent, the beaver structures are interesting and the walk is pleasant and relatively short.

The excursion begins at the northwestern end of the parking lot at the park Visitor Center, which is just off Route 3 in Hulls Cove. A sign at the trailhead explains how, between 1915 and 1933, John D. Rockefeller, Jr. "financed and directed" the building of 50 miles of carriage roads in what is now the national park, as well as the roads' "picturesque gatehouses" and "exquisitely designed stone bridges."

The unusually smooth and wide path is almost level as it curves through a pleasant, open mixed forest that includes many small white birches.

About .2 miles from the parking lot, the path turns left and starts climbing Paradise Hill. Here you'll see a pond through the trees on the right of the trail and a rough path leading to it.

Follow the path to the pond and look at the trees and stumps on both sides of the trail. Many bear the marks of beaver teeth.

About 60 feet from the main trail you'll reach the pond and see what the beavers did with at least a few of the trees. On your right is a large beaver dam—50 feet long and 5 feet high in places. The dam has turned this part of Breakneck Brook into a .2-mile-long pond. The beavers have also built two beaver lodges in the pond; the one closest to you rises at least five feet above the water.

If you'd like to know more about these remarkable builders, inquire at the Visitor Center when you finish your walk.

When you're ready to continue, go back to the main trail and make the gradual but continuous climb up Paradise Hill.

About .5 miles from the parking lot the path ends at a carriage road. Take a left onto the wide, smooth gravelly road, which curves clockwise around the north side of Paradise Hill. (As on all carriage roads, keep an eye out for bicyclists zipping by.) About .7 miles from the parking lot the road reaches the east side of the hill, where suddenly you have a 120-degree view of Frenchman Bay and the eastern shore of Mount Desert Island.

On your left, about .5 miles to the north, is the village of Hulls Cove. Directly below and less than .2 miles away as the gull flies is the park Visitor Center. Almost due east and about four miles away are Burnt Porcupine and Long Porcupine Islands, so close together that from here they look like a single island. To the right of Burnt and Long Porcupine and about

three miles from the road is the smaller Sheep Porcupine Island. To the right of Sheep Porcupine, close to
shore and only two miles from the road, is Bar Island. Eight miles across the bright blue Frenchman
Bay is Schoodic Peninsula.

No other carriage road has an ocean view that
rivals this one. After you've enjoyed it, retrace your
steps to the parking lot.

31 Long Pond

This easy round trip offers an extended, dramatic lake-and-mountain vista from a nearly
level path along Mount Desert Island's largest
body of fresh water. Since the path follows
Long Pond for almost two miles, you can make
this outing as short as one mile (our recommendation) or as long as four miles.

This walk is not a Great Walk because it offers
only one view. We describe it, however, because the
view is long and worth a look and because the pleasant lakeside trail is one of the park's widest, smoothest and most level paths.

The walk begins at the southern end of Long
Pond. To reach the trailhead, take Route 102 to Seal
Cove Road; the intersection is about 4.5 miles south
of Somesville and about .7 miles north of the center
of Southwest Harbor. Turn west on Seal Cove Road
and, about .6 miles from Route 102, turn right onto

Long Pond Road. About 1.8 miles from Route 102, Long Pond Road ends at a white pumping station beside the pond. As the road descends toward Long Pond you'll see the steep slope of Western Mountain ahead.

If you're driving to the trailhead from the north, you can also take a shorter, more scenic but probably slower route that begins at the intersection of Route 233 and the road to the Eagle Lake swimming area. The intersection is on the west side of Route 233, about two miles north of Southwest Harbor and about four miles south of Somesville. A park sign here says "Echo Lake Entrance." Turn onto the Echo Lake Road and, about .3 miles from Route 233, turn onto the unpaved Lurvey Spring Road, which twists through thick, deep evergreen woods; the speed limit is 15 miles per hour. About 1.6 miles from Route 102 the Lurvey Spring Road ends at Long Pond Road. Turn right onto Long Pond Road, which in another .4 miles brings you to the pumping station at the southern shore of the pond.

Even before you get out of your car, you'll enjoy Long Pond's most dramatic view. Here the four-mile-long lake is less than 1,000 feet wide, squeezed on both sides by the steep, forested slopes of two mountains: 949-foot Mansell—the easternmost summit of Western Mountain, which springs up on the left side of the lake—and 849-foot Beech Mountain (Walk No. 24), which sweeps up on the right.

Leave your car in the parking area beside the lake and walk along the shore toward Mansell Mountain. Near the pumping station (the lake is Southwest Harbor's water supply) you'll see a sign beside the path saying "Great Pond Trail" (Long Pond used to be known as Great Pond).

Keep following the trail as it hugs the shore. You'll immediately cross a brook on a wooden bridge and reach a trail junction. The Mansell Mountain Trail goes to the left; the Great Pond Trail goes straight ahead, close to the shore. Keep going straight. On your right, across the pond, you'll see the fire tower on top of Beech Mountain and bare ledge on the slope of the mountain to the right.

About .2 miles from the pumping station you'll come to another trail junction. The Perpendicular Trail, which also ascends Mansell Mountain, climbs steeply away from the shore path, on the left. Keep following the well-groomed Great Pond Trail, which runs easily over rock slides that have tumbled down Mansell's precipitous face. Above the slides are sheer cliffs. You'll also have nearly continuous views of the pond and the sharp slope of Beech Mountain, just a few hundred feet across the water.

About .5 miles from the pumping station — or whenever you've seen enough of the view — turn around and follow the path back to your car.

32
Norumbega Mountain

This moderate 3.8-mile round trip takes you up a 852-foot peak that offers views of Somes Sound and more than a dozen landmarks around it, including Southwest Harbor, Northeast Harbor, Greening Island, the Cranberry Isles and nine summits: Acadia, Beech, Cedar Swamp, Parkman, Sargent, St. Sauveur and Western mountains and Bald and Gilmore peaks. You'll also see Valley Cove and Long and Lower Hadlock ponds.

This trip isn't a Great Walk because its views are only intermittent and you have to walk too long in the woods to see them. We include it, however, because these views are good and the woods are often pleasant.

The trail—the easiest and most scenic route up Norumbega—begins on an unpaved road on the south shore of Lower Hadlock Pond. The road leaves Route 3 and 198 about .3 miles north of the intersection of Route 3 and Route 198 in Northeast Harbor and about four miles south of the intersection of Route 3 and 198 and Route 233 at the north end of Somes Sound. The unpaved road is marked only by a sign saying "No Swimming" (Lower Hadlock Pond is Northeast Harbor's water supply). About .1 miles from Route 3 and 198, the road reaches a gate.

Park off the road, to the left of the gate, and start walking along the road. Lower Hadlock Pond is on your right and the east slope of Norumbega Mountain rises on the other side of the pond. Ahead of you is the Northeast Harbor Water Company's red brick pumping station. Very soon you'll see the well-named 974-foot Bald Peak rising above the north shore of the pond.

Then the road forks twice in quick succession. In each case go right. The second right fork will take you close to the pond, where a sign on your left says "Norumbega Mountain."

The road now goes straight to the pumping station. You'll walk along the top of a handsome earth dam faced on its pond side with rectangular granite stones. Then you'll cross the bridge over Hadlock Brook, which drains the pond, and immediately come to the pumping station.

Now the route divides again; the left fork leads to a golf course, the right one follows the shore. Go right.

You'll walk just a few feet more when, about .2 miles from your car, the path splits yet again. The right fork continues around the pond; the left fork, known as the Shady Hill Trail, goes up the mountain.

Follow the Shady Hill Trail as it climbs away from the pond, through a forest of cedar, spruce and pine. Through the trees on your right you'll glimpse the pond and the mountains beyond it.

The pine needle-carpeted path climbs steadily up the top of Norumbega's south ridge, sometimes passing flat, sunny ledges ringed with blueberry bushes. Then it descends gently, levels off and runs through a shady patch of evergreen trees.

Next it climbs steeply to the top of an open ledge, where you have views in three directions. To the east, on your right, is the long north-south ridge of 942-foot Cedar Swamp Mountain. Behind you is the ocean off Northeast Harbor. On the horizon to the west is 1,071-foot Western Mountain, the park's sixth-highest summit. In front of Western Mountain is 839-foot Beech Mountain (Walk No. 24); you can see the fire tower on its summit. In front of Beech Mountain and slightly to the left of the fire tower is the 679-foot summit of St. Sauveur Mountain (Walk No. 23). To the right of St. Sauveur is 681-foot Acadia Mountain (Walk No. 21).

At this point the trail splits again. The left fork goes to the golf course, the right one to the top of the mountain.

Follow the right fork, which goes into the woods again, then climbs steeply to the top of a picturesque rock garden-like ledge, fringed with thick, tight clumps of blueberry bushes and small, shrublike pitch pines. Here you'll have an even wider view than before. You're now high enough to see Valley Cove (Walk No. 22) at the bottom of St. Sauveur Mountain, in Somes Sound. The cove is walled by the nearly vertical Eagle Cliffs, among the steepest cliffs on the island. Behind you are Southwest Harbor, Northeast Harbor, the Cranberry Isles and Greening Island off the mouth of Somes Sound.

Now the trail rolls easily over ledges surrounded by evergreens. Soon you'll have a view of Cedar Swamp Mountain to the east and the slopes of a trio of summits—Bald Peak, 1,036-foot Gilmore Peak and 941-foot Parkman Mountain—to the northeast and 1,373-foot Sargent Mountain (Walk No. 16), the park's second-highest peak, beyond them.

Then you come to an enormous, five-foot-high cairn on an open ledge where you can see mountains in both directions. On the east side of the ridge are the steep, ledgy slopes of Cedar Swamp, Parkman and Sargent mountains and Bald and Gilmore peaks. To the west, on the other side of Somes Sound, are the even steeper bare ledges of Acadia Mountain. Behind Acadia is Long Pond (Walk No. 31). Left of Acadia are the cliffs of St. Sauveur Mountain.

Walk a bit farther and you'll see Somes Sound, including the white houses in the hamlet of Hall Quarry, to the right of Acadia Mountain, and the village of Somesville, at the northern end of the sound.

About .1 miles north of the giant cairn you'll pass the summit of Norumbega. It's marked by a wooden post set in a cairn about 20 feet to the right of the trail.

A few hundred feet beyond the summit, the trail begins its steep descent down the east side of the mountain. Turn around here and enjoy another look at the views as you follow the path back to Lower Hadlock Pond.

To Our Readers:

Please help us stay current. If you discover that anything described in this guide has changed, let us know so we can make corrections in future editions. Please write to: Great Walks, Box 410, Goffstown, NH 03045. Thank you.

Other Great Walks Guides:

▶ *Great Walks of Southern Arizona:* six Great Walks in the fascinating mountains, canyons, and basins of the surprisingly lush Sonoran Desert near Phoenix and Tucson. Great winter walking. 48 pages; 12 full-color photographs; $3.95.

▶ *Great Walks of Big Bend National Park:* six Walks in the Chisos Mountains, the Chihuahuan Desert, and the deep canyons of the Rio Grande, all at the "big bend" of the Rio Grande in the wild open range of southwest Texas. 44 pages; 12 full-color photographs; $3.95.

▶ *Great Walks of the Great Smokies:* 20 Walks to historic sites, impressive waterfalls and cascades, and exciting mountain vistas in Great Smoky Mountains National Park, which straddles the Appalachian Crest in Tennessee and North Carolina. 120 pages; 20 full-color photographs; $5.95.

▶ *Great Walks of Yosemite National Park:* 28 Walks to giant sequoia trees, beautiful lakes, granite domes and other natural rock sculpture, snowcapped 2½-mile-high peaks, and some of the highest waterfalls in the world—all in America's premier national park, in California's Sierra Nevada. 192 pages; 34 full-color photographs; $8.95.

▶ *Great Walks of Sequoia & Kings Canyon National Parks:* 42 Walks featuring large groves of giant sequoias, awesome canyons, panoramic mountain views, fascinating marble caves, and impressive waterfalls in the Sierra Nevada, just a few hours' drive from Yosemite National Park. 208 pages; 33 full-color photographs; $8.95.

▶ *Great Walks of the Olympic Peninsula:* 62 Great Walks and three Honorable Mentions in Washington's Olympic Peninsula, which has more Great Walks than any other region of its size in America. Forty-two Walks are in Olympic National Park, which has more Great Walks than almost any other national park. The trails take you through wildflower-filled mile-high meadows with uninterrupted views of jagged, glacier-covered Olympic mountains; along wild Pacific beaches adorned with seastacks, arches, and other ocean sculpture; through lush temperate rain forests where trees grow as much as 12 feet thick; and to spellbinding waterfalls, cascading streams, and mountain-rimmed lakes. 336 pages; 42 full-color photographs; $13.95.

You can buy Great Walks guides in bookstores or you can order them directly from the publisher by sending a check or money order for the price of each guide you want, plus $1.50 for mailing and handling the order, to: Great Walks, Box 410, Goffstown, NH 03045.

You can also receive more information on the series by sending $1 (refundable with your first order) to Great Walks at the address above.

Own an Original Oktavec Photograph

You can own an original print of any Eileen Oktavec photograph in this guide.

At your request, we will custom make a high-quality, 9¼- by-14-inch color print of your favorite Acadia & Mount Desert Island photograph(s) by the award-winning Eileen Oktavec. The print will be hand labeled, numbered and signed by the photographer. (Because the photograph will be printed on high-gloss paper and much larger than the photograph in the guide, it will be even clearer and more detailed.)

An original Oktavec photographic print is many things: a treasured memento of Acadia, a masterful depiction of its world-famous scenery, a valuable addition to your collection of visual art and, of course, an excellent gift.

To order, simply tell us what print(s) you would like and enclose a check for $76 for each one, plus $4 for shipping and handling any order. Send your order to Great Walks, PO Box 410, Goffstown, NH 03045. Allow 2-3 weeks for delivery.

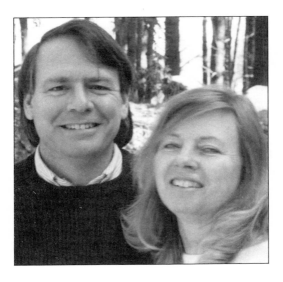

About the Author
And Photographer

Robert Gillmore and Eileen Oktavec have been taking Great Walks throughout the United States and Europe for years. A landscape designer and author, Gillmore graduated cum laude from Williams and holds a Ph.D. from the University of Virginia. His books include *The Woodland Garden* (Taylor Publishing, 1996).

A photographer, painter, author, and cultural anthropologist, Oktavec graduated from the State University of New York at Stony Brook and has a master's degree from the University of Arizona. She is the author of *Answered Prayers: Miracles and Milagros Along the Border* (University of Arizona Press, 1995), which won a Southwestern Book Award in 1996.